ACKNOWLEDGEMENTS

Publication of this manual was facilitated by the work and support of several individuals. The authors would like to thank the following people for their time and dedication. David Robinson Field, MD, Director of Perinatal Services, Kaiser Permanente Medical Center, San Francisco provided expert review and critique of the obstetrical component of the book. Michael P. Hirsch, DC, reviewed and updated the section on backache. Anthony J. Puentes, MD, Medical Director of the Santa Clara County Substance Abuse Services, San Jose, California, generously contributed his newly revised table, "Maternal/Fetal/Neonatal Effects of Substances Commonly Abused by Pregnant Women," for the protocol on substance abuse. Over the years, our trusted teaching assistants, Jenny Shipp, Maria Ruud, Carolyn Muir, and Robin Litt, painstakingly compiled Medline searches and toiled over one copy machine after another. Anja Miller, MA, Senior Administrative Analyst, Office of Research, Evaluation, and Computer Resources, School of Nursing, University of California, San Francisco administered the production of the manual since inception and managed the distribution, correspondence, and general publication aspects. William Holzemer, RN, PhD, FAAN, Director, Office of Research, Evaluation, and Computer Resources, offered us the opportunity to publish and supported the ideation of the manual. Pat Struckman, Administrative Analyst, School of Nursing, University of California, San Francisco edited and prepared this edition for publication.

A special thanks goes to all of our loving family members who supported and encouraged us to endure at times when it may have been easier to quit. Winnie Star would like to offer a very special acknowledgment of her father, Dr. Leon Star, who, throughout his life was a model for her of what stamina and guts and vision are all about. His talents and energy are greatly missed. Maureen Shannon would like to thank her husband, Bob, and children, Matthew, Gregory, and Megan, for providing her with encouragement and understanding whenever needed and for helping her maintain a sense of perspective and humor during her work on this manuscript. Lorrie Sammons offers heartfelt thanks to the three generations who anchor her in life's continuum from past to future: Marion and Max Newmark, and Tim, Julie, and Andy Sammons. Lisa Lommel would like to give special thanks to her husband, Michael, for his relentless optimism and to her family for their constant support. Yolanda Gutierrez would like to thank her husband, Adolfo--"my other self," and Richard and Nancy for their constant support, love, and encouragement.

Finally, we would like to thank the patients and family members, students, clinicians, and others who have shared their lives and visions with us and who have made the practice of obstetrics so enriching.

W. L. S.

M. T. S.

L. N. S.

L. L. L.

Y. G.

PREFACE TO SECOND EDITION

*The authors of **Ambulatory Obstetrics: Protocols for Nurse Practitioners/Nurse-Midwives** are pleased to present the second edition of the manual. We would like to thank all of you who took the time to respond to our questionnaire about the first publication. Many of your suggestions have been incorporated and were extremely helpful in guiding the direction of this edition. As you shall see, the second edition has been expanded to reflect the current standards of obstetrical care and the latest developments in the field. New sections have been added in each chapter of the book. We are also pleased to have a new contributing author, Lisa Lommel, replacing Jean Neeson, who retired this year. We shall miss Jean and thank her for all the contributions she has made to the field of women's health over the years.*

Development of protocols is an ever-growing and changing endeavor. We invite your suggestions and comments. Please address your correspondence to the Office of Research, Box 0604, School of Nursing, University of California, San Francisco, California 94143-0604.

The authors of this manual, Ambulatory Obstetrics: Protocols for Nurse Practitioners/Nurse-Midwives (2nd edition) disavow any responsibility for the outcome of the patients to whom these protocols are applied, both in general treatment/management areas and in the case where specific drug therapy has been delineated.

Ambulatory Obstetrics:

PROTOCOLS FOR
NURSE PRACTITIONERS/NURSE-MIDWIVES

Second Edition

Winifred L. Star, RNC, NP, MS

Maureen T. Shannon, CNM, FNP, MS

Lucy Newmark Sammons, RNC, NP, ACCE, DNS

Lisa L. Lommel, RNC, NP, MPH

Yolanda Gutierrez, MS, RD

School of Nursing
University of California, San Francisco
San Francisco, California

Winifred L. Star, *RNC, NP, MS*
Assistant Clinical Professor
School of Nursing
University of California, San Francisco
Ob/Gyn Nurse Practitioner
Coordinator, Young Mother's Clinic
Kaiser Permanente Medical Center
San Francisco, California

Maureen T. Shannon, *CNM, FNP, MS*
Nurse Clinician
Bay Area Perinatal AIDS Center
San Francisco General Hospital

Lucy Newmark Sammons, *RNC, NP, ACCE, DNS*
Assistant Clinical Professor
School of Nursing
University of California, San Francisco

Lisa L. Lommel, *RNC, NP, MPH*
Assistant Clinical Professor
Coordinator, Young Women's Clinic
School of Nursing
University of California, San Francisco

Yolanda Gutierrez, *MS, RD*
Associate Clinical Professor
School of Nursing
University of California, San Francisco

ISBN 0-943671-07-8

PREFACE TO THE FIRST EDITION

The practice of obstetrical primary care by nurse practitioners and nurse-midwives is legally sanctioned by standardized protocols and procedures defined by the Nurse Practice Act in many states. Nurse Practice Acts vary from state to state as do standards of obstetrical care in the community. In many health care settings it is the nurse who is responsible for the formulation and maintenance of practice protocols. The busy nurse practitioner/nurse-midwife has little time to generate a manual of this magnitude and often looks to outside sources to fulfill the need for written protocols.

Ambulatory Obstetrics: Protocols for Nurse Practitioners/Nurse-Midwives was created as a working manual for health care providers in ambulatory obstetrical care settings. It was collaboratively written by certified nurse practitioners, a certified nurse-midwife, and a registered dietitian, all holding advanced degrees and all with extensive experience in obstetrical care. The manual was originally intended for use in the Young Women's Clinic at the University of California, San Francisco, a clinic serving high-risk pregnant teens. It has been revised for use in other settings with applicability to pregnant populations of all ages. The standards of care delineated reflect integration of the standards of the Ob/Gyn community in San Francisco. Health care practitioners in various practice settings can utilize these protocols as a base from which to adapt and develop a set of standards that meet the needs of the individual practice.

Each protocol contains a succinct definition of the problem followed by a S-O-A-P (Subjective-Objective-Assessment-Plan) format for quick referencing and easy reading. A unique nutrition section offers a comprehensive approach to the obstetrical patients' needs in selected areas of interest. The ring binder assembly allows the NP/NM to revise and update the materials as standards of care change and evolve.

The authors welcome your input, comments, suggestions. Address your correspondence to the individual author, Box 0606, School of Nursing, University of California, San Francisco, California 94143-0606.

TABLE OF CONTENTS

Page

Chapter 1. Routine Prenatal and Postpartum Care

Chapter 2. Prenatal Diagnosis and Surveillance Techniques

Chapter 3. Common Discomforts of Pregnancy

Chapter 4. Obstetrical Complications

Chapter 5. Hematologic Disorders of Pregnancy

Chapter 6. Dermatologic Disorders of Pregnancy

Chapter 7. Infectious Diseases in Pregnancy

Chapter 8. Nutrition Protocol — 361

Bibliography

Chapter 1

Routine Prenatal
and
Postpartum Care

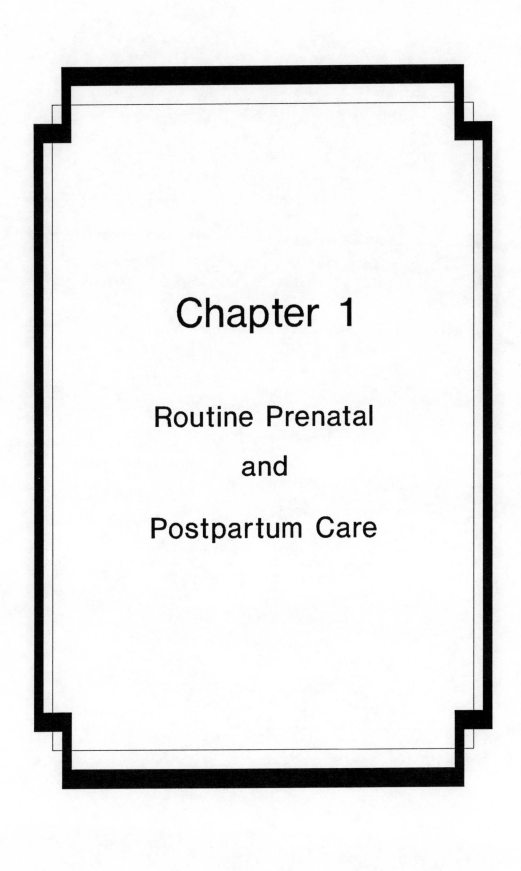

Chapter 1

Routine Prenatal
and
Postpartum Care

INITIAL PRENATAL VISIT

Maureen T. Shannon

Prenatal care is "the evaluation and care of the pregnant woman and her fetus throughout gestation until the onset of active labor" (Whitley, 1985, p. 1). The goals of prenatal care, which begin during a woman's initial obstetrical visit, are: 1) to maintain the health of the woman and her fetus; 2) to establish an accurate gestational age; 3) to screen and monitor the woman and her fetus for the presence and/or development of high-risk conditions that warrant further evaluation and/or referral; 4) to educate the woman (and her partner) regarding the concerns and issues involved in pregnancy, birth, and parenting; 5) to establish rapport with the woman (and her partner); and 6) to refer the woman, as indicated, to appropriate resources available in the practice and community. In order to begin to attain the goals listed above, a woman's initial prenatal visit should include a thorough health history, a complete physical examination, and laboratory testing (routine and additional tests as indicated by the woman's history and physical examination) (ACOG, 1990; Cunningham, MacDonald, & Gant, 1989; Varney, 1987; Whitley, 1985). Women with known medical problems (diabetes, hypertension, thyroid disease, etc.) should be encouraged to have their first prenatal visit with an obstetrician prior to becoming pregnant.

Data Base

Subjective

Menstrual History

- Past menstrual history--including age at menarche, cycle interval, length of flow, amount of flow, intermenstrual bleeding, any associated symptoms

- Last normal menstrual period (LNMP), previous normal menstrual period (PNMP)--include characteristics of LNMP

- Date of ovulation, if known--e.g., basal body temperature chart

- Contraceptive use prior to LNMP

OB/Gyn History

- Pregnancies, abortions (spontaneous and therapeutic), number of living children, length of gestation, type of delivery, sex and birthweight of children, length of labor, anesthesia received

- Past obstetrical complications

- Newborn complications and general health of the child(ren)

- DES exposure, sexual history, contraceptive history, sexually transmitted diseases (e.g., herpes, condylomata, gonorrhea, chlamydia, syphilis, HIV infection), other gynecologic problems, history of sexual assault

General Medical History

- Present medications

- Significant illnesses/accidents/surgeries/transfusions
- Allergies
- Immunizations
- Exposure to environmental toxins/pollutants
- Habits--include use of tobacco, alcohol, caffeine, "social" or "street" drugs, over-the-counter medications, and herbs
- Review of systems

Family History

- Alcoholism or other substance abuse
- Allergies
- Cardiovascular disease
- Cancer
- Congenital anomalies
- Endocrine disorders
- Gastrointestinal disorders
- Genetic/chromosomal disorders
- Hematologic disorders
- Lung disease
- Mental retardation
- Multiple gestations
- Neurological problems
- Psychiatric illness
- Renal disease
- Child abuse, neglect, sexual assault, domestic violence

Social History

- Current living situation
- Educational level of patient
- Occupation, occupational exposure to hazards
- Age and occupation of father of baby
- Relationship with father of baby
- Support persons during pregnancy

Nutritional History

- Pregravid weight
- Weight gain to date

- Adequacy of intake of four food groups
- See Nutrition protocol for further information and/or if specific problems are encountered.

Problems with Current Pregnancy
- Common discomforts of pregnancy (e.g., nausea, vomiting)
- Illnesses, injuries, accidents, surgeries since conception
- Bleeding

Objective (Cunningham et al., 1989; Varney, 1987; Whitley, 1985)
- Height, weight, blood pressure, urine for glucose and protein
- Complete physical examination
- General--note affect, mood
- Skin--note chloasma, striae gravidarum, spider angiomas, linea nigra, increased pigmentation of areola, pallor, jaundice, scars, lesions, pigmented nevi
- Head--note any edema, lesions, deformities, lymphadenopathy, sinus tenderness
- Hair--note consistency, alopecia
- Eyes--determine client's reading ability; check EOMs and pupils; test for lid lag; perform ophthalmoscopic exam and note presence of A-V nicking, papilledema, exudates
- Ears--test for hearing ability; perform otoscopic exam and note presence of serous otitis, otitis media, scarred tympanic membrane, excessive cerumen
- Nose--note pallor, edema, hyperemia, ulcerations, perforation of septum
- Lips--note pallor, cyanosis, presence of lesions, inflammation
- Gums--note gingivitis, epulis, bleeding
- Oral mucosa/palate--note erythema, lesions, ulcerations
- Tongue--note lesions, thrush, hairy leukoplakia
- Teeth--note decay, condition of dental repairs, quality of hygiene
- Posterior pharynx--note presence of tonsils, hyperemia, edema, exudate
- Neck--note position of trachea, lymphadenopathy, tenderness
- Thyroid--note size, consistency, presence of masses/nodules
- Thorax and lungs--note respiratory rate, dullness to percussion, decreased or absent breath sounds, presence of wheezes, rhonchi, crackles, friction rubs
- Heart--note heart rate and rhythm, presence of murmurs, clicks, rubs, extrasystoles
- Breasts--note size, symmetry, masses, puckering, retraction, dimpling, areolar pigment changes, striae, presence of supernumerary nipples; whether nipples are everted, flat, or inverted; lymphadenopathy of axilla or supraclavicular region
- Back--note costo-vertebral angle tenderness (CVAT), scoliosis, kyphosis, lordosis
- Abdomen--note presence of bowel sounds, striae, diastasis recti, rashes, lesions, masses, organomegaly, inguinal lymphadenopathy; measure uterine fundus (if appropriate); auscultate fetal heart tones (if appropriate); determine fetal presentation (if appropriate)
- Musculo-skeletal--note limitation of movement, abnormal gait, swollen/tender joints

- Extremities--note edema, varicosities
- Neuro--note affect, orientation, DTRs; presence of clonus, tics, or tremors; evaluate cranial nerves, sensorimotor and proprioception if indicated
- Pelvic examination
    - External genitalia/perineum--note lesions, warts, varicosities, episiotomy, scars, edema, erythema, discharge
    - Vagina--note rugae, discharge, lesions, hyperemia, masses, quality of muscle tone
    - Cervix--note color, position, consistency, patency, status of os, symmetry, surface characteristics, length, mobility, tenderness, lesions, masses, discharge
    - Uterus--note shape, size, consistency, position, masses, mobility, tenderness
    - Adnexa--If ovaries palpated note size, mobility, tenderness
- Clinical pelvimetry--Assess splay of sidewalls, ischial spines, sacrosciatic notch, curve and length of the sacrum, mobility of coccyx, diagonal conjugate measurement, suprapubic angle, bituberous diameter
- Rectal or rectovaginal examination--confirm uterine examination; note hemorrhoids, masses, lesions

Assessment

- IUP at ___ weeks, size equals dates (S=D)
- Weight gain adequate, poor, excessive
- Problems identified from history or physical examination

Plan

Diagnostic Tests (Cunningham et al., 1989; Varney, 1987; Whitley, 1985)

- CBC
- Hb electrophoresis with quantitative A_2 and F for all Black women
- Blood type, Rh, and antibody screen
- Serology (e.g., VDRL, RPR)
- Rubella titer
- Hepatitis screen
- P.P.D. offered to all clients
- Maternal serum alpha-fetoprotein (MSAFP) if between 15-20 completed weeks of pregnancy
- Urinalysis and urine culture with sensitivities
- Pap smear
- Gonorrhea culture
- Chlamydia culture
- Sonogram if indicated--see Size/Dates Discrepancy and Vaginal Bleeding protocols
- Other lab test as indicated (e.g., herpes culture, 1 hour glucose screen, HIV antibody screen, etc.)

6

Treatment/Management

- Discuss results of physical examination with client.

- Explain about tests that are being ordered.

- Prescribe prenatal vitamins and iron and discuss the importance of taking one vitamin and one iron a day.

- Prescribe other medications as indicated by history and physical exam findings (e.g., vaginitis medications).

- Patient education appropriate to the gestational age of the pregnancy and the concerns of the woman

Consultation

- MD referral is indicated in clients who are in high-risk categories either because of their medical or family histories or because of abnormal findings found during their physical examinations (see below, Guidelines for Medical Consultation).

- MD consultation may be required for the writing or co-signing of prescriptions for medications that not included in the NP/NM's protocols.

Follow-up

- If no problems requiring an MD evaluation exist, then the client should return to see the NP/NM (see Return Prenatal Visit protocol for the recommended schedule for routine prenatal visits).

- Refer for MD evaluation those clients who are in high-risk categories.

- Document any significant historical, chronic or acute problem in the progress notes and problem list.

Guidelines for Medical Consultation

Any patient who falls into a specific high risk category should be referred for an evaluation by a physician. She may be referred back to a NP/NM at the physician's discretion.

Specific high-risk categories include <u>but are not limited to</u> the following:

- Pre-eclampsia

- Diabetes mellitus and glucose intolerance of pregnancy

- Third trimester bleeding

- Previous fetal wastage: greater than 16 weeks gestation

- Habitual abortions: 3 or more serial abortions under 16 weeks gestation

- Known drug abuse

- Rhesus sensitization or other IgG antibody sensitization

- Post-maturity: all patients at 41 weeks or more by menstrual dating

- Hemoglobinopathies--see specific hemoglobinopathy protocol

- Anemias: Hb of less than 10 gm/dl or Hct less than 30%, unresponsive to iron therapy

- Multiple gestation

- Premature rupture of membranes

- Suspicion of intrauterine growth retardation

- High-risk score on preterm labor assessment--see Preterm Birth Prevention protocol

- Polyhydramnios or oligohydramnios

- Severe maternal malnourishment

- Maternal cardiac disease

- Maternal hypertensive disease

- Maternal renal disease, or repeated urinary tract infections

- Maternal collagen disease

- Miscellaneous maternal, gynecological, endocrine, neuromuscular, pulmonary, gastrointestinal, or infectious disease(s)

- Abnormal maternal serum alpha-fetoprotein result (MSAFP)--see MSAFP protocol

- Fetal malpresentation after 34 weeks gestation

- Family or personal history of severe congenital anomalies or chromosomal abnormalities

- Psychiatric illness

- Positive human immunodeficiency virus (HIV) test result

Guidelines for Social Service Consultation

- Family/marital problems

- Difficulty in planning for the care of the baby

- History of being abused as a child or being a child abuser

- History of being a victim of domestic violence

- Financial problems

- Need for other community resources (e.g., adoption, special schools if pregnant adolescent, etc.)

RETURN PRENATAL VISIT

Maureen T. Shannon

The purposes of return prenatal visits are: 1) to evaluate the progress of the woman's pregnancy; 2) to provide the woman with information and support appropriate to her needs; and 3) to make appropriate referrals to an MD, other health care workers or community resources as indicated (Varney, 1987; Whitley, 1985).

Data Base (may include but is not limited to)

Subjective

- Problems or complaints since last visit
- Follow-up of problems identified on preceding visit
- Patient verbalizes preparation for pregnancy, childbirth, and parenting (within cultural context).

Objective

- Weight
- Blood pressure
- Dipstick check of clean catch midstream urine
- Palpation of uterine fundus including McDonald's measurement and Leopold maneuvers when appropriate
- Presence or absence of fetal heart tones and how auscultated

  - By Doppler, 12-20 weeks at provider's discretion

  - By fetoscope or stethoscope when 20 weeks by dates or when fundus at umbilicus

- Assessment of presence/absence of edema
- Other physical exam components as indicated by patient complaints and concerns

Assessment

- IUP at _____ weeks
- Identify any size/dates discrepancy
- Identify any abnormal physical/lab finding
- Determine appropriateness of weight gain/nutritional status
- Evaluate patient's level of acceptance of pregnancy
- Identify social problems and support system
- Update problem list

Plan

Diagnostic Tests

- Tests ordered as indicated by office/institution protocols
- Sonogram if indicated by physical findings
- Other labs as indicated by history or physical findings

Treatment/Management

- Refill prenatal vitamins as necessary.
- Begin therapy for iron deficiency if indicated--see Anemia protocol.
- Calcium supplement given if inadequate dietary intake of calcium
- Treatment of specific problems as indicated (e.g., urinary tract infections, vaginitis, etc.)
- Follow-up on any prior abnormal lab results

Patient Education

- Review lab data with patient.
- Reassure/educate patient in reference to her concerns.
- Inform patient of gestational age and give information regarding fetal growth and development.
- Discuss patient's diet and weight gain with any suggested changes.
- Review danger signs of pregnancy appropriate to gestational age.
- Offer education appropriate to stage of pregnancy and needs of the patient (e.g., common discomforts, breastfeeding, childbirth preparation, child care, contraception).

Consultation

- Refer to/consult with MD about any patients with problems specified in Guidelines for Medical Consultation (see pp. 7-8).

Follow-up (Cunningham et al., 1989; Varney, 1987; Whitley, 1985)

- Routine repeat lab studies

  Weeks Gestation

  - 15-20   Maternal serum alpha-fetoprotein screening (see MSAFP protocol)
  - 24-28   All patients: CBC, 1 hour glucose screen; urinalysis and culture if indicated
  - 26   Rh negative patients: antibody screen and offer Rhogam at 28 weeks if negative screen
  - 34-36   Repeat gonorrhea and chlamydia cultures as indicated

               Repeat serology as indicated

               Repeat CBC on patients who had Hb less than or equal to 11 gm/dl or Hct less than or equal to 33% at 28 weeks

- Routine follow-up visits every 3-4 weeks until 28 weeks; then every 2-3 weeks until 36 weeks; then weekly (ACOG, 1990)

- MD visit required every trimester in normal women; more frequent MD referral(s) as indicated if significant problem(s) develop.

- Document ongoing problem(s) in progress notes and problem list.

POSTPARTUM VISIT

Lucy Newmark Sammons

The postpartum period can be divided arbitrarily into three segments (Novy, 1987). The immediate puerperium is the first 24 hours after delivery, during which time dramatic physiologic changes take place. The early puerperium extends from the second day to the end of the first postpartal week. The remote puerperium is usually considered to be the time from the end of the first postpartal week to the end of the sixth week, the amount of time generally required for healing and restoration of the reproductive organs.

Following delivery, scheduling of maternal visits may depend upon length of hospital/birth center stay, availability and utilization of home nurse visits, procedures for telephone follow-up, complications of delivery, and limitations of provider and family resources for multiple visits. This protocol addresses the nursing assessment, problem-solving, and management aspects of care that should be accomplished by the end of the remote puerperium, regardless of the number and structure of health care contacts. Infant care and care of the mother in the immediate puerperium are not included because the focus is on ambulatory obstetrical care.

Data Base

Subjective

- Review antenatal record for problems identified <u>prenatally</u>.

- Review medical record and labor and delivery summary for <u>intrapartum</u> course, including type of labor and delivery, anesthesia, episiotomy, infant weight, maternal or infant complications, medications required, and discharge orders.

- Elicit <u>interval maternal history</u> of past six weeks including:

  - Any readmissions, calls/visits to providers or emergency care, additional medications, episodic or acute illnesses/fever/pain

    . Abdominal pain: Afterpains caused by uterine contractions, especially in multigravidas and during infant sucking, normally are quite mild after 3 days postpartum. If significant abdominal pain later, consider endometritis--see Endometritis protocol.

    . Headache pain: Headaches occur in 30-40% women in first week postpartum; usually responsive to minor analgesics (Reik, 1988)

  - Breastfeeding: symptoms of mastitis, condition of nipples, nursing pattern, pediatric follow-up of infant status (e.g., weight gain)

  - Bottlefeeding: method/ease of lactation suppression, problems preparing formula, pediatric follow-up of infant status

  - Bowels: pattern of elimination and comparison to norm for client, discomfort, use of medications/aids

    Constipation: Expected puerperal changes predisposing for postpartum constipation include normal mild ileus, perineal discomfort, and postpartum fluid loss. If problematic--see Constipation protocol.

- Hemorrhoids: discomfort, therapeutics--see Hemorrhoids protocol.

- Episiotomy: discomfort, symptomatic treatment

- Intercourse: pattern, discomfort, <u>contraception</u> used or anticipate using, satisfaction with method

- Bladder: voiding pattern (especially if had catheterization), ability to stop flow with Kegel's; urinary frequency and high volume due to diuresis are normal during postpartal days 2-5; for urinary frequency thereafter--see Cystitis protocol.

- Bleeding: amount, color, change with time/activity
  Normal pattern is a continual decrease in amount, with:
  Lochia rubra: red--days 1-3
  Lochia serosa: paler--days 4-10
  Lochia alba: white/yellowish white--days 10-28/35
  Variations in amount during postural change (some increase in amount or clots when rising) and activity is normal.
  Reddish color beyond 2 weeks suggests retained placental parts or subinvolution--see Subinvolution protocol.
  Foul smell suggests infection--see Endometritis protocol
  Resumption of menses (Cunningham et al., 1989):
  Non-nursing--within 6-8 weeks for most women
  Nursing--varies from 2-18 months
  First period postpartally:
  Heavier than normal menstrual period
  Often anovulatory
  Earlier in multipara than primipara

- Elicit <u>general adaptation</u>:

  - Rest/sleep: patterns, aids, hindrances

  - Activity/exercise: type and amount

  - Nutrition: assessment with attention to special needs, (e.g., lactation, anemia); check appetite

  - Progress with future plans: e.g., moving, continued education, work re-entry, child care arrangements, social services support

- Elicit maternal and family behavioral and psychological <u>responses to childbearing/childrearing</u>:

  - Global response to birthing experience

  - Note infant's name.

  - Responses of self, significant others, and siblings to infant's personality/temperament; identify mother's greatest strengths, her most important need for continued assistance

  - Maternal experience of "postpartum blues", crying spells, or depression; for severe or prolonged postpartum depression--see Depression-Postpartum protocol.

  - Maternal sense of social isolation vs connectedness; sense of self and worthiness

  - Extent of maternal return of functional ability (resumption of household, social, community and occupational activities); only 72% of vaginally-delivered women and 34% of cesarean-delivered women reported having regained usual energy level at six weeks (Tulman & Fawcett, 1988).

- Family accommodation to household tasks while new mother recuperating and acquainting with infant

Objective

- Vital signs: within normal limits (WNL); temperature elevations associated with breast engorgement normally confined to first 2-3 days postpartum; bradycardia (50-70 bpm) normal first 6-10 days (Weber, 1988).

- BP: Compare to range in pregnancy.

- Weight: Compare to prepregnant weight and weight at delivery. Normal to retain 60% of weight gain in excess of 24 lb beyond puerperium (Novy, 1987)

- Urine: Dipstick (obtain clean-catch midstream specimen to reduce faulty results due to lochia/menstrual contamination)

- Check previous lab work as indicated: e.g., prenatal and postpartum Hb/Hct, Rubella immunity and documentation of Rubella vaccine given postpartally, and Rh factor.

- Breast examination: Note size, shape, consistency, masses, galactorrhea, nipple condition, lactation status, and axillary and supra-clavicular nodes. Distension, firmness, tenderness, warmth are normal with engorgement days 3-4 postpartum; beyond that consider mastitis-- see Mastitis protocol.

- Thyroid exam; 6% incidence of transient thyrotoxicosis or hypothyroidism after delivery (Novy, 1987)

- Back: Assess costo-vertebral angle tenderness (CVAT), and/or pain and tenderness along paraspinous muscles.

- Abdominal examination: Assess diastasis in fingerbreadths, tenderness, masses, cesarean section incision (operative patients are often evaluated at 2 weeks and 6 weeks postpartum), striae, and inguinal lymph nodes. Abdominal musculature involution may require 6-7 weeks.

- Pelvic examination:

  - Perineum/external genitalia: Check episiotomy healing for edema, inflammation, hematoma, suppuration, wound dehiscence, and ecchymosis. If lochia present, check appearance and odor. Red, brawny, swollen, gaping opposing episiotomy edges, with serous, serosanguinous, or purulent exudate indicate localized infection of episiotomy.

  - Vagina: Check lacerations, rugae, coloration, dryness, inflammation, leukorrhea, and odor. Assess pelvic muscle tone by requesting "Kegel's" during digital exam. Palpate episiotomy scar on posterior vaginal septum for tenderness and integrity. Vaginal epithelium appears thin and smooth until ovaries function to produce estrogen; lactation extends hypoestrogenic condition. Rugae reappear by third week postpartum.

  - Cervix: Check for lacerations, healing, normal changes of parity with vaginal delivery, and tenderness. Cervical canal reformed by 10-13 days postpartum. External os converted to transverse slit after vaginal birth.

  - Uterus: position, size, shape, tenderness, consistency; normal size:
    1 week postpartum--12 week gestation size
    6 weeks postpartum--near complete involution

  - Adnexa: size, shape, tenderness, masses

- Rectum: Assess sphincter tone, check recto-vaginal septum for episiotomy scar, palpate sacrospinous ligaments, and assess masses, fistulas, external or internal hemorrhoids, and presence/absence of stool.

  - General muscle tone: Check for cystocele or rectocele.

- Extremities: edema, varicosities, calf tenderness, increased warmth, erythema, Homan's sign

- Observe affect and mood; check for alteration/disturbance.

Assessment

- Normal _____ week postpartum exam

- Non-lactating, non-problematic suppression; or breastfeeding, lactation well-established

- Episiotomy or cesarean section incision well-healed

- Maternal-infant interactions appropriate; progressing social and emotional adaptations

- Contraception method in use/planned: _____

- Nutritional status appropriate; weight appropriate/high/low

- Identified problems: e.g., episiotomy or cesarean section incision problems, dyspareunia, pyelonephritis, postpartum depression or maternal maladaptation, unstable social situation, hemorrhoids, history of recurrent asymptomatic bacteriuria, cystitis, gestational diabetes, anemia--see pertinent protocols

Plan

Diagnostic Tests

- Pap smear

- CBC or Hb/Hct if history of anemia

- Urine culture if bacteriuria in pregnancy--see Cystitis protocol

- Other tests as indicated by data base and assessments

Treatment/Management

- Contraceptive method of choice

- Continue vitamin/folate/iron supplementation x 3-4 months

- Calcium supplement if dietary sources inadequate for lactation

- Specific treatment(s) for identified problem(s)

- See Patient Education.

Consultation

- Medical consultation for prescriptions and the following variations from normal: infection or abnormal healing of surgical site; abnormal vaginal bleeding; suspected breast abscess or mass; suspected pelvic infection or subinvolution; postpartum depression

- Nutritional consultation if nutritional status severely compromised

- Social services, public health nursing services, or child protective services referrals as needed

Patient Education

- Sleep/rest: Provide practical, concrete suggestions to enhance maternal rest and recuperation, sensitive to the client's lifestyle and cultural milieu.

- Contraception/sexual adaptation: Provide specific guidelines explaining when healthy to resume intercourse if not yet done. Provide anticipatory guidance regarding postpartal differences in sensation, lubrication, elasticity, etc., and strategies for increasing satisfaction. Assist patient in selecting and implementing contraceptive measures best-suited to her lifestyle.

- Nutritional counseling: lactation and/or recuperative diet, with attention to any special problems

- Lactation support: anticipatory guidance, helpful suggestions, recommended reading; see Nutrition protocol for lactation diet.

- Exercise/activity/weight guidance: Describe average weight loss pattern and assist woman in determining realistic, healthy short and long-term goals. Provide postpartum exercise instructions, emphasizing gradual return of muscle tone and weight while focusing on recuperation first in early postpartum. Teach/reinforce Kegel's exercise.

- Parenting: Support realistic expectations for parenting and parent-infant interaction. If the infant is present, identify characteristics of this infant, reinforce mother's strengths in dealing with infant, and use self as a role model when possible.

- Infant care concerns: feeding, pediatric care, infant safety

- Health maintenance: Instruct woman in self-breast examination techniques. Provide anticipatory guidance regarding continued postpartal recuperation, e.g., timing of return of menses. Encourage regular gynecologic care/Pap smears.

- Immunization update: Address questions about Rubella immunization as needed. Women at risk for inadequate measles (Rubeola) protection may seek vaccination combining Rubella-Rubeola. Tetanus toxoid boosters may be part of postpartal vaccination routine.

- Explain findings: Review laboratory results as needed. Clarify questions about Rho(D) Immune Globulin (RhIG) given postpartally. Discuss findings from current examination.

- Additional problems: Discuss comfort/recuperative measures for any identified problems. See also particular protocols.

Follow-up

- Health maintenance: Pap smear/gyn exam at 6 or 12 months as indicated

- Infant to be followed by a primary care provider

- Return for specific contraceptive method as needed

- Antenatal condylomata to be followed by colposcopic/dysplasia services as available

- Referrals for special interest groups: La Leche League, single mothers, parent-infant classes, play groups, etc.

- Referral to lactation specialist if indicated for nursing dyad problems

- For identified problems as necessary, document in progress notes and problem list.

Chapter 2

Prenatal Diagnosis

and

Surveillance Techniques

ALPHA-FETOPROTEIN SCREENING

Maureen T. Shannon

Alpha-fetoprotein (AFP) is a protein produced in the fetal yolk sac during the first trimester and later in pregnancy by the fetal liver. In pregnant women AFP is found in both the amniotic fluid and maternal serum in significantly lower concentrations than is found in fetal serum. The highest concentration of AFP in fetal serum and amniotic fluid occurs at approximately the 13th gestational week, after which time these levels decrease rapidly. In maternal serum, the AFP concentration remains at low levels, but does exhibit a gradual increase in concentration until 30-32 weeks gestation (Burton, 1988). Abnormally elevated levels of AFP (either from amniotic fluid or maternal serum samples) have been associated with several fetal disorders including open neural tube defects (NTDs), abdominal wall defects, congenital nephrosis, and other birth defects (Main & Mennuti, 1986). Elevated AFP levels are also noted in multiple gestations. Abnormally low AFP levels have recently been associated with Down's Syndrome (Knight, Palomaki, & Haddow, 1988) and other chromosomal abnormalities (Drugan et al., 1989).

In order for the test to be accurate, a woman must have her blood sample drawn between the 15th and 20th gestational weeks. Women who are having an amniocentesis (e.g., women who are 35 years or older) do not need to have MSAFP testing done since AFP levels can be determined from the amniotic fluid sample obtained during amniocentesis. Prior to a woman's consent or refusal for testing she should be educated about the incidence of NTDs in the general population (approximately 1/1000 - 1/1500), the cost of the testing, and what services are included for this fee (e.g., repeat MSAFP samples, ultrasonography, amniocentesis). See Table 2.1, *"Time Window" for MSAFP Blood Collection*, pp. 22-23, for optimum AFP testing times based on a woman's LNMP.

Data Base

Subjective

- No physical complaints
- May report a family history positive for NTD, abdominal wall defect, etc.

Objective

- MSAFP result = 2.5 - 3.0 multiples of the mean (M.o.M.) is considered "a little high."
- MSAFP result greater than 3.0 M.o.M. is considered "high."
- "Low" MSAFP result (value calculated from maternal age and M.o.M.) indicates a second trimester risk of Down's Syndrome equal to or greater than 1/270 (Knight et al., 1988).
- "Normal" MSAFP result = less than 2.5 M.o.M. at more than 15 weeks gestation.

Assessment

A positive MSAFP result is not diagnostic--it is only a screening tool. Therefore, the assessment is simply "elevated," "low," or "normal" MSAFP result.

Plan

Diagnostic Tests (see Figure 2.1, *Alpha-fetoprotein Screening*, p. 24)

- MSAFP initial screening must be done between 15-20 weeks' gestational age (105 - 140th day from LMP). When filling out the AFP forms, only one method of determining the gestational age should be used (e.g., first trimester pelvic exam or ultrasound results). Ideally, the most reliable method of determining gestational age should be used.

- Initial MSAFP result of 2.5 - 3.0 M.o.M.--repeat the MSAFP test.

- Initial MSAFP result greater than 3.0 M.o.M.--refer to regional Prenatal Diagnostic Center for counseling, sonogram, and possibly amniocentesis.

- Initial MSAFP result is "low"--refer to regional Prenatal Diagnostic Center for a sonogram (to confirm gestational age).

- If second MSAFP result is still elevated--refer to regional Prenatal Diagnostic Center.

Treatment/Management

- Continue routine prenatal care on clients with normal MSAFP results.

- Clients who have been found to have a fetus with an NTD, abdominal wall defect, Down's Syndrome, etc., are referred to MD care.

- Clients who have "low" MSAFP results, without having a fetus affected with Down's Syndrome, should be co-managed with an MD secondary to a possible increased incidence of adverse pregnancy outcomes (e.g., spontaneous abortion, fetal demise, hydatidiform mole, and choriocarcinoma [Knight et al., 1988]).

- Clients who have "high" MSAFP results and normal amniocentesis results should be co-managed with an MD because of an increased risk of IUGR, spontaneous abortion, preterm labor, stillbirth, and neonatal death.

Consultation

- Required that all clients with initial MSAFP results greater than 3.0 M.o.M., initial "low" MSAFP results, or repeat MSAFP results equal to or greater than 2.5 M.o.M. be referred to the regional Prenatal Diagnostic Center for further testing. Follow-up is based upon the results of the sonogram and amniocentesis done there.

Patient Education

- Advise client regarding the MSAFP screening and what fetal problems it can help delineate (e.g., open neural tube defects, abdominal wall defects, etc.).

- Must discuss the fee ($49.00 in California) for MSAFP screening, especially for those clients who are not on Medi-Cal (Medicaid) or whose health insurance does not cover the cost of this testing.

- Clients with initial MSAFP results which are "a little high" (2.5 - 3.0 M.o.M.) can be told that the majority of the time this result is due to incorrect dating of the pregnancy.

- Clients with elevated repeat MSAFP results and correct dates have only a 6% chance of having a fetus with an open neural tube defect (this can reassure some women).

- MSAFP screening will not help in the prenatal diagnosis of closed neural tube defects (which constitutes about 10% of all NTDs).

Follow-up

- See Treatment/Management.
- Document MSAFP results in progress notes and problem list.

Table 2.1

"Time Window" for MSAFP Blood Collection Based on the 1st Day of Last Normal Menstrual Period (LNMP). "Time Window" is from 105th Through 140th Day.

LNMP DATE	DRAW BLOOD BETWEEN	
14FEB	30MAY	04JUL
15FEB	31MAY	05JUL
16FEB	01JUN	06JUL
17FEB	02JUN	07JUL
18FEB	03JUN	08JUL
19FEB	04JUN	09JUL
20FEB	05JUN	10JUL
21FEB	06JUN	11JUL
22FEB	07JUN	12JUL
23FEB	08JUN	13JUL
24FEB	09JUN	14JUL
25FEB	10JUN	15JUL
26FEB	11JUN	16JUL
27FEB	12JUN	17JUL
28FEB	13JUN	18JUL
01MAR	14JUN	19JUL
02MAR	15JUN	20JUL
03MAR	16JUN	21JUL
04MAR	17JUN	22JUL
05MAR	18JUN	23JUL
06MAR	19JUN	24JUL
07MAR	20JUN	25JUL
08MAR	21JUN	26JUL
09MAR	22JUN	27JUL
10MAR	23JUN	28JUL
11MAR	24JUN	29JUL
12MAR	25JUN	30JUL
13MAR	26JUN	31JUL
14MAR	27JUN	01AUG
15MAR	28JUN	02AUG
16MAR	29JUN	03AUG
17MAR	30JUN	04AUG
18MAR	01JUL	05AUG
19MAR	02JUL	06AUG
20MAR	03JUL	07AUG
21MAR	04JUL	08AUG
22MAR	05JUL	09AUG
23MAR	06JUL	10AUG
24MAR	07JUL	11AUG
25MAR	08JUL	12AUG
26MAR	09JUL	13AUG
27MAR	10JUL	14AUG
28MAR	11JUL	15AUG
29MAR	12JUL	16AUG
30MAR	13JUL	17AUG
31MAR	14JUL	18AUG

LNMP DATE	DRAW BLOOD BETWEEN	
01APR	15JUL	19AUG
02APR	16JUL	20AUG
03APR	17JUL	21AUG
04APR	18JUL	22AUG
05APR	19JUL	23AUG
06APR	20JUL	24AUG
07APR	21JUL	25AUG
08APR	22JUL	26AUG
09APR	23JUL	27AUG
10APR	24JUL	28AUG
11APR	25JUL	29AUG
12APR	26JUL	30AUG
13APR	27JUL	31AUG
14APR	28JUL	01SEP
15APR	29JUL	02SEP
16APR	30JUL	03SEP
17APR	31JUL	04SEP
18APR	01AUG	05SEP
19APR	02AUG	06SEP
20APR	03AUG	07SEP
21APR	04AUG	08SEP
22APR	05AUG	09SEP
23APR	06AUG	10SEP
24APR	07AUG	11SEP
25APR	08AUG	12SEP
26APR	09AUG	13SEP
27APR	10AUG	14SEP
28APR	11AUG	15SEP
29APR	12AUG	16SEP
30APR	13AUG	17SEP
01MAY	14AUG	18SEP
02MAY	15AUG	19SEP
03MAY	16AUG	20SEP
04MAY	17AUG	21SEP
05MAY	18AUG	22SEP
06MAY	19AUG	23SEP
07MAY	20AUG	24SEP
08MAY	21AUG	25SEP
09MAY	22AUG	26SEP
10MAY	23AUG	27SEP
11MAY	24AUG	28SEP
12MAY	25AUG	29SEP
13MAY	26AUG	30SEP
14MAY	27AUG	01OCT
15MAY	28AUG	02OCT
16MAY	29AUG	03OCT

LNMP DATE	DRAW BLOOD BETWEEN	
17MAY	30AUG	04OCT
18MAY	31AUG	05OCT
19MAY	01SEP	06OCT
20MAY	02SEP	07OCT
21MAY	03SEP	08OCT
22MAY	04SEP	09OCT
23MAY	05SEP	10OCT
24MAY	06SEP	11OCT
25MAY	07SEP	12OCT
26MAY	08SEP	13OCT
27MAY	09SEP	14OCT
28MAY	10SEP	15OCT
29MAY	11SEP	16OCT
30MAY	12SEP	17OCT
31MAY	13SEP	18OCT
01JUN	14SEP	19OCT
02JUN	15SEP	20OCT
03JUN	16SEP	21OCT
04JUN	17SEP	22OCT
05JUN	18SEP	23OCT
06JUN	19SEP	24OCT
07JUN	20SEP	25OCT
08JUN	21SEP	26OCT
09JUN	22SEP	27OCT
10JUN	23SEP	28OCT
11JUN	24SEP	29OCT
12JUN	25SEP	30OCT
13JUN	26SEP	31OCT
14JUN	27SEP	01NOV
15JUN	28SEP	02NOV
16JUN	29SEP	03NOV
17JUN	30SEP	04NOV
18JUN	01OCT	05NOV
19JUN	02OCT	06NOV
20JUN	03OCT	07NOV
21JUN	04OCT	08NOV
22JUN	05OCT	09NOV
23JUN	06OCT	10NOV
24JUN	07OCT	11NOV
25JUN	08OCT	12NOV
26JUN	09OCT	13NOV
27JUN	10OCT	14NOV
28JUN	11OCT	15NOV
29JUN	12OCT	16NOV
30JUN	13OCT	17NOV
01JUL	14OCT	18NOV

LNMP DATE	DRAW BLOOD BETWEEN	
02JUL	15OCT	19NOV
03JUL	16OCT	20NOV
04JUL	17OCT	21NOV
05JUL	18OCT	22NOV
06JUL	19OCT	23NOV
07JUL	20OCT	24NOV
08JUL	21OCT	25NOV
09JUL	22OCT	26NOV
10JUL	23OCT	27NOV
11JUL	24OCT	28NOV
12JUL	25OCT	29NOV
13JUL	26OCT	30NOV
14JUL	27OCT	01DEC
15JUL	28OCT	02DEC
16JUL	29OCT	03DEC
17JUL	30OCT	04DEC
18JUL	31OCT	05DEC
19JUL	01NOV	06DEC
20JUL	02NOV	07DEC
21JUL	03NOV	08DEC
22JUL	04NOV	09DEC
23JUL	05NOV	10DEC
24JUL	06NOV	11DEC
25JUL	07NOV	12DEC
26JUL	08NOV	13DEC
27JUL	09NOV	14DEC
28JUL	10NOV	15DEC
29JUL	11NOV	16DEC
30JUL	12NOV	17DEC
31JUL	13NOV	18DEC
01AUG	14NOV	19DEC
02AUG	15NOV	20DEC
03AUG	16NOV	21DEC
04AUG	17NOV	22DEC
05AUG	18NOV	23DEC
06AUG	19NOV	24DEC
07AUG	20NOV	25DEC
08AUG	21NOV	26DEC
09AUG	22NOV	27DEC
10AUG	23NOV	28DEC
11AUG	24NOV	29DEC
12AUG	25NOV	30DEC
13AUG	26NOV	31DEC

SOURCE:

California Department of Health Services, Genetic Disease Branch. California AFP Screen Program (1986).

Table 2.1 (continued)

LNMP DATE	DRAW BLOOD BETWEEN	
14AUG	27NOV	01JAN
15AUG	28NOV	02JAN
16AUG	29NOV	03JAN
17AUG	30NOV	04JAN
18AUG	01DEC	05JAN
19AUG	02DEC	06JAN
20AUG	03DEC	07JAN
21AUG	04DEC	08JAN
22AUG	05DEC	09JAN
23AUG	06DEC	10JAN
24AUG	07DEC	11JAN
25AUG	08DEC	12JAN
26AUG	09DEC	13JAN
27AUG	10DEC	14JAN
28AUG	11DEC	15JAN
29AUG	12DEC	16JAN
30AUG	13DEC	17JAN
31AUG	14DEC	18JAN
01SEP	15DEC	19JAN
02SEP	16DEC	20JAN
03SEP	17DEC	21JAN
04SEP	18DEC	22JAN
05SEP	19DEC	23JAN
06SEP	20DEC	24JAN
07SEP	21DEC	25JAN
08SEP	22DEC	26JAN
09SEP	23DEC	27JAN
10SEP	24DEC	28JAN
11SEP	25DEC	29JAN
12SEP	26DEC	30JAN
13SEP	27DEC	31JAN
14SEP	28DEC	01FEB
15SEP	29DEC	02FEB
16SEP	30DEC	03FEB
17SEP	31DEC	04FEB
18SEP	01JAN	05FEB
19SEP	02JAN	06FEB
20SEP	03JAN	07FEB
21SEP	04JAN	08FEB
22SEP	05JAN	09FEB
23SEP	06JAN	10FEB
24SEP	07JAN	11FEB
25SEP	08JAN	12FEB
26SEP	09JAN	13FEB
27SEP	10JAN	14FEB
28SEP	11JAN	15FEB

LNMP DATE	DRAW BLOOD BETWEEN	
29SEP	12JAN	16FEB
30SEP	13JAN	17FEB
01OCT	14JAN	18FEB
02OCT	15JAN	19FEB
03OCT	16JAN	20FEB
04OCT	17JAN	21FEB
05OCT	18JAN	22FEB
06OCT	19JAN	23FEB
07OCT	20JAN	24FEB
08OCT	21JAN	25FEB
09OCT	22JAN	26FEB
10OCT	23JAN	27FEB
11OCT	24JAN	28FEB
12OCT	25JAN	01MAR
13OCT	26JAN	02MAR
14OCT	27JAN	03MAR
15OCT	28JAN	04MAR
16OCT	29JAN	05MAR
17OCT	30JAN	06MAR
18OCT	31JAN	07MAR
19OCT	01FEB	08MAR
20OCT	02FEB	09MAR
21OCT	03FEB	10MAR
22OCT	04FEB	11MAR
23OCT	05FEB	12MAR
24OCT	06FEB	13MAR
25OCT	07FEB	14MAR
26OCT	08FEB	15MAR
27OCT	09FEB	16MAR
28OCT	10FEB	17MAR
29OCT	11FEB	18MAR
30OCT	12FEB	19MAR
31OCT	13FEB	20MAR
01NOV	14FEB	21MAR
02NOV	15FEB	22MAR
03NOV	16FEB	23MAR
04NOV	17FEB	24MAR
05NOV	18FEB	25MAR
06NOV	19FEB	26MAR
07NOV	20FEB	27MAR
08NOV	21FEB	28MAR
09NOV	22FEB	29MAR
10NOV	23FEB	30MAR
11NOV	24FEB	31MAR
12NOV	25FEB	01APR
13NOV	26FEB	02APR

LNMP DATE	DRAW BLOOD BETWEEN	
14NOV	27FEB	03APR
15NOV	28FEB	04APR
16NOV	01MAR	05APR
17NOV	02MAR	06APR
18NOV	03MAR	07APR
19NOV	04MAR	08APR
20NOV	05MAR	09APR
21NOV	06MAR	10APR
22NOV	07MAR	11APR
23NOV	08MAR	12APR
24NOV	09MAR	13APR
25NOV	10MAR	14APR
26NOV	11MAR	15APR
27NOV	12MAR	16APR
28NOV	13MAR	17APR
29NOV	14MAR	18APR
30NOV	15MAR	19APR
01DEC	16MAR	20APR
02DEC	17MAR	21APR
03DEC	18MAR	22APR
04DEC	19MAR	23APR
05DEC	20MAR	24APR
06DEC	21MAR	25APR
07DEC	22MAR	26APR
08DEC	23MAR	27APR
09DEC	24MAR	28APR
10DEC	25MAR	29APR
11DEC	26MAR	30APR
12DEC	27MAR	01MAY
13DEC	28MAR	02MAY
14DEC	29MAR	03MAY
15DEC	30MAR	04MAY
16DEC	31MAR	05MAY
17DEC	01APR	06MAY
18DEC	02APR	07MAY
19DEC	03APR	08MAY
20DEC	04APR	09MAY
21DEC	05APR	10MAY
22DEC	06APR	11MAY
23DEC	07APR	12MAY
24DEC	08APR	13MAY
25DEC	09APR	14MAY
26DEC	10APR	15MAY
27DEC	11APR	16MAY
28DEC	12APR	17MAY
29DEC	13APR	18MAY

LNMP DATE	DRAW BLOOD BETWEEN	
30DEC	14APR	19MAY
31DEC	15APR	20MAY
01JAN	16APR	21MAY
02JAN	17APR	22MAY
03JAN	18APR	23MAY
04JAN	19APR	24MAY
05JAN	20APR	25MAY
06JAN	21APR	26MAY
07JAN	22APR	27MAY
08JAN	23APR	28MAY
09JAN	24APR	29MAY
10JAN	25APR	30MAY
11JAN	26APR	31MAY
12JAN	27APR	01JUN
13JAN	28APR	02JUN
14JAN	29APR	03JUN
15JAN	30APR	04JUN
16JAN	01MAY	05JUN
17JAN	02MAY	06JUN
18JAN	03MAY	07JUN
19JAN	04MAY	08JUN
20JAN	05MAY	09JUN
21JAN	06MAY	10JUN
22JAN	07MAY	11JUN
23JAN	08MAY	12JUN
24JAN	09MAY	13JUN
25JAN	10MAY	14JUN
26JAN	11MAY	15JUN
27JAN	12MAY	16JUN
28JAN	13MAY	17JUN
29JAN	14MAY	18JUN
30JAN	15MAY	19JUN
31JAN	16MAY	20JUN
01FEB	17MAY	21JUN
02FEB	18MAY	22JUN
03FEB	19MAY	23JUN
04FEB	20MAY	24JUN
05FEB	21MAY	25JUN
06FEB	22MAY	26JUN
07FEB	23MAY	27JUN
08FEB	24MAY	28JUN
09FEB	25MAY	29JUN
10FEB	26MAY	30JUN
11FEB	27MAY	01JUL
12FEB	28MAY	02JUL
13FEB	29MAY	03JUL

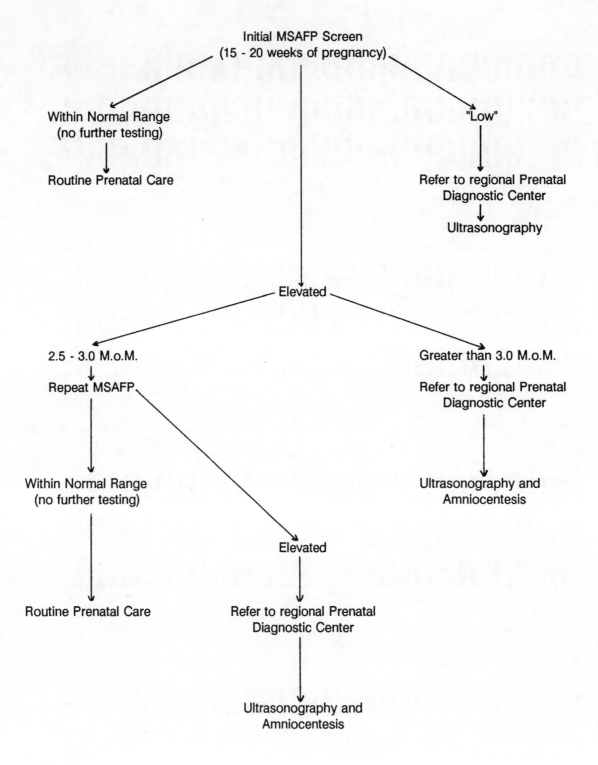

Initial MSAFP Screen
(15 - 20 weeks of pregnancy)

Within Normal Range
(no further testing)

Routine Prenatal Care

"Low"

Refer to regional Prenatal
Diagnostic Center

Ultrasonography

Elevated

2.5 - 3.0 M.o.M.

Repeat MSAFP

Within Normal Range
(no further testing)

Routine Prenatal Care

Elevated

Refer to regional Prenatal
Diagnostic Center

Ultrasonography and
Amniocentesis

Greater than 3.0 M.o.M.

Refer to regional Prenatal
Diagnostic Center

Ultrasonography and
Amniocentesis

© 1990 M. T. Shannon

Figure 2.1. Alpha-fetoprotein screening

AMNIOCENTESIS

Lisa L. Lommel

Amniocentesis is the removal of a sample of amniotic fluid from the amniotic sac. There are a variety of indications for amniocentesis including: 1) assessment of fluid for presence of bilirubin secondary to erythroblastosis fetalis, 2) assessment of lecithin and sphingomyelin ratio indicating level of fetal lung maturity, and 3) analysis of fluid for genetic fetal abnormalities. Depending upon the indication, amniocentesis may be completed at varying times during the pregnancy. Amniocentesis for genetic diagnosis may be completed between 15 and 21 weeks gestation. It is most commonly performed between 15 and 18 weeks gestation. Presently, several studies are focusing on genetic amniocentesis at 14 weeks or less that will enable the patient to receive results earlier in the pregnancy (Johnson & Godmilow, 1988; Evans et al., 1988; Evans et al., 1989).

The amniocentesis protocol includes an ultrasound, performed immediately prior to the procedure, to determine the following: fetal age, position of the placenta, location of amniotic fluid, fetal cardiac movement, and number of fetuses. Ultrasound is also utilized during the amniocentesis to help avoid puncturing the placenta, fetus, and umbilical cord. After the patient has emptied her bladder, a 19 to 22 gauge needle is passed through the lower abdomen into the uterus and amniotic sac. Approximately 15 to 30 ml of fluid is aspirated. Amniotic cells that originate from fetal skin, amnion, and fetal mucous membranes are grown in culture for analysis (Knuppel & Drukker, 1986). Karyotype results are usually available within 10 days to 3½ weeks depending upon cell development and the laboratory.

The overall risk for pregnancy loss following amniocentesis is 0.50% to 0.90% or less (Gold et al., 1989). Most centers counsel that risk of abortion secondary to amniocentesis is 1/200 or less (ACOG, 1987). These rates are related to the amniocentesis procedure alone and do not include the background rate of miscarriage.

Maternal complications associated with amniocentesis include puncture of the bladder or gut, amnionitis, vaginal bleeding, amniotic fluid leakage, and Rh sensitization. Maternal organ puncture is very rare and can be avoided with concurrent ultrasound visualization and an experienced clinician. Symptomatic amnionitis occurs very rarely. Transient vaginal bleeding occurs more often and usually is not associated with fetal complications. Amniotic fluid leakage occurs in approximately 1.7% of patients after amniocentesis (Gold et al., 1989). Most cases of fluid leakage are transient, with only a few continuing until delivery and requiring hospitalization. The rate of Rh sensitization after second trimester genetic amniocentesis is between 2.1% and 5.4%. Although routine administration of Rh immune globulin is controversial, most centers recommend prophylactic treatment in the Rh-negative, antibody screen negative patient (Brandenburg, Pipers, & Wladimiroff, 1989).

Fetal complications associated with amniocentesis are rare. Only a small number of cases of damage to the fetus and placenta by needle injury have been reported. The preterm birth rate, stillbirth rate, perinatal mortality rate, and physical growth and neurological development of the infant have not been affected by genetic amniocentesis (Tabor, 1988).

Second trimester amniocentesis has some major advantages and disadvantages when compared to chorionic villus sampling (see Chorionic Villus Sampling protocol). Advantages include the following: the ability to detect neural tube defects through alpha-fetoprotein analysis, visualization of fetal anatomy and function during the procedure-related second trimester ultrasound, and well-established maternal-fetal risks and laboratory analysis. Disadvantages center on the timing of the procedure. Since most amniocenteses are completed at 15 to 18 weeks' gestation, the results are usually not available until approximately 17 to 21 weeks' gestation. An elected termination at that time would pose a greater risk to the mother than an earlier termination done after chorionic villus sampling. Due to the later availability of results, studies show that maternal anxiety is maintained and "maternal attachment to the fetus" is delayed in patients who undergo amniocentesis (Robinson et al., 1988; Sjögren & Uddenberg, 1989; Spencer & Cox, 1988).

Data Base

Subjective

- Common indications for amniocentesis include (ACOG, 1987):

  - Advanced maternal age: standard practice is to offer prenatal diagnosis to women who will be 35 or older when their infant is born. Flexibility is recommended when women under 35 years of age request prenatal diagnosis. See Table 2.2, *Chromosomal Abnormalities in Liveborns*, p. 29.

  - Previous child with chromosomal abnormality

  - Parental chromosomal abnormality (balanced translocations and inversions are most common)

  - Family history of neural tube defect

  - Elevated level of maternal serum alpha-fetoprotein

  - Mother who is a carrier for a X-linked disease (i.e. hemophilia, Duchenne muscular dystrophy)

  - Parents who are both known to be carriers of certain autosomal recessively inherited disorders (i.e. inborn errors of metabolism, Tay-Sachs disease, cystic fibrosis)

  - History of ≥ 3 successive spontaneous abortions

- The most common difficulties associated with performing an amniocentesis are maternal obesity and an anteriorly-placed placenta.

- Common effects related to the procedure include local discomfort and deep pelvic pressure during needle insertion. Cramping may be experienced immediately following the procedure but is usually self-limiting.

Objective

- Data review for accurate dating of pregnancy

- Pre-procedure ultrasound confirming viable pregnancy at 15 to 21 weeks gestation and documentation of placental position, location of amniotic fluid, and number of fetuses

- Karyotype result:

  - normal 46 XX chromosomes or

  - normal 46 XY chromosomes or

  - abnormal chromosomes

- Alpha-fetoprotein result:

  - elevated for gestational age

- normal for gestational age

- low for gestational age

- Bloody amniotic fluid is aspirated in 2% of amniocenteses. It is often maternal in origin and does not adversely affect cell growth. Brown, dark-red, or wine-colored amniotic fluid is associated with an increased likelihood of adverse pregnancy outcome. Greenish amniotic fluid has not been associated with adverse pregnancy outcome (ACOG, 1987).

Assessment

- Normal 46 XX or XY chromosomes

- Abnormal chromosomes with diagnosed condition

- Abnormal alpha-fetoprotein level with diagnosed condition

Plan

Diagnostic Tests

- Amniocentesis performed by a physician trained in the procedure

- Ultrasound to confirm viable fetus between 15 and 21 weeks gestation, location of placenta, location of amniotic fluid, and number of fetuses

Treatment/Management

- Continue routine prenatal care on patients whose fetus has a normal karyotype and alpha-fetoprotein level.

- Patients whose fetus has an abnormal karyotype and/or abnormal alpha-fetoprotein level should be referred to a physician.

- Administer 300μg of Rh immune globulin to Rh-negative, antibody screen negative patients after the procedure.

Consultation

- Patients who are at risk of delivering an infant with a genetic disorder should be referred to a geneticist as early as possible in their pregnancy.

- Patients who desire an amniocentesis should be referred to a physician for the procedure.

- Patients whose fetuses have an abnormal karyotype and/or abnormal alpha-fetoprotein level should be referred to a physician.

Patient Education

- Genetic counseling should be completed by a geneticist and should include the woman's risk of delivering an infant with a genetic disorder.

- Provide a thorough explanation of the procedure.

- Discuss the common discomforts associated with the procedure.

- Advise the patient to call her provider for persistent uterine cramping, vaginal bleeding, or leakage of amniotic fluid.

- Teach the patient common signs of infection including temperature elevation, flu-like symptoms, and/or change in vaginal discharge.

- Advise the patient to refrain from strenuous activity and intercourse for the remainder of the day following the procedure.

- Provide emotional support to the patient and her partner. This will be most important after the procedure while waiting for the results. This is a time of increased anxiety for the patient and her family.

- Provide emotional support to the patient and her family when an abnormal result is obtained.

Follow-up

- Refer women with an abnormal result to a social worker or counselor as appropriate.

- Document karyotype result in progress notes and problem list.

Table 2.2

Chromosomal Abnormalities in Liveborns*

Maternal Age	Risk for Down's Syndrome	Total Risk for Chromosomal Abnormalities**
20	1/1,667	1/526
21	1/1,667	1/526
22	1/1,429	1/500
23	1/1,429	1/500
24	1/1,250	1/476
25	1/1,250	1/476
26	1/1,176	1/476
27	1/1,111	1/455
28	1/1,053	1/435
29	1/1,000	1/417
30	1/952	1/385
31	1/909	1/385
32	1/769	1/322
33	1/602	1/286
34	1/485	1/238
35	1/378	1/192
36	1/289	1/156
37	1/224	1/127
38	1/173	1/102
39	1/136	1/83
40	1/106	1/66
41	1/82	1/53
42	1/63	1/42
43	1/49	1/33
44	1/38	1/26
45	1/30	1/21
46	1/23	1/16
47	1/18	1/13
48	1/14	1/10
49	1/11	1/8

*   Because sample size for some intervals is relatively small, 95% confidence limits are some-times relatively large. Nonetheless, these figures are suitable for genetic counseling.

** 47 XXX excluded for ages 20-32 (data not available)

SOURCE:

American College of Obstetricians and Gynecologists (1987). *Antenatal diagnosis of genetic disorders* (Technical Bulletin No. 108). Washington, DC: Author. Reprinted with permission.

CHORIONIC VILLUS SAMPLING

Lisa L. Lommel

Chorionic villus sampling (CVS) is the removal of a small sample of chorionic (placental) tissue for prenatal genetic diagnosis. The two most common methods of CVS are the transcervical and transabdominal techniques. The transcervical method is the most widely used. Both techniques are completed at 9 to 12 weeks' gestation when the chorionic villi are abundant enough to be easily sampled while avoiding the gestational sac. Under ultrasound guidance, and with the patient's bladder full, a catheter is passed through the vagina and cervix into the uterine cavity (transcervical technique). The transabdominal technique usually requires an empty bladder while the catheter is passed through the abdominal wall into the uterine cavity under ultrasound guidance. When the chorionic villi is located and visualized, approximately 5-30 mg weight of villi is removed by applying suction to the end of the catheter with a syringe. Karyotype results can be available within 3 to 4 days when using the direct method of tissue analysis. It is recommended that a tissue culture also be completed on the same sample to confirm the results (available in 2 to 3 weeks in most labs) (Wapner & Jackson, 1988).

The overall risk for pregnancy loss following transcervical CVS has been found to be between 2.0% and 4.6% (Blakemore, 1988) and 2.2% and 5.4% (Wapner & Jackson, 1988). These rates include the background rate of miscarriage for patients who did not undergo CVS and the frequency of miscarriages attributed to the sampling procedure. Current large scale studies are focusing on procedure-related spontaneous abortion rates. Presently, total miscarriage rates following the transabdominal procedure have been found to be comparable to those after the transcervical method (Blakemore, 1988; Wapner & Jackson, 1988).

Additional complications associated with CVS include bleeding, infection, and Rh isoimmunization. Vaginal spotting or light bleeding is rare following transabdominal CVS but has a 10% to 25% incidence rate after the transcervical method. Vaginal spotting is usually resolved in 10 to 14 days and does not persist or recur in later pregnancy (Jackson & Wapner, 1987). Heavy vaginal bleeding is infrequent and rarely presents serious complications.

The risk of intrauterine infection poses a threat to the woman and her fetus. It is believed that the risk for infection using the transcervical method is higher than the transabdominal method. Risk of infection has been found to be 0.2% for the transcervical method. Many providers require a negative *N. gonorrhoea* culture before the procedure. Careful patient education regarding signs and symptoms of infection is important in reducing the risk of serious sequelae.

Rh sensitization has been of concern following CVS because of a reported rise in maternal serum alpha-fetoprotein following 50% of the procedures, implying a fetal maternal hemorrhage. Prophylactic use of 50μg of Rh immune globulin is recommended in Rh negative patients who have a negative antibody screen. A review of the literature has not substantiated an increase in perinatal complications following CVS. Pre-term deliveries, intrauterine growth retardation, placental abnormalities, rupture of membranes and congenital structural defects have not been proven to be associated with CVS.

Chorionic villi sampling has some major advantages and disadvantages when compared to second trimester amniocentesis for genetic diagnosis. The primary advantage is the availability of results early in the pregnancy. Because of early availability of results, studies have shown that maternal anxiety is reduced and "maternal attachment to the fetus" is enhanced in patients who undergo CVS (Robinson et al., 1988; Sjögren & Uddenberg, 1989; Spencer & Cox, 1988). Additionally, if termination was elected by the patient, the termination procedure would pose less risk at 11 to 14 weeks' gestation compared to 20 to 22 weeks' after amniocentesis. Disadvantages to CVS include a higher total loss rate of 0.8% when compared to amniocentesis (Rhoads et al., 1989), the inability to screen for neural tube defects with amniotic fluid alpha-fetoprotein analysis, and the inability to visualize fetal anatomy via ultrasound at the earlier weeks of gestation.

Data Base

Subjective

- Common indications for CVS include (ACOG, 1987):

  - Advanced maternal age: standard practice is to offer prenatal diagnosis to women who will be 35 or older when their infant is born. Flexibility is recommended when women under 35 years of age request prenatal diagnosis. See Table 2.2, *Chromosomal Abnormalities in Liveborns*, p. 29.

  - Previous child with chromosomal abnormality

  - Parental chromosomal abnormality (balanced translocations and inversions are most common)

  - Mother who is a carrier for an X-linked disease (i.e. hemophilia, Duchenne muscular dystrophy)

  - Parents who are both known to be carriers of certain autosomal recessively inherited disorders (i.e., inborn errors of metabolism, Tay-Sachs disease cystic fibrosis)

  - History of ≥3 successive spontaneous abortions

- Absolute contraindications for CVS include (Blakemore, 1988):

  - Presence of intrauterine device

  - Active bleeding

  - Cervical stenosis (transabdominal technique may be utilized)

  - Untreated endocervicitis or pelvic inflammatory disease

  - Positive *N. gonorrhoeae* culture of the cervix

  - Active genital herpes simplex

- Common effects related to the procedure include discomfort attributed to a full bladder, cramping associated with placement of the tenaculum, and insertion and removal of the catheter.

Objective

- Data review for accurate dating of pregnancy

- Pre-procedure ultrasound confirming viable pregnancy at 9 to 12 weeks' gestation and absence of uterine anomalies

- Karyotype result:

  - normal 46 XX chromosomes or

  - normal 46 XY chromosomes or

  - abnormal chromosomes

- *N. gonorrhoeae* culture negative

Assessment

- Normal 46 XX or 46 XY chromosomes

- Abnormal chromosomes with diagnosed condition

Plan

Diagnostic Tests

- Chorionic villus sampling is done by a physician who is trained in this procedure.

- Cervical culture for *N. gonorrhoeae*

- Culture for herpes simplex if suspicious lesion is present or if the patient has a history of herpes simplex lesion within previous 6 months

- Ultrasound to confirm viability of fetus and date pregnancy between 9 and 12 weeks

- Ultrasound to rule out uterine abnormalities, presence of intrauterine device, and presence of multiple gestation. CVS can be accomplished in a twin gestation with an experienced clinician.

Treatment/Management

- Continue routine prenatal care on patients whose fetus has a normal karyotype.

- Patients whose fetuses have an abnormal karyotype should be referred to a physician.

- Administer 50μg of Rh immune globulin to Rh-negative, antibody screen negative patients.

Consultation

- Patients who are at risk of delivering an infant with a genetic disorder should be referred to a geneticist as early as possible in their pregnancy.

- Patients who desire CVS should be referred to a physician for the procedure.

- Patients whose fetuses have an abnormal karyotype should be referred to a physician.

Patient Education

- Genetic counseling should be completed by a geneticist and should include the woman's risks of delivering an infant with a genetic disorder.

- Explain that CVS cannot evaluate for neural tube defects. Women should be offered maternal alpha-fetoprotein screening at 16-18 weeks' gestation.

- Provide explanation of the procedure.

- Discuss the common discomforts that are associated with the procedure.

- Explain that spotting is common after the procedure but should subside within 3 days. Advise patient to contact her care provider if bleeding persists or increases in amount.

- Teach the patient common signs of infection including temperature elevation, flu-like symptoms, or change in vaginal discharge. Advise the patient to contact her care provider if any of the symptoms are present.

- Advise the patient to refrain from strenuous activity for the remainder of the day following the procedure and to avoid intercourse until one week after vaginal spotting has stopped.

- Provide emotional support to the patient and her partner. This will be most important after the procedure while waiting for the results. This is a time of increased anxiety for the patient and her family.

- Provide emotional support to the patient and her family when an abnormal result is obtained.

Follow-up

- Offer maternal alpha-fetoprotein screening to women at 16 to 18 weeks to screen for neural tube defects.

- Many CVS programs recommend a second-trimester ultrasound to evaluate the fetus for malformations and organ function.

- Refer women with an abnormal result to a social worker or counselor as appropriate.

- Document karyotype result in progress notes and problem list.

ANTEPARTUM FETAL SURVEILLANCE

Lisa L. Lommel

The major goal of antepartum fetal surveillance is to detect potential fetal compromise (ACOG, 1987). By instituting specific surveillance tests, the clinician is better able to diagnose potential fetal abnormalities and can more confidently pronounce a fetus normal. Previously utilized indirect biochemical tests have been replaced by direct biophysical testing of the fetus. Most recently, there has been the introduction of newer fetal surveillance techniques including Doppler blood flow studies. At the same time, the contraction stress test (CST) is being used less often, replaced by the nonstress test (NST) and biophysical profile (BPP). Although these tests are widely used and accepted, interpretation of results, testing schemes, and management strategies vary greatly (Schifrin & Clement, 1990).

The primary indication for antepartum surveillance testing of fetal well-being is the high-risk pregnancy. There are a variety of conditions that would require testing. They include (ACOG, 1987; Freeman, 1987):

- Hypertensive disorders
- Diabetes mellitus (insulin dependent)
- Suspected oligohydramnios
- Intrauterine growth retardation
- Prolonged pregnancy (≥42 weeks)
- Isoimmunization
- Chronic renal disease
- Maternal cyanotic heart disease
- Hemoglobinopathies (SS, SC, S-Thal)
- Multiple gestation
- Previous unexplained fetal demise
- Decreased fetal movement (maternal perception)
- Preterm labor
- Premature rupture of membranes
- Vaginal bleeding

The choice of surveillance test to evaluate fetal well-being will vary, but there are important points that should be considered when choosing the most appropriate test. These include availability, patient compliance, early predictability of fetal compromise, rate of false-positive results, and rate of false-negative results.

The initiation of testing will depend upon the prognosis for neonatal survival. The frequency of testing will depend upon the severity, timing, and number of clinical conditions. Generally, with multiple or severe high-risk conditions, testing may begin as early as 26-28 weeks when there is a possibility of extrauterine survival and with the understanding that interpretation of results at this gestation may be unclear. In most high-risk pregnancies, testing usually begins at 32 to 34 weeks gestation or when evidence of fetoplacental compromise is found. The frequency of testing will vary with the specific test techniques and clinical condition. Generally, the frequency for repeating tests is every 7 days unless the previous test was abnormal or specific conditions necessitate more frequent surveillance (i.e., prolonged pregnancy, insulin-dependent diabetes, or intrauterine growth retardation) (ACOG, 1987). Refer to protocols of specific conditions for antepartum surveillance management recommendations.

Pregnancies monitored by surveillance tests should be co-managed by a physician. For specific conditions, such as insulin-dependent diabetes, management may be provided primarily by the physician. Management of abnormal tests requires further evaluation or delivery as appropriate. In the absence of obstetric contraindications, delivery of a fetus with an abnormal test is usually attempted by induction of labor. Cesarean delivery may be indicated for obstetric complications or with abnormal fetal heart rates.

The following are descriptions of each of the common antepartum fetal surveillance tests.

Fetal Movement Counts

The majority of women feel fetal movements beginning at the fifth month of pregnancy. Early fetal movements are weak, infrequent, and are sometimes difficult to distinguish from abdominal movements of the intestines. Fetal activity increases in strength and is most frequent between 28 and 34 weeks gestation (Rayburn, 1987). A decline in the number of fetal movements is expected to occur within weeks of delivery but maternally perceived fetal movement does not significantly change in the healthy fetus (Rayburn, 1987). The average number of recorded daily fetal movements vary between 4 and 1440. Most women will perceive a certain number of movements daily that will stay fairly constant throughout the pregnancy (Sadovsky & Polishuk, 1977). Fetal movement is greatest during the late night hours (between 9:00 P.M. and 1:00 A.M.), when compared to the rest of the day (Patrick, Campbell, Carmichael, & Probert, 1982).

Fetal movements may be altered by maternal ingestion of medications and cigarette smoke. Sedatives such as barbiturates, narcotics, methadone, and alcohol cross the placenta, causing a reduction in the number and duration of fetal movements. Nicotine has a depressant effect on the fetal nervous system causing a temporary reduction in fetal gross body movement and breathing (Goodman, Visser, & Dawes, 1984). Altered fetal body movement will usually reverse after drug clearance (Rayburn, 1987).

Maternally perceived fetal activity is used as an indicator of fetal well-being. Maternal recording of fetal activity near term correlates with approximately 85% of motions recorded by ultrasound (Rayburn, 1987). A drop or decrease in fetal activity is associated with fetal distress, especially when chronic uteroplacental insufficiency is present (Rayburn, 1987). If the fetal distress is severe enough to cause intrauterine fetal demise, fetal movements may rapidly diminish and stop 12 to 48 hours before death (Pearson & Weaver, 1976).

Fetal movement monitoring is used as a generally acceptable, non-invasive, cost effective method of fetal surveillance in high- and low-risk pregnancies. Because a large proportion of stillbirths occur at term in pregnancies that are not classified as high-risk, it is recommended that monitoring be done on all pregnant women starting at 28 weeks' gestation (Neldman, 1980; Moore & Piacquadio, 1989).

The techniques and quantification for evaluating fetal movements vary. The count-to-ten method has been generally accepted. It proposes that less than 10 fetal movements in 2 hours is inadequate and should be followed by additional fetal surveillance (Moore & Piacquadio, 1989). Education includes advising patients at 28 weeks gestation to record daily the time it takes to count 10 fetal movements (rolling, stretching, kicking, jabbing, punching, hiccuping, or flutters). In the healthy fetus, 10 movements are usually felt within 10 to 60 minutes. Advise the patient to monitor movements at the same time every day, preferably after eating a meal. Teach her to rest in the lateral recumbent position with her hands extending over the abdomen. External stimuli should be reduced so she can concentrate on the movements. The patient should call her health care provider if 10 movements have not been felt within a two-hour period. See Table 2.3, *Example of Kick Count Record*, p. 43.

Nonstress Test

It has been well established and accepted that fetal heart rate increases during periods of fetal movement. The premise for the nonstress test (NST) is that the normal fetus will demonstrate movement at varying intervals and that the fetal central nervous system and myocardium will respond to this movement in a reflex action by demonstrating fetal heart rate accelerations (Keegan, 1987). An increase in fetal heart rate during movement is accepted as a sign of fetal well-being. A fetus that fails to show fetal heart rate accelerations may be at risk for or suffering from hypoxemia.

The NST is performed with the patient in the semi-Fowler's position. The patient should be non-fasting and have not smoked recently. The fetal heart rate is monitored with an ultrasound transducer for approximately 20 minutes. If no accelerations occur, the monitoring is continued for 40 minutes to account for the fetal sleep-wake cycles. Various techniques have been used to stimulate the fetus to achieve reactivity. Fetal acoustic stimulation has recently been employed by applying a vibratory device on the maternal abdomen overlying the fetus. Sound and vibration are used to startle the fetus, thereby accelerating its heart rate. The relative safety of these devices has not been established (Gagnon, Hunse, & Patrick, 1988; Polzin, Blakemore, Petrie, & Amom, 1988; Paine, Johnson, & Alexander, 1988).

Interpretation of criteria for reactivity of the NST vary widely. The most commonly accepted criteria are as follows (Keegan, 1987):

> Reactive pattern (normal NST) is defined as the presence of two accelerations, lasting ≥ 15 seconds and reaching a zenith ≥ 15 bpm, within a 20 minute period.

> Non-reactive pattern (abnormal NST) fails to meet any one criterion over a 40-minute period.

Non-reactive tests should be followed immediately by a contraction stress test or biophysical profile. Reactive NSTs are usually repeated in seven days and twice weekly in patients with insulin-dependent diabetes, prolonged pregnancy, or intrauterine growth retardation (Keegan, 1987).

The NST is the most commonly used antepartum fetal surveillance test. When compared to other test techniques, the NST has many advantages including: 1) less time consuming, 2) less costly, 3) no contraindications, 4) easier to interpret, 5) does not require frequent repeat testing for suspicious or hyperstimulation test results, 6) can be employed in an outpatient setting, and 7) is reassuring when it is reactive (less than 1% chance of fetal death within one week of reactive NST) (Field, 1989).

The major disadvantage of the NST is its high false-positive rates (nonreactive NST with a normal outcome). The false-positive rates exceed 50% in studies of neonatal morbidity and 80% in studies of neonatal mortality (Keegan, 1987). The major reason for high false-positive rates is the non-uniformity of what represents normal fetal reactivity. Other factors that increase the false-positive rates include: 1) gestational age less than 30 weeks, 2) relative sleep-wake cycles of the fetus, and 3) maternal ingestion of depressant drugs including alcohol and nicotine.

Contraction Stress Test

The contraction stress test (CST) is based on the observation of fetal heart rate response to uterine contractions. The premise for the test is that the fetus beginning to develop marginal basal oxygenation, with the ordinary hypoxic stresses of normal uterine contractions, will manifest late decelerations (Huddleston & Quinlan, 1987). Recurrent late decelerations indicate that the fetus has suboptimal oxygenation of its blood. The absence of late decelerations is considered to be a sign of fetal well-being.

The CST is performed with the patient in the semi-Fowlers or lateral tilt position to prevent maternal hypotension and decrease of uterine blood flow (ACOG, 1987). The fetal heart rate is obtained with an ultrasound transducer, and contraction activity is monitored with a tocodynamometer. A baseline tracing is obtained for 15 to 20 minutes. No uterine stimulation is needed if adequate uterine contractions are present spontaneously. Adequate contractions are defined as at least three contractions within a 10 minute period of time. If fewer than three contractions are observed, uterine stimulation can be produced by oxytocin infusion (Oxytocin Challenge Test, OCT) or manual nipple massage (Breast Self-Stimulation Test, BSST). Breast self-stimulation is generally more acceptable than OCT because of the increased discomfort and cost associated with the OCT. If BSST is inadequate in producing the desired contractions, an intravenous oxytocin infusion is given at a rate of 0.5 mU/minute and is slowly increased as necessary to achieve adequate contractions (Huddleston & Quinlan, 1987). The BSST is accomplished by instructing the patient to rub one nipple, through her clothing, in a to and fro motion with the palmar surface of her fingers, rapidly but gently for 2 minutes or until contractions begin. Stimulation is then stopped for 5 minutes to evaluate uterine activity. If three 40 to 60-second contractions do not occur within ten minutes, another cycle of 2 minutes of stimulation and 5 minutes of rest is started. Stimulation should be discontinued if contractions begin. It takes approximately 40 minutes to complete the BSST including a baseline tracing of 15 to 20 minutes. The success rate of adequate uterine activity with the BSST is 80% to 100% (Huddleston, Sutliff, & Robinson, 1984).

Interpretation and management of the CST is as follows (Field, 1989):

Negative CST (normal): There are no late decelerations. Repeat test in one week.

Positive CST (abnormal): Late decelerations are seen after every contraction. Requires further evaluation or delivery.

Suspicious CST: Late decelerations are seen with some but not all contractions. Requires further evaluation and repeat within 24 hours. Repeat suspicious tests are most often negative. Only 10% to 15% become positive in repeated testing (Huddleston & Quinlan, 1987).

Hyperstimulated CST: There are late decelerations and the uterine contractions are closer together then every two minutes or last longer than 90 seconds. Repeat test within 24 hours.

Unsatisfactory CST: The quality of the tracing is inadequate for accurate interpretation or adequate uterine activity cannot be achieved.

The major advantages of the CST are: 1) low false-negative rate of 1% (Huddleston & Quinlan, 1987), 2) false-positive rate of 50%, which is lower than that of the NST (80%), 3) false-positive rate that does not increase at gestational ages less than 33 weeks (Gabbe, Freeman, & Goebelsman, 1978), 4) negative CST which is associated with a lower antepartum fetal death rate within one week after testing compared to the NST (Freeman, 1987), and 5) the CST appears to be a more sensitive indicator of fetal hypoxia and acidosis making it a better long-range predictor of uteroplacental deterioration (Freeman, 1987).

Contraindications to the CST include clinical conditions that would preclude stimulating uterine contractions: 1) placenta previa, 2) previous vertical uterine scar, and 3) conditions for which risk of preterm delivery is increased (i.e., premature rupture of the membranes, multiple gestation, incompetent cervix, hydramnios, previous preterm delivery) (Huddleston & Quinlan, 1987). Additional disadvantages of the CST include: 1) need for I.V. infusion if OCT is performed, 2) need for hospital based setting in which to perform the test, 3) increased cost compared to the NST, 4) large number equivocal results (10% to 25%) (Porto, 1987), 5) difficulty in interpreting the results, and 6) length of time required to complete the test. The OCT can take one to two hours but the BSST has shortened test time to an average of 40 minutes, reducing the cost of testing.

Biophysical Profile

The biophysical profile (BPP) was developed based on the premise that observing multiple biophysical variables will identify nearly all fetuses with chronic asphyxia in utero, the majority of fetuses with congenital anomalies, and a proportion of fetuses at risk for acute asphyxia (Manning, Morrison, Lange, & Harman, 1982).

The components of the BPP include the nonstress test (NST) and four ultrasound parameters: fetal breathing movements (FBM), body movement (FM), tone (FT), and amniotic fluid volume (AFV) (Manning et al., 1982). Placental grading has been included in a more recent scoring system (Vintzileos, Campbell, Ingardia, & Nochimson, 1983). The NST is performed and interpreted according to the criteria outlined in the protocol for NST. Real-time ultrasound is used to evaluate the remaining variables. Ultrasound observation is continued until the variable becomes normal or 30 minutes elapse. There are currently two types of scoring systems: 1) each variable is either normal (score=2) or abnormal (score=0) (Table 2.4, *Technique of Biophysical Profile Scoring*, p. 44), and 2) each variable receives a score of 0, 1, or 2 (Table 2.5, *Criteria for Scoring Biophysical Variables*, p. 45).

Guidelines for obstetric management based on the BPP score have been developed. It is recommended to use this protocol as a guide and to individualize management according to the patient and her presenting condition. See Table 2.6, *Biophysical Profile Scoring: Management Protocol*, p. 46 for the BPP management protocol.

The major advantage of the BPP is a lower false-positive rate when compared to the single variable tests. The single variable tests (NST, CST) are accurate predictors of normal fetal condition (false-negative rate of 1%) but are relatively inaccurate in predicting the fetus at risk for poor outcome (50% to 80% false-positive rate). Using a combination of variables, the BPP has a greater ability to accurately identify the sick fetus. The BPP provides other useful information with regard to fetal number and position, placental location and grading, risks of IUGR where oligohydramnios is common, and identification of major congenital anomalies (Brar, Platt, & Devore, 1987). The BPP may be used as a confirmatory test for the fetus with an abnormal NST or CST. This may prevent unnecessary intervention when well-being is assured. When performed by trained personnel, the BPP can be completed in as little as 20 minutes.

Limitations of the BPP include: 1) lack of knowledge regarding the sequelae of fetuses with low scores, 2) how the duration and frequency of hypoxia will affect the fetus, and 3) the relative weight of each of the scoring criteria (i.e., does the absence of fetal movement or amniotic fluid volume have the same significance as the absence of fetal breathing movements and a non-reactive NST?) (Manning et al., 1982). A major disadvantage of the BPP is that it requires sonographic skills for interpretation and it may be more costly and time consuming than the single variable tests. These factors may make it too cumbersome for use as a primary mode of fetal surveillance in some settings. The modified BPP (NST and amniotic fluid assessment) has been shown to be quicker and at least as effective as a full BPP or a CST (Clark, 1990). With the modified BPP, assessment of fetal breathing, body movement, and tone are reserved for cases when the NST is nonreactive (Vintzileos, Campbell, Nochimson, & Weinbaum, 1987).

Ultrasound

Perinatal ultrasound imaging is used to obtain information about the fetus and mother that will aid in diagnosis and patient management. Ultrasound is defined as any sound with a frequency of greater than 20,000 hertz (Hz) (undetectable by the human ear). A frequency of 3 to 5 megahertz (Mhz) (3 to 5 million cycles per second) is most commonly used in obstetric examinations (ACOG, 1988). The two basic types of ultrasound equipment are called static and real-time. Static scanners produce a "frozen" image from several different points of the examining field. Real-time scanners are able to detect fetal movement, heart activity, and breathing movement. The real-time scanners are used almost exclusively in the obstetric setting because of their obvious advantages over static scanners (ACOG, 1988).

Obstetric ultrasound instrumentation functions by emitting sound waves into the maternal abdomen. The sound waves are reflected when they interface with tissue or structures of varying densities. The reflected sound waves' frequency, length, speed, amplitude, and intensity are analyzed to produce a visible image of the internal structures (Modica & Timor-Trisch, 1988).

The two techniques for ultrasound imaging in obstetrics are the transabdominal and transvaginal procedures. The transabdominal procedure usually requires the patient to drink six 8-ounce glasses of clear fluid (no milk) one hour prior to the exam to fill the bladder. The patient is instructed not to urinate and that the exam will take approximately 30 to 60 minutes. A full bladder is necessary to elevate the uterus into the abdomen, permitting optimal visualization of the fetus. A full bladder may not be necessary in the third trimester when the fetus is out of the pelvis. The ultrasound probe, covered with coupling gel, is placed on the maternal abdomen and slowly passed through all four quadrants. The only discomfort associated with the procedure may be from a full bladder.

The transvaginal procedure is performed by inserting the probe, covered with a condom and coupling gel, into the vagina. Insertion may be performed by the ultrasonographer or the patient. The benefit of the transvaginal technique is its clearer image resolution, enhanced by a higher sound frequency and by the fact that the sound waves travel to a depth of only 1 to 2 cm before reaching the area under examination. The primary advantage of the transvaginal ultrasound is its ability to diagnose early tubal pregnancies. Diagnosis of cervical incompetence, ovarian lesions, low-lying placentas, early intrauterine pregnancies, and a pregnancy in an obese patient are also made easier with the transvaginal approach (Timor-Tritsch & Rottem, 1988).

Indications for use of ultrasound during pregnancy include (National Institutes of Health Consensus Development Panel, 1984):

- Estimation of gestational age for patients with uncertain dates
- Evaluation of fetal growth when intrauterine growth retardation is suspected
- Significant uterine size/date discrepancy
- Evaluation of fetal condition in late registrants
- Suspected ectopic pregnancy
- Vaginal bleeding of unknown origin
- Suspected hydatidiform mole
- Presence of a pelvic mass
- Determination of fetal presentation

- Suspected fetal demise

- Polyhydramnios or oligohydramnios

- Possible abruptio placenta or previa

- Estimation of fetal weight

- History of previous congenital anomaly

- Abnormal maternal serum alpha-fetoprotein value

- Suspected uterine anomaly

- Suspected cervical incompetence

- IUD localization

- Ovarian follicle surveillance

- Adjunct to special procedures such as cervical cerclage, external version, manual removal of the placenta, intrauterine transfusion, percutaneous umbilical blood sampling, amniocentesis, chorionic villus sampling, *in vitro* fertilization, biophysical profile

The safety of ultrasound has been supported in the low Mhz frequency range (obstetric instrument outputs are well below this range). There are no studies to date that confirm significant biological effects in human tissue (American Institute of Ultrasound in Medicine, Bioeffects Committee, 1988). Because of the possibility of unknown risk, it is recommended that ultrasound imaging be used only when medically indicated with minimum exposure to the patient and fetus. At this time, routine scanning is not recommended.

Percutaneous Umbilical Blood Sampling

Percutaneous umbilical blood sampling (PUBS) is performed at 16 to 40 weeks' gestation by inserting a needle into the fetal umbilical vessel for fetal evaluation and/or intrauterine treatment. Prior to the sampling, an ultrasound is performed to confirm gestational age, to estimate fetal weight, and to exclude fetal anatomical malformation. Ultrasound is then used to guide a 10 to 16 cm, 22 gauge needle through the maternal abdomen into the umbilical vessel. The umbilical cord is punctured 1 to 2 cm from its placental insertion where it is more stable. An artery or vein can be sampled, although the artery has greater advantage for fetal transfusion. A vein is used most frequently because it has a larger diameter and is easily punctured. A sample of 0.5 to 3cc of blood is removed and assayed by a Kleihauer-Betke test to evaluate sample purity. Maternal blood contamination is more common when samples are taken closer to the placenta.

Percutaneous umbilical blood sampling is primarily used for rapid fetal karyotyping and to evaluate fetuses at risk for isoimmune hemolytic disease. Other indications for PUBS include evaluation of: 1) intrauterine infection, 2) hemoglobinopathies, 3) coagulation factor deficiencies, 4) nonimmune hydrops fetalis, 5) fetal blood gases and acid base status, 6) immune deficiencies, 7) platelet abnormalities, and for fetal drug therapy (Seeds, 1988).

The major treatment indication for using PUBS is to correct fetal anemia. Percutaneous umbilical blood sampling is preferred to intraperitoneal transfusion because it can be performed 4 to 5 weeks earlier and because the red cells are transfused directly into the fetal circulation. Platelets can also be transfused into a fetus with severe thrombocytopenia. Transfusion therapy can be started as early as 19 weeks gestation or when PUBS reveals a Coomb's positive fetus to have a hematocrit of less than 30% (Ludomirski & Weiner, 1988).

Complications of the PUBS procedure include chorioamnionitis, premature labor, rupture of amniotic membranes, abruptio placenta, bleeding, laceration or thrombus of the umbilical vessel, and transient fetal arrhythmias (Dunn, Weiner, & Ludomirski, 1988). To reduce the incidence of chorioamnionitis, a broad spectrum antibiotic can be administered after the procedure. Infection has occurred in 1% and rupture has been reported in 0.2% of PUBS procedures (Dunn et al., 1988). Cord bleeding is common (18.3%) but is usually self-limiting and stops after 10 to 60 seconds (Dunn et al., 1988).

A nonstress test is usually performed immediately after the PUBS procedure. An ultrasound and Doppler flow studies may also be performed. Postprocedure education should include premature labor precautions and the signs and symptoms of infection.

Doppler Flow Studies

Doppler ultrasound is used to measure the speed of blood in the vessels or chambers through which it flows. It has been used in the adult and pediatric populations for assessment of blood vessels and the myocardium. Recently, Doppler ultrasound has been found to be an important tool for assessment of the fetus.

Doppler ultrasound is performed by applying a transducer to the maternal abdomen and directing an ultrasound beam at a maternal or fetal blood vessel. The beam is reflected from the red cells moving within the vessel which causes a change in frequency of the ultrasound beam. These changes in frequency are proportional to the velocity of the reflecting red cells moving at various rates within the vascular channels (Watson, Young, & Hegge, 1987).

There are three types of Doppler ultrasound: 1) continuous-wave, 2) pulsed-wave, and 3) color-flow imaging. Continuous-wave ultrasound emits a continuous beam that records the velocity of blood cells moving in its path. This form of Doppler is used for fetal heart rate monitoring and determination of fetal heart rate via the pocket Doppler system. The disadvantages of the continuous-wave Doppler is that there is no real-time imaging of the vessels. Parameters of flow velocity and total blood flow cannot be determined.

The pulsed Doppler system uses real-time ultrasound to locate and measure a specific vessel or specific area of the fetal heart. The pulsed-wave Doppler system is more expensive and more difficult to operate, although it allows for precise velocity and flow determinations.

Doppler color-flow imaging is a new technology in which a sample of an entire image is taken as opposed to a selected area. The image is color coded so that it looks like an angiogram of blood flow with velocity superimposed upon a real-time image (Platt, DeVore, Schulman, & Wladimiroff, 1989).

The Doppler system has a variety of clinical uses for fetal assessment. Early in the first trimester, the continuous-wave system is used to detect a fetal heart beat. Color-flow imaging is used in the first half of pregnancy to diagnose and assess congenital heart defects and circulation of the growth-retarded fetus. During the second half of pregnancy, the Doppler system has been used to evaluate the fetus at risk for intrauterine compromise or fetal death by assessing blood flow changes in the fetal heart, aorta, cerebrum, and maternal uterine and umbilical arteries. Doppler studies are also beneficial in assessing blood flow in monochorionic twins where shared circulation places at least one of the twins at risk for growth retardation.

Currently, Doppler flow studies are being utilized as an adjunctive surveillance technique in pregnancies at risk for growth retardation. An abnormal flow study does not indicate an immediate change of management protocol but indicates further fetal evaluation (Platt et al., 1989). There is no evidence to date that shows Doppler ultrasound to be harmful to the fetus (Watson et al., 1987; Platt et al., 1989).

Table 2.3

Example of Kick Count Record

DATE:

An easy way to check the health of your baby is once each day to count the number of times the baby kicks. At the same time every day, after you have eaten, record the amount of time it takes for your baby to kick 10 times.

For example, on Monday, you begin to count your baby's kicks at 7:00 P.M. By 7:30 P.M. your baby has kicked 10 times. You fill in the chart like this.

Remember that every baby is an individual. It has times when it sleeps and times when it is active. If you start counting and the baby is not kicking, stop, walk around for 5 minutes, and then count again. (Helpful hint: count baby's kicks after you have eaten). If, at the end of two hours, your baby has not kicked 10 times, call the Delivery Room.

Kicks = movements, twists, turns.

40th Week							
	M	T	W	T	F	S	S
MINUTES 10							
20							
30	X						
40							
50							
HOURS 1							
1 ½							
2							

DATE:

	28th WEEK							29th WEEK							30th WEEK							31st WEEK						
	M	T	W	T	F	S	S	M	T	W	T	F	S	S	M	T	W	T	F	S	S	M	T	W	T	F	S	S
MINUTES 10																												
20																												
30																												
40																												
50																												
HOURS 1																												
1 ½																												
2																												

(Charting would continue through end of pregnancy)

SOURCE:

Adapted from: UCSF Department of Obstetrics (1988).

Table 2.4

Technique of Biophysical Profile Scoring

Biophysical Variable	Normal (Score=2)	Abnormal (Score=0)
1. Fetal breathing movements	At least 1 episode of at least 30 seconds' duration in 30 minutes' observation	Absent or no episode of ≥ 30 seconds in 30 minutes
2. Gross body movement	At least 3 discrete body/limb movements in 30 minutes (episodes of active continuous movement considered as a single movement)	Two or fewer episodes of body/limb movements in 30 minutes
3. Fetal tone	At least 1 episode of active extension with return to flexion of fetal limb(s) or trunk. Opening and closing of hand considered normal tone	Either slow extension with return to partial flexion, or movement of limb in full extension, or absent fetal movement
4. Reactive fetal heart rate	At least 2 episodes of acceleration of ≥ 15 bpm and at least 15 seconds' duration associated with fetal movement in 30 minutes	Less than 2 accelerations or acceleration < 15 bpm in 30 minutes
5. Qualitative amniotic fluid volume	At least 1 pocket of amniotic fluid that measures at least 2 cm* in two perpendicular planes	Either no amniotic fluid pockets or a pocket < 1 cm in two perpendicular planes

SOURCE:

Manning, F. A., Morrison, I., Lange, J. R., & Harman, C. (1982). Antepartum determination of fetal health: Composite biophysical profile scoring. *Clinics in Perinatology, 9*(2), 285-296. Reprinted with permission.

*Chamberlain, P. F., Manning, F. A., Morrison, J., Harman, C. R., & Lange, J. R. (1984). Ultrasound evaluation of amniotic fluid volumes. I. The relationship of marginal and decreased amniotic fluid to perinatal outcome. *American Journal of Obstetrics and Gynecology, 150*(3), 245-249.

Table 2.5

Criteria for Scoring Biophysical Variables

Nonstress Test
  Score 2 (NST 2): ≥ 5 FHR accelerations of at least 15 bpm in amplitude and at least 15 seconds duration associated with fetal movements in a 20-minute period.
  Score 1 (NST 1): 2-4 acceleration of at least 15 bpm in amplitude and at least 15 seconds duration associated with fetal movements in a 20-minute period.
  Score 0 (NST 0): ≤ 1 acceleration in a 20-minute period.

Fetal movements
  Score 2 (FM 2): ≥ 3 gross (trunk and limbs) episodes of fetal movements within 30 minutes. Simultaneous limb and trunk movements counted as a single movement.
  Score 1 (FM 1): 1-2 fetal movements within 30 minutes.
  Score 0 (FM 0): Absence of fetal movements within 30 minutes.

Fetal breathing movements
  Score 2 (FBM 2): ≥ 1 episode of fetal breathing of at least 60 seconds duration within a 30-minute observation period.
  Score 1 (FBM 1): ≥ 1 episode of fetal breathing lasting 30-60 seconds within 30 minutes.
  Score 0 (FBM 0): Absence of fetal breathing or breathing lasting < 30 seconds within 30 minutes.

Fetal Tone
  Score 2 (FT 2): ≥ 1 episode of extension of extremities with return to position of flexion and 1 episode of extension of spine with return to position of flexion.
  Score 1 (FT 1): ≥ 1 episode of extension of extremities with return to position of flexion or 1 episode of extension of spine with return to position of flexion.
  Score 0 (FT 0): Extremities in extension. Fetal movements not followed by return to flexion. Open hand.

Amniotic fluid volume
  Score 2 (AF 2): Fluid evident throughout the uterine cavity. A pocket that measures ≥ 2 cm in vertical diameter.
  Score 1 (AF 1): A pocket that measures < 2 cm but > 1 cm in vertical diameter.
  Score 0 (AF 0): Crowding of fetal small parts. Largest pocket < 1 cm in vertical diameter.

Placenta grading
  Score 2 (PL 2): Placental grading of 0, 1, or 2.
  Score 1 (PL 1): Placenta posterior difficult to evaluate.
  Score 0 (PL 0): Placental grading 3.

Legend:

NST, nonstress test	FHR, fetal heart rate	bpm, beats per minute;
FM, fetal movements	FBM, fetal breathing movements	FT, fetal tone
AF, amniotic fluid	PL, placental grading	

Maximal score, 12	Minimal score, 0.

SOURCE:

Vintzileos, A. M., Campbell, W. A., Ingardia, C. J., & Nochimsom, D. J. (1983). The fetal biophysical profile and its predictive value. *Obstetrics and Gynecology, 62*(3), 271-278. Reprinted with permission.

Table 2.6

Biophysical Profile Scoring: Management Protocol

Score	Interpretation	Recommended management
10	Normal infant, low risk for chronic asphyxia	Repeat testing at weekly intervals. Repeat twice weekly in diabetic patients and patients ≥ 42 wk
8	Normal infant, low risk for chronic asphyxia	Repeat testing at weekly intervals. Repeat twice weekly in diabetic patients and patients ≥ 42 wk. Indication for delivery = oligohydramnios
6	Suspected chronic asphyxia	Repeat testing within 24 hr. Indication for delivery = oligohydramnios or remaining ≤ 6
4	Suspected chronic asphyxia	Indication for delivery = ≥ 36 wk and favorable cervix. If < 36 wk and lecithin/sphingomyelin ratio < 2.0, repeat test in 24 hr. Indication for delivery = repeat score ≤ 6 or oligohydramnios
0-2	Strong suspicion of chronic asphyxia	Extend testing time to 120 min. Indication for delivery = persistent score ≤ 4, regardless of gestational age

SOURCE:

Adapted from: Manning, F. A., Morrison, I., Lange, J. R., Harmon, C. R., & Chamberlain, P. F. (1985). Fetal assessment based on fetal biophysical scoring: Experience in 12,620 referred high-risk pregnancies. *American Journal of Obstetrics and Gynecology*, *151*(3), 343-350. Reprinted with permission.

Chapter 3

Common Discomforts
of Pregnancy

BACKACHE

Winifred L. Star

Lordosis (anterior convexity of the spine) is a characteristic of a normal lumbar spine that becomes exaggerated during pregnancy as the weight of the enlarging uterus shifts the woman's center of gravity, causing stretching and strain of the muscles in this area. Lack of support from lax abdominal muscles may contribute to compensatory lordosis. Relaxation of the pelvic joints (secondary to hormonal changes of pregnancy), inadequate rest, or strain due to improper body mechanics are factors that may also contribute to low backache. Pain in the cervicothoracic as well as the sternocostal and costovertebral areas may occur as a result of the increased weight of the breasts during pregnancy. Pathologic causes of pain such as sprain due to trauma, intervertebral disc herniation, vertebral fractures, pyelonephritis, and radicular pain should be evaluated as indicated. Obstetric causes of backache such as premature labor should be ruled out.

Data Base

Subjective

- History of back problems/injury/surgery

- Obesity

- Excessive weight gain in pregnancy

- High-heeled or improperly fitting shoes

- Recent trauma

- History of excessive exercise, bending, lifting, twisting, sitting, or walking

- Improper use of body mechanics

- Fatigue

- Weight loss

- Symptoms may include: pain, aching, tightness, or spasm in upper or lower back; numbness, tingling, weakness in back, buttocks, or extremities. Pain may be aggravated by coughing, sneezing, laughing. May have associated gastrointestinal or genitourinary symptomatology.

- May report signs and symptoms of premature labor. See Preterm Birth Prevention protocol.

Objective

- Lax abdominal musculature

- Lordotic curve

- Abnormal gait

- Patient may have tenderness/spasm along paraspinous muscles.

- Patellar, ankle or plantar deep tendon reflexes may be decreased, uneven or absent (indicates neurological deficit).

- Straight leg raising may cause or increase pain in back, buttocks, or legs (indicates disc/neurological involvement).

- Abdominal exam may reveal tenderness or decreased bowel sounds.

- Costovertebral angle tenderness may be present.

- Vaginal exam may reveal abnormal lesions/discharge.

- If in labor, uterine contractions may be palpable by examiner.

Assessment

- Physiologic backache
- R/O Lumbar, cervicothoracic, sternocostal, or costovertebral muscle strain/sprain
- R/O Sciatica
- R/O Intervertebral disc herniation
- R/O Vertebral tumor/fracture
- R/O Pyelonephritis
- R/O Gastrointestinal disorder/disease
- R/O Genital infection
- R/O Premature labor

Plan

Diagnostic Tests

- Perform physical exam as indicated by history and symptom assessment.

- X-rays are to be avoided in pregnancy except per MD consult.

- Labs may include: CBC, urinalysis with culture and sensitivities, cervical cultures.

Treatment/Management

Physiologic Causes or Strain:

- Apply ice to affected area(s) for first 24 hours after an acute injury. Application may be for 10-20 minutes at a time, 20 minutes/hour, or as indicated (M. P. Hirsch, personal communication, 1990).

- Apply local, moist heat with proper padding or toweling to affected area(s) if there is no acute injury or if pain is due to physiologic cause. Dry heat (i.e., heating pad) is not recommended as the heat from this source is non-penetrating and does not reach the deep muscles of the back (M. P. Hirsch, personal communication, 1986).

- Warm (not hot) tub baths not to exceed 30 minutes

- Rest on firm supportive surface; a bed board may be necessary.

- Massage and relaxation

- Supportive brassiere

- Low-heeled, supportive, and comfortable shoes

- Pelvic rocking exercise -- about 10-12 times a day

- Proper body mechanics; avoidance of heavy lifting

- Abdominal muscle strengthening exercises

- Maternity girdle -- especially useful in obese women, multiparas, or women with extreme lordosis

- Analgesics such as acetaminophen 325 mg two tablets q 4 hours prn pain. Long-term use of analgesics may indicate more serious pathology and would require MD evaluation.

- General fitness exercise 3-4 times a week for at least 30 minutes (e.g., stretching, walking, swimming, prenatal exercise class)

- Physiotherapy as indicated by MD consult

Pathologic Causes:

- Refer to either orthopedic specialist, neurologist, or internal medicine physician for significant pathologic back pain, or if physical exam findings indicative of pathology.

- Physiotherapy as indicated by MD consult

- Treat genitourinary infections as indicated. See protocols.

- See also Preterm Birth Prevention protocol.

Consultation

- Not required for cases of physiologic back pain

- Required for acute strain/sprain or other pathologic causes of back pain

- Discuss appropriateness of referrals to alternative sources of care such as chiropractic, acupuncture, or acupressure.

Patient Education

- Stress avoidance of sitting, standing, or walking for long periods of time; encourage patient to wear low-heeled, comfortable shoes.

- Discuss need for adequate rest periods, avoidance of fatigue, and excess stress.

- Teach patient pelvic rock exercise, abdominal exercises, and use of proper body mechanics for lifting, moving, standing, etc.

- Encourage general fitness; suggest formal prenatal exercise class.

- Suggest that a friend or partner give a back massage.

- Suggest incorporation of relaxation techniques into daily living.

- Give hints for support to lower back area while resting/sleeping (e.g., use of pillows under knees and between legs).

- Offer suggestions for reading materials related to relaxation, exercise in pregnancy, massage, etc.

- Encourage maintenance of well-balanced diet and give suggestions for meal planning if on bed rest. See Nutrition protocol.

Follow-up

- Refer to MD all patients with significant pathologic causes of back pain.

- Refer to MD those patients whose pain is not responding to routine conservative therapies.

- Give referrals for prenatal exercise class in your facility or community.

- Encourage patient compliance with suggested treatment modalities.

- Evaluate response to therapy as indicated; may need to see patient more frequently for return visits.

- If patient on restrictive bed rest, refer to social services for assistance with child care arrangements as indicated.

- Document in problem list and in progress notes if a significant ongoing problem.

CONSTIPATION

Lucy Newmark Sammons

Constipation is defined as defecation that is difficult, infrequent, or marked by unduly hard and dry stool (Thomas, 1989). Decreased bowel motility during pregnancy may be caused by: 1) progesterone, a smooth muscle relaxant, acting on the bowel; 2) changes in dietary habits; 3) mechanical compression and displacement of the bowel by the gravid uterus; 4) relaxation of abdominal musculature; 5) increased fluid absorption from the large intestine; 6) change in activity/exercise patterns; 7) tension and anxiety; or 8) constipating effect of supplemental iron.

Data Base

Subjective

- Reports decreased frequency of defecation and/or increased hardness of stool with difficulty emptying bowels

- Client may report:

  - History of irregular/difficult bowel movements

  - History of laxative habit

  - Diet lacking adequate roughage and fluids; high in refined carbohydrates

  - Sedentary activity level or bedrest

  - Complaints of abdominal cramping and flatulence

  - Complaint of hemorrhoids or other local anorectal problem contributing to suppression of defecation

  - Emotional tension, inability to relax

  - Use of drugs that increase constipation: antacids with aluminum hydroxide or calcium, iron supplements, anticholinergies, tricyclic antidepressants, codeine analgesics, or cough medicine (Seller, 1986).

- Patient reports NO severe abdominal pain or passing of blood, pus, or mucus per rectum.

Objective

- May palpate fullness in large intestines abdominally

- May detect unevacuated stool on rectal exam

Assessment

- Constipation

- R/O Pathologic causes of abdominal pain if warranted by data base (e.g., appendicitis, irritable colon)

- R/O Alternative causes of abdominal cramping, e.g., labor, Braxton-Hicks contractions

- R/O Intestinal obstruction

53

- R/O Fecal impaction
- R/O Irritable bowel syndrome

Plan

Diagnostic Tests

- No further diagnostic tests indicated in absence of other suspected pathology

Treatment/Management

- See Patient Education for modifications of diet, activity, and lifestyle.
- If necessary, bulk laxative such as Psyllium hydrophilic mucilloid (Metamucil) <u>Sig</u>: i rounded teaspoon in 8 oz liquid po qd to tid x 2-3 days prn followed by additional 8 oz liquid (higher dosages may be considered). Other bulk laxatives are methylcellulose, malt soup extract, and polycarbophil (Brucker, 1988).
- If necessary, stool softener such as Docusate Sodium (dioctyl sodium sulfosuccinate, DSS, DOSS, Colace, Doxinate), 100 mg capsules, <u>Sig</u>: caps ii po stat, then cap i-ii po qd prn; or Docusate Calcium 240 mg capsule, <u>Sig</u>: cap i po qd x 2-3 days
- If necessary in severe cases, magnesium hydroxide (milk of magnesia, MOM) <u>Sig</u>: ii-iv Tbsp po, followed by glass of water
- In extreme cases, may consider senna concentrate natural laxative (Senekot) <u>Sig</u>: tabs i-ii po at HS prn, but caution necessary because may stimulate gravid uterus and cause discomfort with abdominal cramping.
- Correct any perianal problems interfering with bowel evacuation
- If administering iron supplement, advise taking with prune juice or consider interrupting use until severe constipation resolves. Re-evaluate use of other constipating medications.

Consultation

- For impaction or failure to respond to conservative treatment consult MD.

Patient Education

- Explain multiple causes of constipation in pregnancy and rationale for treatment approaches.
- Explore variety of treatment approaches (modification of diet and activities), maintaining sensitivity to the lifestyle and habits of the woman.
    - Modify dietary intake to include sufficient roughage (e.g., bran--3 Tbsp daily; fruits and vegetables; whole grain products).
    - Avoid or reduce constipating foods.
    - Improve hydration by drinking 6-8 glasses of water daily in addition to mealtime beverages.
    - Drink warm beverages upon rising.
    - Establish regular time for bowel evacuation.
    - Increase abdominal muscle tone by walking or other exercise, and maintaining good posture.
- Avoid reliance on laxatives and enemas.

- Avoid prolonged attempts to empty bowels with exertion, which predisposes to hemorrhoids. Support feet on stool or box to reduce straining.

Follow-up

- Reassess bowel activity and related lifestyle habits in subsequent visits.

- Document in progress notes and problem list while an active problem.

COUGH

Lucy Newmark Sammons

A cough is defined as a forceful expiratory effort, preceded by a preliminary inspiration (Thomas, 1989). The main purpose of coughing is to clear the airway. A cough in which mucus or an exudate is expectorated is described as productive, moist, or effective; a cough without expectoration is dry or nonproductive.

Coughing is caused by a large variety of conditions, most often irritation of the upper or lower airways (Seller, 1986). Acute coughing is most often caused by infections (i.e., viral upper respiratory tract infection (URI), bronchitis, or laryngitis), allergic responses, or postnasal drip. Chronic coughing is usually caused by bronchitis (especially in smokers), postnasal drip, chronic obstructive pulmonary disease (COPD), asthma, environmental irritants, allergies, postnasal drip, heart failure, tuberculosis, lung tumor, or habit (Seller, 1986). The treatment approach will be based on the causative factors.

Data Base

Subjective

- Client complains of coughing

- History and symptoms may suggest cause (Seller, 1986):

  - Viral: Sudden onset of cough, accompanied by fever or acute infection symptoms; cough noisy, productive of minimal sputum or dry and hacking, often worse at night, lasting 7-10 days

  - Bacterial/mycoplasma: Cough prominent; onset over hours or days; sputum thick, yellowish; persistence beyond 14 days suggests secondary bacterial infection of viral URI; coughs from mycoplasma infections may continue for months after other symptoms gone

  - Asthma: Cough accompanied by shortness of breath, bilateral wheezing; if productive, only small amount clear mucus, precipitated by exercise

  - Postnasal drip: Frequent swallowing of mucus; cough worse in morning

  - Allergy: Cough occurs at night without dyspnea; associated with exposure to allergens (e.g., pollens), has seasonal variation; accompanied by itching on roof of mouth or eyes

  - Congestive heart failure/paroxysmal nocturnal dyspnea: Cough occurs at night with shortness of breath

  - Tobacco smoke: Woman is cigarette smoker, or cough associated with passive exposure to tobacco smoke; chronic cough may be worse in morning, produces minimal sputum

  - Bronchogenic carcinoma: chronic cigarette smoker, long-standing cough with recent change in pattern; hemoptysis; chest pain

Objective

- Observe for systemic and localized signs of infectious processes in ears, nose, throat, mouth, sinuses, neck, and chest.

- Observe for allergic responses in nasal mucosa and conjunctiva.

- Observe for mucoid secretion (postnasal drip) in posterior pharynx.

- Observe for signs of cardiopulmonary diseases; tachypnea with respiratory rate greater than 20 breaths per minute is hallmark of respiratory disease (Noble, Lavee, & Jacobs, 1988).

- Examine sputum characteristics.

Assessment

Cough, secondary to:

- Upper respiratory system infection, e.g., sinusitis, chronic bronchitis

- Asthma

- Postnasal drip

- Allergic response

- Tobacco smoke, other irritants

- Cardiac or pulmonary diseases as identified, e.g., pneumonia

- Habit/psychogenic factors

- Reflex (ear-cough) mechanism, caused by irritation of external auditory canal or tympanic membrane (e.g., cerumen, foreign body)

- R/O Pneumocystis carinii pneumonia (PCP), Human immunodeficiency virus (HIV)

- R/O Bronchogenic carcinoma, tuberculosis, ornithosis (from contact with fowl or pet birds), coccidioidomycosis (fungal infection common in southwestern United States)

Plan

Diagnostic Tests

- Purified protein derivative (PPD) intradermal test for tuberculosis, followed by chest radiograph if positive and patient is symptomatic (Noble, Lavee, & Jacobs, 1988)

- Sputum cytologic or microscopic examination, if indicated

- See Dyspnea protocol and Upper Respiratory Infection protocol as indicated. Tests ordered on consultation with physician may include complete blood count, eosinophil count, sinus radiograph, chest radiograph (for fever with productive cough, persistent cough of 2 weeks, hemoptysis, pleural rub, or evidence of pulmonary edema of pneumothorax), pulmonary function tests

Treatment/Management

- Identify and treat underlying cause of coughing, as needed.

- Antitussive/expectorant combination: Dextromethorphan and Guaifenesin (Robitussin-DM), available without prescription

- If acetaminophen indicated, additional Codeine acts as antitussive: Tylenol with Codeine #3 30 mg tab <u>Sig</u>: tab i po q 4 hrs, prn pain and cough; try to avoid codeine first trimester (Vintzileos, Deaton, & Campbell, 1986).

- Decongestant: Pseudoephedrine HCl (Sudafed) 30 mg tab <u>Sig</u>: tab i po q 4 hrs

- For additional symptom relief and preventive strategies, see Patient Education.

Consultation

- Medical consultation for evaluation and management of suspected underlying pathology beyond scope of practice

- Consultation for prescriptions as needed

Patient Education

- Explain causes of coughing and rationale for treatment approach.

- If factors can be identified which cause/increase coughing, advise woman to try to avoid situations in which they occur, e.g., avoid or reduce exposure to allergens (pets, pollens) or irritants (chemicals, smoke).

- Advise smoking cessation if woman a smoker, emphasizing relief from coughing as an additional motivator.

- Advise maintaining good hydration by drinking plenty (8 glasses or more) of fluids per day.

- Use of vaporizer may help loosen secretions and promote comfort.

- Client to contact provider if treatment approach not successful or if symptoms become worse.

Follow-up

- Follow-up will be based on underlying cause of cough. Generally, patient to contact provider if symptom relief not obtained in 48 hours.

- Document in progress notes and problem list if a significant ongoing problem.

DIZZINESS

Lucy Newmark Sammons

Complaints of dizziness may represent true vertigo or dizziness/lightheadedness (Seller, 1986). True vertigo refers to the feeling of a disturbed relation to space, while lightheadedness/dizziness refers to the sensation of being about to faint without true syncope or feeling of movement. Pregnancy related syncopal episodes are most common after taking a large meal or upon quickly rising from a lying or sitting position (Morrison & Palmer, 1987). Fainting episodes are usually accompanied by sweating, pallor, and a drop in pulse rate. Both vertigo and lightheadedness are considered in this discussion of dizziness.

Dizziness has many causes, including central nervous system disorders, disturbances affecting vestibular function (middle ear disease, impacted cerumen, Meniere's disease), or ocular disease or strain. Central vertigo may be caused by head trauma, brain tumors, migraine headaches, seizure disorders, or multiple sclerosis (Morrison & Palmer, 1987). Additional causes include substance toxicity (e.g., drugs or alcohol), sunstroke, hyperventilation or emotional distress, endocrine disorders, or hypoglycemia.

Circulatory system problems causing dizziness include anemia, cardiac insufficiency, hypovolemia (especially in hot weather), and postural hypotension. Syncope and faintness during pregnancy related to vasomotor instability occur because blood pools in the lower extremities, splanchnic, and pelvic areas, resulting in transient cerebral ischemia. Supine hypotensive syndrome is caused by compression of the vena cava by the gravid uterus in the recumbent position.

Data Base

Subjective

- Reports occasional lightheadedness, especially upon changing to upright or standing position, with onset during pregnancy

- History negative for exposure to possible toxic agents (e.g., drugs)

- History negative for middle ear or central nervous system disease, visual problems, endocrine disorders, seizure disorders, or migraine headaches

- May report erratic food intake patterns

Objective

- Middle ear, central nervous system (CNS), cardiac, and thyroid examination within normal limits (WNL)

- Differential between lying and standing BP and pulse rate may be observed.

- Hb/Hct WNL

Assessment

- Dizziness/disequilibrium--benign

- R/O Orthostatic hypotension/systemic hypotension/vena caval syndrome

- R/O Cardiac insufficiency or arrhythmia
- R/O Hyperventilation
- R/O Middle ear disease
- R/O Ocular strain/refractive error
- R/O Substance toxicity
- R/O Anemia--see Anemia protocol
- R/O CNS pathology
- R/O Endocrine disorders, hypoglycemia
- R/O Anxiety/psychological disturbance
- R/O Migraine headaches
- R/O Head trauma
- R/O Multiple sclerosis
- R/O Mass lesion

Plan

Diagnostic Tests

- No specific laboratory test is diagnostic for benign dizziness.

Treatment/Management

- See Patient Education.

Consultation

- Medical consultation for severe symptoms not responsive to palliative treatment or if underlying pathologic condition is suspected

Patient Education

- Explain vascular changes usually responsible for dizziness in pregnancy when no underlying pathology exists.
- Suggest use of elastic stockings or vigorous pumping leg motions to reduce pooling of blood in lower extremities.
- Advise avoiding prolonged periods of standing or sitting.
- Change positions (to rising) slowly.
- Structure activities so that loss of balance would be of minimal danger (e.g., do not climb ladders).
- Identify anxiety-provoking situations and counsel in relation to these, if psychological component apparent.
- Avoid prolonged periods with no food intake; take 5-6 small meals if needed.
- Increase fluid intake, if low.
- To avoid compression of vena cava, rest on left side rather than on back when recumbent.

Follow-up

- Re-evaluate number and circumstances of dizzy episodes on subsequent visits.

- Further evaluation and consultation needed if dizziness is not responsive to therapeutic measures and is interfering with patient safety/activities of daily living.

- Document in progress notes and problem list if a significant ongoing problem.

DYSPNEA

Maureen T. Shannon

Dyspnea is "air hunger" requiring a conscious effort to breathe (Neeson & Stockdale, 1981). In pregnant women, dyspnea is often experienced secondary to the anatomic and physiologic changes associated with pregnancy. However, since respiratory diseases can be more serious during pregnancy, it is important to rule out the possibility of a pathologic cause for a pregnant woman's complaint of dyspnea (Cunningham, MacDonald, & Gant, 1989).

Data Base

Subjective

Non-pathologic dyspnea

- Increased awareness of the need to breathe--may or may not be associated with exercise
- Dizziness
- Lightheadedness
- May need an extra pillow at night during the 3rd trimester

Pathologic Dyspnea

- Chest pain
- History of cardiac problems, asthma, or other respiratory problems
- Smoker
- Dyspnea on exertion--if woman cannot carry out routine household chores
- Severe fatigue
- Signs and symptoms of a URI--rhinorrhea, sore throat, headache, fever, coughing (productive or non-productive)
- Hemoptysis

Objective

Non-pathologic

- No clinical signs are found when client is examined.

Pathologic

- Presence of rhonchi, wheezes or crackles that do not clear after 2-3 deep breaths or coughs
- Fever greater than 100°F (37.7°C)
- Cyanosis
- Intercostal retractions

- Cardiac arrhythmias
- Diastolic, presystolic, or continuous heart murmur
- Loud, harsh systolic murmur with a thrill
- Unequivocal cardiac enlargement

Assessment

- Dyspnea secondary to anatomic/physiologic changes of pregnancy
- R/O URI
- R/O Pulmonary diseases (e.g., bronchitis, pneumonia, asthma, etc.)
- R/O Cardiac disorders

Plan

Diagnostic Tests

Non-pathologic dyspnea

- No further diagnostic tests needed

Pathologic dyspnea: Some of the following tests may be ordered after consultation with an MD:

- EKG
- Respiratory function studies
- Chest x-ray
- Sputum cultures

Treatment/Management

Non-pathologic dyspnea

- Symptomatic treatment--see Patient Education below

Pathologic dyspnea

- Treatment of underlying condition after consultation with MD and appropriate referrals

Consultation

- Required for suspected pathologic causes of dyspnea with referral to MD care if long-term follow-up is necessary (e.g., cardiac disease)

Patient Education

Non-pathologic dyspnea

- Educate client about anatomic and physiologic changes that contribute to this problem.
- Advise client to sit and stand up straight, not to overexert herself, to rest after exercise, and to avoid restrictive clothing.
- Advise client to turn onto her side if dyspnea occurs when resting on her back.
- Suggest using an additional pillow for her head and upper torso when sleeping.

<u>Pathologic dyspnea</u>

- Educate client about the need for consultation and possible follow-up by MD.

- Educate client about tests that will be ordered.

Follow-up

<u>Non-pathologic dyspnea</u>

- No specific follow-up indicated--continue routine prenatal care.

- Document in problem list and in progress notes if a significant ongoing problem.

<u>Pathologic dyspnea</u>

- Follow-up by MD until problem resolves.

EDEMA--PHYSIOLOGIC

Lucy Newmark Sammons

Edema is defined as an increase in the extravascular or interstitial fluid volume. Several liters of fluid may accumulate in the interstitial space before swelling in the extremities or face is clinically evident (Friedlander, 1987).

During normal pregnancy, salt and water retention increases. Thirty-five to 83% of healthy pregnant women demonstrate clinical edema (Friedlander, 1987). Despite the increased vascular volume of pregnancy, renal salt handling and maintenance of salt balance are unimpaired. Cardiac output, renal blood flow, glomerular filtration rate, and levels of renin, aldosterone, and angiotensin II are all increased during pregnancy. There is normally no increase in blood pressure. Estrogen increases vascular capacity by causing vasodilation. In pregnancy, local edema is caused by alteration of the near-equilibrium (Starling equilibrium) maintained at the capillary membrane, where fluid filtered outward through arterial capillaries no longer approximates the amount reabsorbed at the venous end of the capillaries. Extremely decreased plasma proteins contribute to edema by lowering colloid-osmotic pressure of the plasma (Guyton, 1986).

Impeded venous return from the lower extremities commonly contributes to dependent edema late in pregnancy (Taylor & Pernoll, 1987). However, generalized edema seen in the hands and face requires further evaluation, as it may be a sign of pre-eclampsia/eclampsia.

Data Base

Subjective

- Client describes swelling in lower extremities, particularly after periods of standing or sitting

- Client free of other complaints related to pre-eclampsia. See Hypertensive Disorders of Pregnancy protocol.

- Client in mid- to third trimester of pregnancy

- Client may report:

    - low protein intake, high intake of salty foods

    - recent weight gain

    - exposure to warm/hot weather

Objective

- Edema of the lower extremities. Extent of the edema may be quantified by gently pressing the affected area (e.g., pretibial area) with examiner's thumb for 5 seconds. If a depression persists, edema is described as pitting and may be ranked (Fuller & Schaller-Ayres, 1990):

    - 1+: slight indentation, normal contour

    - 2+: pitting is deeper and more persistent, fairly normal contour

    - 3+: deeper pit of several seconds duration, obvious swelling

    - 4+: deeper pit possibly lasting minutes, frank swelling

- Client may exhibit <u>mild</u> swelling in hands and fingers.
- Absence of signs suggestive of pre-eclampsia:
    - no significant increase in BP
    - no proteinuria
    - no increase in deep tendon reflex (DTR) tonicity
    - absence of periorbital or generalized edema
- Client may exhibit recent weight gain.

Assessment

- Edema of pregnancy--physiologic
- R/O Pre-eclampsia/eclampsia and related disorders--see Hypertensive Disorders of Pregnancy protocol
- R/O Renal disease
- R/O Localized inflammatory response, trauma
- R/O Varicosities, thrombosis--see varicosities protocol
- R/O Carpal tunnel syndrome

Plan

Diagnostic Tests

- No laboratory test is diagnostic.
- Urine dipstick for protein is negative.

Treatment/Management

- See Patient Education.

Consultation

- Medical and nutritional consultation if failure to respond to conservative therapeutics and client is in discomfort

Patient Education

- Explain basis of edema and distinction between dependent and generalized edema, review signs and symptoms of pre-eclampsia.
- Advise elevation of affected extremities 1-2 hours 1-2 times per day as needed, using left lateral recumbent position when possible.
- Avoid prolonged standing or sitting.
- Nutritional counseling to include instruction to:
    - avoid excessive sodium intake, but do not overly restrict; maintain minimum of 2 to 3 grams of sodium per day (Worthington-Roberts, 1989)
    - avoid excessive carbohydrate intake
    - maintain high protein diet

- maintain high fluid intake, to 8 glasses/day, especially water.

- Explain that diuretics may be dangerous and should be avoided.

- Avoid wearing constricting garters, socks, etc.

- Wear supportive hose with adequate room abdominally, if helpful.

- Explain increased susceptibility of swollen tissues to injury and the consequent need to be careful (e.g., wear protective foot covering, even though difficult because of enlarged size).

Follow-up

- Re-evaluate edema in 1-2 weeks.

- Patient to contact provider if she gains 2 or more pounds in less than 2 weeks.

- Document in progress notes and problem list if a significant ongoing problem.

EPISTAXIS

Lucy Newmark Sammons

Epistaxis, or nasal bleeding, originates most often from the rich network of veins on the antero-inferior portion of the nasal septum, labelled Kiesselbach's plexus. Posteriorly, bleeding often occurs at the back third of the inferior meatus. Because of the highly vascular nature of the nasal turbinates and mucosa, bleeding may be profuse. Factors contributing to nosebleeds are local infections such as sinusitis, systemic infections, drying of nasal mucous membranes, local trauma, arteriosclerotic changes, hypertension, bleeding disorders, ulcerative disease or malignancy, overheating, and cocaine use. During pregnancy, nosebleeds are more common because of the vasodilating effects of estrogen on mucous membranes, relaxing effects on venous walls of progesterone, and engorgement of the blood vessels of the nasal passages.

Data Base

Subjective

- Client describes nosebleeding incident(s).
- Client may describe:
  - history of nosebleeds prior to pregnancy
  - precipitating event, such as nose picking, overexertion
- Able to control nosebleeds within 10-15 minutes
- History negative for other local or systemic disease, trauma

Objective

- Vital signs, BP, blood count, and indices within normal limits
- Physical examination otherwise normal relevant to local or systemic disease
- Nasal mucosa pink or dull red. May see residual clotted blood. May see superficial vessels, particularly in triangular area on antero-inferior nasal septum of affected side.
- Absence of visible nasal growths or polyps

Assessment

- Epistaxis of pregnancy, uncomplicated
- R/O Acute or chronic local infections: rhinitis, sinusitis, vestibulitis
- R/O Systemic infections: scarlet fever, infectious mononucleosis, influenza, measles, etc.
- R/O Elevated BP
- R/O Anemias and bleeding disorders
- R/O Local ulcerative disease, malignant polyp
- R/O Cocaine abuse

Plan

Diagnostic Tests

- No diagnostic test indicated

Treatment/Management

- Immediate care:
  - Loosen clothing around neck.
  - Woman to sit with head tilted forward or lie with head and shoulders elevated, and use mouth breathing
  - Apply pressure by pinching nostrils for 10-15 minutes.
  - Apply ice packs or cold compresses across nose.
  - May pack affected nostril with small sterile pad.
- Continued care:
  - Treat any concomitant local infections as indicated.
  - Application of topical antibiotic ointment (e.g., Neosporin) tid may combat local inflammation if needed and moisturize mucous membranes.
  - Increase moisture to dry mucous membranes by use of humidifier, aerosol moisturizer, or topical application of petroleum jelly.
  - See also Patient Education.

Consultation

- Medical consultation required for bleeding not relieved by above measures, or suspicion of underlying related pathology

Patient Education

- Explain that, in the absence of identified pathology, nosebleeds may be considered normal in pregnancy.
- Explain the physiologic basis for nosebleeds in pregnancy and the rationale and techniques of management described above. Client is to contact health care provider immediately for nosebleeds not responsive to described treatment approaches.
- Avoid trauma to nasal mucosa, e.g., avoid nose picking, forceful nose blowing, coughing, or sneezing.
- Avoid overheating or excessive exertion which may precipitate nosebleed.
- Advise woman who is prone to nosebleeds that they may occur with change in atmospheric pressure (e.g., when flying).

Follow-up

- Client to contact provider if nosebleeds not responsive to described treatments
- Re-evaluate pattern and management of nosebleeds at next regularly scheduled appointment.
- Document in progress notes and problem list if a significant ongoing problem.

FATIGUE/INSOMNIA

Lucy Newmark Sammons

Fatigue, feelings of tiredness or weariness, may be caused by insufficient rest, inadequate nutrition, circulatory problems, hematologic problems, respiratory problems, infections, hormonal influences, emotional factors, or postural factors in pregnancy. The normative fatigue of pregnancy may be caused by increased progestational levels and energy depletion from a myriad of physiological changes including increased oxygen consumption, fetal growth demands, increased cardiac output, and increased tidal volume (Poole, 1986). In addition, tremendous psychological changes take place as the woman redefines her own role and family relationships. Late in pregnancy, fatigue may be increased by additional weight gain, physical discomforts because of the growing baby, increased metabolic demands of pregnancy, and difficulty falling asleep or staying asleep.

Insomnia, which is difficulty in initiating or maintaining sleep, may have multiple causes in pregnancy. These include disturbance from fetal movement, inability to assume a position of comfort because of the enlarging abdomen, interruption by the need to urinate, discomfort from gastric reflux or other gastrointestinal changes, feelings of shortness of breath, or psychological concerns and thoughts.

Data Base

Subjective

- Complaints of tiredness

- Reports of difficulty sleeping that may be aggravated by fetal movement or nocturia

- Perceptions of fatigue often increase:

    - with multiparity (Sammons, 1986)

    - during the first and third trimesters

- Negative history of circulatory, respiratory, endocrine, infectious, or emotional problems

- Reports of adequate (or inadequate) nutritional intake

Objective

- Lethargic or droopy appearance

- Possible poor posture

- Respiratory impairment--refer to Dyspnea protocol

- Vital signs are within normal limits (WNL).

- CBC and indices are WNL.

Assessment

- Fatigue--physiologic fatigue of pregnancy

- R/O Respiratory disorder--see Dyspnea protocol

- R/O Circulatory/hematologic disorder--see Anemia protocol
- R/O Pre-eclampsia--see Hypertensive Disorders of Pregnancy protocol
- R/O Inadequate nutritional intake--see Nutrition protocol
- R/O Depression, anxiety, or stress
- R/O Infectious process

Plan

Diagnostic Tests
- Consider CBC if warranted by data base.
- No further diagnostic tests indicated

Treatment/Management
- See Patient Education.

Consultation
- None required without evidence of pathology

Patient Education
- Explain that in the absence of identified pathology, feelings of fatigue are a normal part of the pregnancy experience.
- Encourage adequate periods for sleep, which may extend to 8-12 hours.
- Encourage periods for napping/resting during the day as work/school/child care arrangements permit.
- If difficulty sleeping at night, explore comfort measures (pillows, bladder emptying in late evening, relaxation techniques) or suggest toleration of awakening at night while maintaining physical rest.
- Suggest sleep inducing aids (warm milk, outdoor exercise, music, reading, love-making, shower) if difficulty falling asleep.
- Reinforce adequate nutritional intake.
- Instruct in relaxation techniques or refer to resource.
- Use good posture to relieve fatigue.
- Explore possible sources of anxiety/emotional discomfort that may be increasing fatigue; counsel appropriately; refer to psychological health care provider if indicated by emotional status.
- Realistic planning may require alterations in scheduling commitments to employment and activities that were manageable prior to pregnancy.
- Avoid use of sleeping medications.
- Avoid use of central nervous system stimulants or heavy meals in late evening.

Follow-up
- Re-evaluate degree of fatigue and effectiveness of therapeutics on following visit.
- Document in progress notes and problem list if a significant ongoing problem.

HEADACHE

Lucy Newmark Sammons

Headache, defined as any pattern of pain in a portion of the head, is common in pregnancy. The experience of pre-existing headaches may be affected by pregnancy. Migraine headaches occur in 20% of all women, with greatest occurrence during the reproductive years; therefore, it is not surprising that they are common during pregnancy. Pre-existing migraines usually improve (60%), with 13% getting worse, and the balance unchanged (Reik, 1988). Possible reasons for improvement of migraines in pregnancy are the loss of hormonal fluctuation and the protective effect of beta-endorphins (Martignoni, Sances, & Nappi, 1987). Cluster headaches occur predominantly in men. They may improve in women during pregnancy, but this is not consistent. Chronic paroxysmal hemicrania (CPH) is a rare category of clusterlike headaches, which tend to abate during late pregnancy. Tension (psychogenic) headaches are common during pregnancy, but the pattern in pregnancy is not established.

Headaches with an initial onset during pregnancy may be reported. The most common type of headache with onset during pregnancy is migraine (Reik, 1988). The other commonly occurring benign headache of pregnancy is nonmigrainous vascular headache of early pregnancy, which usually occurs in the first trimester and spontaneously resolves after several days to weeks. Other physiologic changes of pregnancy may increase the occurrence of other types of headaches. Vasodilation of the sinus passages may contribute to sinusitis and resultant headache. Ocular changes of pregnancy may lead to headaches caused by eye strain or refractive changes.

Headaches first occurring during pregnancy may also be caused by serious illnesses. Headaches in pregnancy may be symptoms of pre-eclampsia/eclampsia, pseudotumor cerebri, subarachnoid hemorrhage from an aneurysm or arteriovenous malformation, a rapidly growing solid brain lesion, thrombosis of the cortical vein, or Listeria meningitis (Reik, 1988).

Data Base

Subjective

- Client complains of mild to moderate diffuse pain in the head

- Description of the headache (nature, frequency, onset, prodrome or associated symptoms, severity, location, relief measures attempted, and relief obtained) is elicited to allow categorization by standard classification (Reik, 1988; Seller, 1986):

  - Tension: dull, not throbbing, steady, of low persistent intensity; usually occipital, suboccipital and bilateral, like a constrictive band or tightness of the scalp, may radiate to neck; constant or persisting several days

  - Migraine: severe, throbbing, or boring; common migraine usually unilateral in frontotemporal or supraorbital region, lasting 12 hours to several days; classic migraines are proceeded by aura and prodrome, occur unilaterally, lasting 2-8 days; improvement in women with pre-existing migraine common in second trimester if previous episodes were menstrual

  - Cluster: unilateral and periorbital, felt in the eye and radiating to face or temporal regions, lasting 20-60 minutes

- Sinus: pain over involved sinuses (maxillary, ethmoid, frontal)

- Benign vascular headache of pregnancy: mild, throbbing, bifrontal; usually limited to first trimester, occurring daily for days to weeks, then spontaneously resolves

- Personal or family history may be positive for migraines or other headache categories

- Client may report visual changes or difficulty using glasses

- General health history otherwise unremarkable. In particular, history negative for:

  - recent trauma to head

  - symptoms suggesting disease or trauma to paranasal sinuses, teeth, eye, ear, nose, or throat

  - exposure to toxic chemicals or agents

  - association of symptoms with consumption of alcohol or wine with high histamine content

  - constipation

  - sunstroke

  - fatigue

  - motion sickness

Objective

- BP, opthalmic examination, weight pattern, fluid retention, urine laboratory values are within normal limits (WNL)

- Afebrile, free of signs of infection

- Nasal sinuses non-tender, absence of abnormal drainage

- Physical examination, with particular attention to neurologic assessment, head, and neck (e.g., palpation, range of motion, assessment of meningeal irritation, etc.), WNL

Assessment

- Headache--physiologic vascular headache of early pregnancy, benign

- Migraine headache, classic or common

- Tension headache, R/O Muscle tension, trapezius muscle spasm, temporomandibular joint (TMJ) dysfunction, bruxism (teethgrinding), stress, psychological tension

- Sinus headache, R/O Sinusitis, allergies

- Other standard headache syndromes, as indicated

- R/O Pre-eclampsia/eclampsia--see Hypertensive Disorders of Pregnancy protocol

- R/O Eye strain/refractive changes

- R/O Infectious disease, e.g., meningitis

- R/O Cerebrovascular disease, e.g., cortical thrombosis

- R/O Space-occupying lesion, e.g., cerebral tumor

Plan

Diagnostic Tests

- No diagnostic test indicated in absence of neurologic abnormalities, if signs and symptoms conform to standard headache syndromes.

Treatment/Management

- Vascular headache of early pregnancy:

    - Rest and reassurance of absence of serious neurologic problem

    - Acetaminophen (Tempra, Tylenol) 325 mg tabs <u>Sig</u>: tab i-ii po q 4° prn.

    - Consider caffeine if severe.

- Migraine:

    - Acute episode: (Usual agent, ergotamine, contraindicated in pregnancy, Reik, 1988).
      Analgesic, e.g., acetaminophen
      Antiemetics, e.g., antihistamines
      Sedatives, e.g., barbiturates
      Consider narcotics, e.g., codeine or meperidine

    - Preventive therapy:
      May be able to await improvement in later pregnancy
      Consider propranolol if needed

- Cluster headache. Management per Reik (1988):

    - Intranasal lidocaine

    - Oxygen inhalation

    - Avoidance of alcohol and afternoon naps

    - Consider preventive therapy with prednisone, if needed

- Tension headache:

    - Acetaminophen

    - Relaxation techniques

    - Consider biofeedback

- Treat contributing disorders as needed.

- See also Patient Education.

Consultation

- Consultation for prescription as needed

- Medical consultation for headaches accompanied by neurologic abnormalities or not conforming to standard headache syndromes, for headaches not relieved by treatment approaches within scope of practice, or for suspicion of underlying pathology

- Referral to eye care specialist as needed for relief of headache caused by visual strain/difficulty

- Referral to psychologic health care provider as needed for stress and anxiety management

Patient Education

- Explain the physiologic basis of headaches during pregnancy and the rationale for the treatment approaches selected.

- Explain that, in the absence of identified pathology, mild, transient headaches may be considered normal in pregnancy.

- Explore tension reduction techniques with client (e.g., progressive relaxation, use of imagery, meditation).

- Massage, moist heat, or cold application to neck muscles may relax muscles in spasm.

- Delete foods and beverages from diet if strongly associated with symptom occurrence. Particular foods may be nitrites, monosodium glutamate, or chocolate.

- Eat at regular intervals, avoiding skipping meals (hypoglycemia) or overeating carbohydrates at one time (hyperglycemia).

- Explore and identify environmental factors that precipitate headaches. Structure activities to avoid these stimuli when possible. Examples are bright lights, loud noises, intense odors, cigarette smoke, stuffy rooms, sleeping late.

- Suggest plenty of rest and sleep.

Follow-up

- Patient to contact provider if headache not relieved with rest and analgesic in 24 hours, or if marked increase in severity of headache

- If good relief obtained, no additional follow-up is required.

- Document in progress notes and problem list if a significant ongoing problem.

HEMORRHOIDS

Lucy Newmark Sammons

Hemorrhoids are now understood to be normal features of the anal canal and consist of: 1) the lining, made up of mucosa or anoderm; 2) the stroma, with blood vessels, smooth muscle, and supportive connective tissue; and 3) the anchoring connective tissue (Dennison, Whiston, Rooney, & Morris, 1989). There are two types of hemorrhoids. Internal hemorrhoids are made up of the redundant mucus membrane above the dentate line, the border separating pink mucosa from the modified squamous lined anoderm (Smith, 1987). External hemorrhoids lie below the dentate line. Hemorrhoids may be classified clinically from first degree to fourth degree, with increasing protrusion of the mucosa (Dennison et al., 1989). Hemorrhoids become clinically significant as they cause symptoms. Symptoms are produced by protrusion of the vascular submucosa through an increasingly congested anal canal.

Theories of etiology of hemorrhoids have included those factors that cause hemorrhoidal veins to become distended, such as portal hypertension. Constipation and straining at defecation have traditionally been associated with hemorrhoidal symptoms. Dennison et al. (1989) give importance to family history and increasing age. Pregnancy and labor increase hemorrhoidal symptoms, whether due to hormonal influences, impeded venous circulation, or increased constipation.

Other clinical entities occurring in people with symptomatic hemorrhoids are anal fissures, perianal hematomas, skin tags, and mucosal prolapse, although cause and effect relationships are difficult to establish. Clot formation within a hemorrhoidal vessel can occur in the internal or external portion.

Data Base

Subjective

- Complaints of perianal prolapse or "lump," pruritis, discomfort, swelling, or discharge

- Client may describe perianal bleeding:

  - Painless, bright red bleeding on surface of stool at time of defecation (suggests internal hemorrhoids)

  - Spontaneous bleeding (suggests large internal and external hemorrhoids)

- Pain should not be major complaint if no thrombosis present (Smith, 1987).

- History may include:

  - Family history of symptomatic hemorrhoids

  - Personal history of symptomatic hemorrhoids

  - Multiparity

  - Increased age

  - Constipation or straining during defecation

Objective

- External hemorrhoids visible on examination, at rest, or when bearing down
- Internal hemorrhoids may be palpable on digital examination of anal canal; visible externally when prolapsed.
- Thrombosis (shiny blue or purple masses; subcutaneous clots adjacent to anus) or infection (inflamed appearance) may be evident.
- Fecal soiling may be noted where swelling of the external component makes hygiene difficult.
- Increased mucus may be seen, as mucus production increases with traumatic proctitis.

Assessment

- Hemorrhoids
- R/O Anal fissures, skin tags, fibrous anal polyps
- R/O Condyloma acuminata
- R/O Abscess
- R/O Idiopathic pruritus ani
- R/O Cancerous lesions
- R/O Inflammatory bowel disease

Plan

Diagnostic Tests

- Check hematocrit if bleeding has been substantial and continued.

Treatment/Management

- Attempt to replace hemorrhoids.
- Topical anesthetic: Hemorrhoidal suppositories and ointment (e.g., Anusol)
  - Suppositories--<u>Sig</u>: insert i per rectum q AM and q HS, and i post q BM;
  - Ointment--<u>Sig</u>: apply freely and gently rub into anal area q 3-4° prn
- Topical anesthetic: Hemorrhoidal suppositories and ointment (e.g., Preparation H)
  - Suppositories--<u>Sig</u>: insert i per rectum prn (3-5 per day, especially q AM, q HS, and i post q BM);
  - Ointment--<u>Sig</u>: apply freely to affected area (3-5 x per day, especially q AM, q HS, and post q BM).
- Sitz baths (warm or cool) x 15-20 minutes prn for comfort, when bleeding absent
- Apply ice pack; apply cold compress, or use epsom salt bath to aid reduction.
- Astringent compresses--witch hazel pads (Hamamelis water, Tucks)
- Stool softeners/laxatives--see Constipation protocol.
- See Patient Education.

Consultation

- For extremely painful, large, strangulated or thrombosed hemorrhoids, or continued bleeding, refer to medical consultant for evaluation and intervention.

Patient Education

- Explain to patient the cause and treatment approaches for hemorrhoids in pregnancy.

- Correct and avoid constipation--see Constipation protocol for education and therapeutics (includes high fiber diet, adequate hydration).

- Teach digital replacement, if possible.

- Careful anal hygiene

- Petroleum jelly may be placed inside rectum.

- Elevate hips while sidelying to reduce discomfort; elevate foot of bed if tolerated.

Follow-up

- Client to call provider if pain increases severely, if bleeding continues, or if no relief from therapeutic measures in one week. Otherwise reassess at next regular appointment.

- Document in progress notes and problem list if a significant ongoing problem.

LEG CRAMPS

Lucy Newmark Sammons

Leg cramps are spasmodic, usually painful contractions of leg muscles, most often affecting the gastrocnemius. Although the etiology in pregnancy is uncertain, they may be caused by a reduced level of diffusible serum calcium or elevation of serum phosphorus (Taylor & Pernoll, 1987). An imbalance in the calcium/phosphorous ratio appears related to the spasms; however, rigorous investigation has failed to support the correlation between leg cramps and dairy/calcium intake (Worthington-Roberts, 1989). Intake of either excessive or inadequate amounts of dairy/calcium may be related to leg cramps. Impairment of circulation to the area or nerve compression by the uterus may be contributing factors.

Data Base

Subjective

- Complaints of painful cramping in calf, thigh, or buttock, often at night or in early morning

- Client may report:

    - Previous history of muscle cramping

    - Fatigue in extremities

    - Diet may be very high or very low in calcium sources

Objective

- No evidence of dehydration, hyperthyroidism, hypothyroidism, hypomagnesemia, salt depletion, uremia, or nerve root compression

- Absence of local warmth, redness, or positive Homan's sign

Assessment

- Leg cramps, physiologic

- R/O Varicose veins or deep vein thromboembolic disease. See Varicosities protocol.

Plan

Diagnostic Tests

- No diagnostic test indicated.

Treatment/Management

- Extend calf muscle by dorsiflexion of the foot, compress muscle, apply heat, and massage for immediate relief.

- First, modify grossly excessive or inadequate dairy/calcium intake.

- Second, increase calcium intake without phosphorus and then reduce phosphate intake.

    - Calcium carbonate (Os-Cal 500, Titralac) 1250 mg tabs <u>Sig</u>: tab i po bid or tid

- Trial of reduction of phosphate intake: reduce milk, reduce excessive sources of phosphates (e.g., sodas), and reduce nutritional supplements containing calcium phosphate

Consultation

- No consultation necessary if symptoms mild and responsive to treatment

Patient Education

- Explain causes of leg cramps and rationale for therapeutics.
- Dietary modifications as indicated above
- Teach patient to:
  - Avoid pointing toes when stretching or walking, which may trigger a cramp.
  - Avoid fatigue in legs.
  - Keep legs warm (with knee socks or leg warmers) and use leg massage if helpful.
  - Use relief measures above (dorsiflexion, compression, massage, warmth) as needed.
  - Maintain good circulation through exercise, posture, and positioning.

Follow-up

- Re-evaluate symptoms and calcium/phosphate intake on next visit, or sooner if symptoms severe or non-responsive to treatment.
- Document in progress notes and problem list if a significant ongoing problem.

LEUKORRHEA--PHYSIOLOGIC

Winifred L. Star

Physiologic leukorrhea is an increased amount of normal vaginal discharge without signs or symptoms of infection. The amount and duration of leukorrhea varies from woman to woman and from pregnancy to pregnancy. The presence of coexisting vaginitis or cervicitis or other cervical pathology should be ruled out.

Data Base

Subjective

- Client may complain of increased amount of vaginal discharge or sensation of increased wetness in vulvar area without symptoms of vulvo/vaginal itching, irritation, burning, or odor.

Objective

- Pelvic exam within normal limits; presence of increased amount of normal vaginal discharge. Note color and amount.

- Wet mounts: NaCl--normal amount of lactobacilli present, normal squamous epithelium, lack of WBCs, no clue cells or trichomonads. KOH--no yeast, negative amine odor.

Assessment

- Physiologic leukorrhea

- R/O Rupture of membranes

- R/O Onset of labor/preterm labor

- R/O Vaginitis/Cervicitis

- R/O Condyloma acuminata

- R/O Cervical intraepithelial neoplasia (CIN)

Plan

Diagnostic tests

- Pap smear as indicated by history and physical exam

- Wet mounts to be performed to R/O infection

- Chlamydia and gonorrhea cultures to be done as indicated by physical exam

- Other tests as indicated (e.g., herpes culture)

Treatment

- Symptomatic relief; see Patient Education section in Vaginitis protocol.

- If vulvar, vaginal, and/or cervical pathology identified, treat accordingly.

Consultation

- Not required

Patient Education

- See Vaginitis protocol.

Follow-up

- As necessary for signs/symptoms of infection
- Refer patients with CIN for colposcopy.
- Document in progress notes and problem list if a significant ongoing problem.

NAUSEA/VOMITING

Lucy Newmark Sammons

Nausea and vomiting of pregnancy (NVP) are among the most common complaints of pregnancy, occurring in about 60-80% of women in Western societies (Nuwayhid, 1986). Emesis gravidarum is defined as nausea alone, or nausea with retching and occasional vomiting, in early pregnancy (Jarnfelt-Samsioe, 1987). Symptoms will resolve for most women with conservative treatment and the passage of time. The more serious condition of intractable nausea and vomiting leading to dehydration, acidosis, and weight loss is labelled hyperemesis gravidarium.

Numerous theories are suggested to explain NVP (reviewed in DiIorio, 1988; Jarnfelt-Samsioe, 1987). Elevated levels of serum human chorionic gonadotropin (HCG) have been implicated, bolstered by the higher HCG levels in pregnancies with greater vomiting, such as twin gestation and molar pregnancy (Nuwayhid, 1986). Smooth muscle relaxation from progestational effects retards stomach emptying. Decreased gastric acidity also contributes to gastric hypofunction. Mechanical stretching and stimulation by the gravid uterus may also be a factor. New evidence suggests women with NVP have a lower "functional reserve" of their liver capacity and may be hypersensitive to estrogens or catecholestrogens. These steroids may act directly on the area postrema of the brain. Other possible etiological factors include adrenal and pituitary dysfunction, hypoglycemia, hyponatremia, and hyperthyroxinemia. Psychological factors may also contribute to NVP. Emotional stress and fatigue appear to increase symptom occurrence. Cultural and dietary factors have also been explored, particularly in relation to Vitamin B_6 intake.

Data Base

Subjective

- Client complains of loss of appetite; sensations of nausea; aversion to sight, smell or thought of food; "queasy stomach"; retching; and/or vomiting.

- Symptoms may be limited to the morning or persist throughout the day, particularly increasing with fatigue.

- Symptoms most freqeunt during weeks 4-14 of pregnancy

- Client may report history of nausea when using oral contraceptives.

- Data inconclusive to support any greater risk for NVP due to parity, maternal age, fetal gender, racial or ethnic group, intendedness of pregnancy, or socio-economic status

- Remainder of history unremarkable; particularly noting absence of abdominal pain, diarrhea, or fever

Objective

- Mucous membranes, skin turgor, and urine specific gravity indicate absence of dehydration.

- Urine multi-dipstick/urinalysis is negative for ketones, indicating absence of ketosis. (If patient has ketonuria, see Ketonuria protocol.) Negative or trace proteinuria

- Serum electrolytes, if obtained, are within normal limits, indicating absence of severe dehydration or acidosis.

- CBC, if done, is within normal limits, indicating absence of severe hemoconcentration (e.g., relative elevation of Hb, Hct, and RBCs).

- Uterine size is appropriate for dates, and ultrasound shows normal intrauterine pregnancy, indicating absence of molar or multiple pregnancy.

- Mucosal surfaces are free of bleeding, indicating absence of severe vitamin C and B complex deficiency or hypoprothrombinemia.

- Fetal heart tones audible at appropriate gestation, indicating fetal well-being and absence of molar pregnancy (in almost all cases)

- Vital signs normal

- Fundoscopic exam is within normal limits, indicating absence of retinal hemorrhage.

- Weight may show increase, stability, or decrease, depending on severity of symptoms.

- Abdominal exam: no pain or tenderness, no organomegaly

Assessment

- Nausea/vomiting of pregnancy
- R/O Hyperemesis gravidarum
- R/O Multiple gestation--see Multiple Gestation protocol
- R/O Molar pregnancy--see Gestational Trophoblastic Neoplasia protocol
- R/O Gastrointestinal influenza
- R/O Acute infectious disease, e.g., appendicitis, pancreatitis, or pyelonephritis
- R/O Hiatal hernia, peptic ulcer, gastric carcinoma, or other disorders of the alimentary tract, biliary system, pancreas and peritoneum
- R/O Eating disorders (anorexia, bulimia)
- R/O Pica--see Pica protocol
- R/O Food poisoning
- R/O Migraine headache--see Headache protocol
- R/O Pre-eclampsia/eclampsia--see Hypertensive Disorders of Pregnancy protocol
- R/O Anemia--see Anemia protocol
- R/O Diabetic ketosis
- R/O Hyperthyroidism
- R/O Irritation of the external acoustic meatus
- R/O Torsion of an ovarian cyst
- R/O Increased intracranial pressure

Plan

Diagnostic Tests

- No test is diagnostic for nausea/vomiting.
- See laboratory tests in Objective Data.

Treatment/Management

- Obtain accurate dietary history to assess quality, quantity, and pattern of food intake and food loss by vomiting.

- Administer iron and vitamin supplementation after meals, rather than on an empty stomach. If iron still causing distress, woman may defer iron supplementation until symptoms resolve.

- If necessary, pyridoxine HCl (vitamin B_6, Hexa-Betalin) 50 mg tabs <u>Sig</u>: i tab po tid - qid, not to exceed 200 mg qd (Vitamin B_6 dependency has been induced in adults with 200 mg/day intake [Scherer, 1985].)

- Consider Emetrol 15 ml or 30 ml on arising, repeated q 3 hours prn nausea. Emetrol, a hyperosmolar carbohydrate solution with phosphoric acid, appears to reduce smooth muscle contraction and delay gastric emptying time (Scherer, 1985).

- If necessary, use an upper gastrointestinal tract stimulant, e.g., Metoclopramide hydrochloride (Reglan) 10 mg tab <u>Sig</u>: tab i po tid.

- If necessary consider an antihistamine, Doxylamine succinate (Unisom, Sleep-Aid) 25 mg tab <u>Sig</u>: ½ tab po tid and HS.
  NOTE: A combination of this and vitamin B_6 reproduces the effective elements of Bendectin, which is no longer available because of earlier concerns of fetal safety. The evidence supporting Bendectin's safety in pregnancy is "impressive" (Briggs, Freeman, & Yaffe, 1986). Client and provider may discuss implications of relevant litigation and controversy.

- If necessary, temporarily rest gastrointestinal tract with clear liquid diet only for 24 hours, then advance to full liquid, then add complex carbohydrates. Avoid dairy and fats for 48 hours.

- If necessary, with medical consultation as needed, treat with antiemetics, either oral or rectal suppository.

- For extreme cases, may be hospitalized under medical supervision for rehydration and parenteral nutrition.

- See also Patient Education.

Consultation

- Consultation for prescription as needed

- Nutritional consultation may be indicated where strong food preferences, food allergies, or other dietary restrictions compound the problem of maintaining adequate intake, or where intake is seriously compromised.

- Medical consultation required for ketonuria greater than or equal to 1+; for documented weight loss of four or more pounds or 5% of body weight attributable to nausea and vomiting; for hyperemesis gravidarum; or for suspicion of other underlying pathology.

- Referral to mental health professional as indicated for contributory extreme anxiety, psychological disturbance, or evidence of eating disorder

Patient Education

- Explain possible causes of nausea and vomiting in pregnancy, the therapeutic plan, and signs or symptoms requiring early return contact with provider.

- Provide reassurance that mild symptom levels do not appear to have negative effects on fetal growth and development.

- Encourage additional rest, sleep, and relaxation--see Fatigue protocol. Lying down has been found to be the most frequently used relief measure with adolescents (Dilorio, 1985) and adult women (Dilorio & van Lier, 1989), and the most effective self-care measure among adults (Jenkins & Shelton, 1989).

- Explore alterations in solid and liquid nutritional intake patterns, food preparation techniques, and activity patterns that may be helpful, considered with patient's lifestyle and preferences. Although rigorous evidence of their effectiveness has not been established in all cases, the following self-help measures may provide relief (Coalition for Medical Rights of Women, 1987; Dilorio & van Lier, 1989; Jenkins & Shelton, 1989).

  - Eat a small amount of a dry, complex carbohydrate in the morning before rising, e.g., crackers, toast, or cereal.

  - Avoid letting the stomach become overly full or empty for too long; try small, frequent meals.

  - Snacks of high protein foods (yogurt, nuts) may reduce NVP.

  - Try taking fluids between meals instead of with meals.

  - Nausea may be relieved by sipping carbonated beverages or clear juices.

  - Avoid food preparation if upsetting; avoid offensive odors; maintain good ventilation when preparing foods and sleeping.

  - Gastric acid may be neutralized by taking milk, apples, or potatoes.

- Avoid foods/substances that irritate the stomach, e.g., coffee, alcohol and cigarettes; iron and vitamins; fried foods and spices.

- Acupressure at the P6 (Neiguan) acupuncture point near the wrist crease (effective per Dundee, Sourial, Ghaly, & Bell, 1988)

- Receive extra attention from partner (Jenkins & Shelton, 1989)

- Alternative remedies, which may be helpful but lack rigorous medical testing, include:

  - Herbal/spice teas: spearmint, peppermint, chamomile, ginger root, raspberry leaf, and cinnamon (Ehudin-Pagano, Paluzzi, Ivory, & McCartney, 1987; Streitfeld, 1986).

  - Hypnosis

  - Cold compresses to forehead or throat

- If woman employed, consider degree of disability and responsibilities of the job. Discuss alternative strategies for coping.

- Advise avoidance of constrictive clothing around abdomen.

- Advise avoidance of reclining immediately after eating, when the relaxed cardiac sphincter may more readily allow reflux regurgitation.

- Consider maintaining a diary to monitor food intake, identify precipitating factors, and evaluate effectiveness of relief measures.

Follow-up

- Client to contact provider if unable to retain minimum of liquids only, for 12 hours or more, or for continued weight loss after identification of problem.

- If client able to maintain weight, recheck weekly (weight, urine ketones, signs and symptoms of dehydration) in first trimester until symptoms subside.

- If symptoms mild, respond well to therapeutics, and weight gain pattern appropriate, recheck at 2-4 week intervals of routine prenatal care.

- Document in progress notes and problem list if a significant ongoing problem.

PICA

Lucy Newmark Sammons

Pica (cissa) has more than one definition. A narrow definition refers just to the persistent eating of non-nutrient substances. A broader definition encompasses cravings and ingestion of both food and non-food items. Pica may also include sucking or mouthing objects beyond 18 months of age. Related terms describe the substance that is craved, such as amylophagia (cornstarch or laundry starch), geophagia (earth or clay), lithophagia (gravel), and pagophagia (ice or frost scraped from a refrigerator). Many other substances have been involved in pica, including cigarette ashes, mothballs, powdered bricks, wood, antacid tablets, and coffee grounds.

The incidence of pica during pregnancy is not clearly established. Although it has occurred in all ethnic and socioeconomic groups across the United States, it appears to be most common among pregnant Black women in the Southeast. Surveys reveal occurrence varies from 7% to as high as 75% among different groups (Worthington-Roberts, 1989).

There are multiple theories of the etiology of pica (McLoughlin, 1987). The homeostatic theory supports an attempt to restore minerals that are lacking in the diet. Physiologic disorder theories are based on neurotransmitter substance malfunction or damage to the lateral or ventral medial areas of the hypothalamus. Some picas may have psychological origins based in reinforced behaviors of learning theory, modelling, compulsive disorders, or addictive behaviors. Strong cultural components are recognized. Certain picas are associated with protective beliefs for the welfare and comfort of the mother and baby.

Numerous medical complications are associated with pica (McLoughlin, 1987; Worthington-Roberts, 1989). The cause-and-effect relationship between pica and commonly co-existing iron and zinc deficiencies and the related anemias is still unclear (McLoughlin, 1987). Other biochemical problems encountered are hypercalcemia and lead intoxication. Gastrointestinal problems include vomiting, obstruction, perforation, intussusception, parotid enlargement, and constipation. Additional possible sequelae are obesity, parasitic infection, congenital lead poisoning, or fetal hemolytic anemia (from mothballs or air freshener).

Data Base

Subjective

- Client reports cravings for/ingestion of non-food items such as starch, clay, ashes, plaster, antacids, ice, coffee grounds, or paraffin.

- Client states non-food items (e.g., clay, cornstarch, flour) relieve discomforts of pregnancy and delivery or promote well-being of infant, while denial of such items causes birthmarks.

- Client may have history of having eaten clay or dirt as a child.

- Client may also complain of:

    - fatigue, dyspnea on exertion, or other symptoms of anemia

    - constipation, fecal impaction, persistent vomiting, or anorexia

    - ptyalism

Objective

- Client may demonstrate any of the following:

    - low serum iron values and iron deficiency anemia

    - maternal weight gain below ideal, equal to ideal, or in excess of ideal

    - severe abrasion to teeth

- BP and urine protein/ketones within normal limits (WNL)

- Fetal growth parameters WNL

Assessment

- Pica

- R/O Nutritional deficiency

- R/O Anemia--see Anemia protocol

- R/O Ketonuria--see Ketonuria protocol

- R/O Parasitic infections--common concomitant problem

- R/O Maternal intestinal and pyloric obstruction, toxemia, or chronic constipation

- R/O Emotional problems

- R/O Hypercalcemia

- R/O Lead intoxication

Plan

Diagnostic Tests

- Check serum iron/TIBC or ferritin for concomitant iron deficiency anemia if indicated--see Anemia protocol.

Treatment/Management

- Thoroughly evaluate nutritional status, maternal weight gain pattern, and fetal status.

- See also Patient Education.

Consultation

- Nutritional consultation may be needed if food intake is markedly distorted.

- Medical consultation needed if pathology from malnutrition or complications of pica develop.

- Social services referral needed if warranted by socio-economic situation.

Patient Education

- Explain need for well-balanced and adequate nutritional intake during pregnancy, with sensitivity to the beliefs of the client. Reinforce nutritional counseling.

- Demonstrate tolerance towards cravings if nutrition is otherwise adequate and ingested substances are not harmful.

- Provide additional education for related problems (e.g., constipation, obesity) as needed.

Follow-up

- Reassess food and non-food intake patterns at subsequent visits. If nutritional deficiencies are minimal, progress of pregnancy and fetal growth is unremarkable, and there are no signs of complications of pica, routine scheduling is adequate.

- Document in progress notes and problem list if a significant ongoing problem.

UPPER RESPIRATORY INFECTION, MILD

Lucy Newmark Sammons

An upper respiratory infection (URI) is defined as an infectious disease process involving the nasal passages, pharynx, or bronchi (Thomas, 1989). Upper respiratory infections are the most common illnesses in adults (Seller, 1986), and pregnant women are more susceptible to the common cold than nonpregnant women (Laros, 1987). A variety of viruses cause common colds, mild URIs, and flu-like symptoms. Complications of these illnesses often take the forms of sinusitis, bronchitis, or pneumonia after a secondary bacterial infection is superimposed on the original viral infection.

The most common causes of rhinitis during pregnancy are allergic rhinitis, bacterial rhinosinusitis, rhinitis medicamentosa, structural abnormalities, eosinophilic non-allergic rhinitis, nasal polyps, and vasomotor rhinitis of pregnancy (Incaudo, 1987). Physiological changes of pregnancy, specifically estrogenic effects on nasal mucosa, have been associated with nasal congestion and swelling of the nasal turbinates. Progestationally induced smooth muscle relaxation may increase nasal congestion. This "rhinitis of pregnancy" appears to be caused by direct cholinergic action affecting increased local acetylcholine production. Whether the incidence of rhinitis is truly increased during pregnancy, or attributable to pre-existing or newly-developed causative factors comparable to the non-pregnant population has been questioned (Incaudo, 1987; Mabry, 1986). The effect of pregnancy on pre-existing allergic rhinitis varies, with reports of both exacerbation and improvement (Mabry, 1986). Stress or stopping use of topical antihistamine nasal products may contribute to rhinitis of pregnancy.

Data Base

Subjective

- Common viral upper respiratory infection (Seller, 1986):

    - Nasal discharge, congestion, "stuffy nose," sneezing, postnasal drip, cough, sore throat

    - May include: headache, fever, malaise, hoarseness

- Influenza viral infections:

    - Symptoms as common cold above, but may also include sudden onset of chills, shivering, aching in extremities and back, malaise, loss of appetite, dry cough (Seller, 1986)

- Allergic rhinitis:

    - Perennial: persistent nasal obstruction with watery mucoid discharge

    - Seasonal: seasonal variation in symptoms, which include sneezing, itchy and watery eyes, and watery nasal discharge

- Vasomotor/idiopathic/rhinitis of pregnancy:

    - Continued nasal passage blockage and watery discharge

- Women at high risk for complications report history of

    - Recurrent sinusitis

- Smoking

- Underlying cardiac or pulmonary disease

- Diabetes

- Chronic anemia

- Altered immune response

Objective

- Rhinitis of pregnancy: nasal mucosa are edematous, hyperemic, and hypersecretory

- Mild URI may include:

  - Oropharyngeal vesicles, pharyngeal mucosa dull red, faucial pillars slightly edematous

  - Lymphadenopathy

  - Nasal turbinates pale, boggy, or occasionally dull red (perennial allergic rhinitis)

- Septal deflection and nasal polyps contribute to nasal obstruction

- Client <u>free</u> of signs of bacterial complications or more severe pathology:

  - Fever to 103° F. (39.5° C.) or above

  - Severe sore throat; pharyngeal mucosa bright red and swollen, with yellow or white follicles

  - Pain on percussion over nasal or maxillary sinuses, mucopurulent nasal discharge, opaque maxillary or frontal sinuses on transillumination

  - Tachypnea (rate greater than 20 breaths/minute)--hallmark of respiratory disease (Noble et al., 1988)

  - Other abnormalities of ears, eyes, cranial nerves, nose, mouth, throat, neck, pharnyx, lungs, or generalized disease signs suggesting more serious pathology

Assessment

- Common viral URI, "cold"

- Influenza-like viral infection

- Allergy, seasonal or perennial

- Vasomotor rhinitis, rhinitis of pregnancy

- Rhinitis medicamentosa (rebound from continued use of topical nasal vasoconstricting drugs)

- R/O Sinusitis, streptococcal pharyngitis, bronchitis, pneumonia, meningitis

- R/O Infectious mononucleosis

- R/O Measles, mumps

- R/O Otitis media

Plan

Diagnostic Tests

- Throat culture, if done, negative for streptococcal infection

92

- Monospot, if done, negative for infectious mononucleosis

- Nasal smear, if done, showing that greater than 4% of polymorphonuclear leukocytes are eosinophils, indicates allergic rhinitis.

- Radiographs of sinuses, if done, can support diagnosis of sinusitis.

Treatment/Management

- See related symptomatology: Cough and Dyspnea protocols.

- Treatment based on symptom relief for mild URIs

- Decongestant: Pseudoephedrine HCl (Sudafed) 30 mg tab <u>Sig</u>: tab i po q 4 hrs

- Analgesic/Antipyretic: Acetaminophen 325 mg tab or cap <u>Sig</u>: tab i-ii q 4 hrs

- Antihistamine, if required: Tripelennamine HCl 50 mg tab <u>Sig</u>: tab ½-i q 6 hrs, prn rhinorrhea and sneezing, not to exceed 200 mg per day, terminating prior to delivery (Incaudo, 1987)

- Buffered saline nose spray to reduce nasal dryness, bleeding, and vascular congestion

- Gargle or soothing (honey, lemon juice, warm liquids) beverages for relief of sore throat

- Influenza vaccine may be given in second or third trimester for women at high risk for epidemic influenza A respiratory infections (CDC, 1984).

- See Patient Education.

Consultation

- Medical consultation for evaluation and management of suspected pathology beyond scope of practice

- Consultation for prescriptions as needed

Patient Education

- Explain causes of symptoms and rationale for treatment approach.

- If environmental factors cause/increase symptoms, advise woman to reduce exposure to allergens (e.g., pets, pollens) or irritants (e.g., chemicals, smoke).

- Nasal congestion may be relieved by breathing steam from a vaporizer, hot shower, or heated pot of water; general humidification.

- Warm, moist compresses placed on face may soothe sinuses.

- Camphor/menthol ointment (Vicks) may provide relief of head and chest cold symptoms when applied topically or in vaporizer.

- Warm non-caffeine teas may be soothing.

- Massage or pressure over sinuses may give relief.

- If stopping topical nasal vasoconstrictors, combat bilateral rebound nasal congestion by stopping one side at a time, allowing 1-2 weeks for untreated nostril to adjust.

- General restorative measures ease recovery from minor illnesses: plenty of rest/sleep, good hydration, diet as tolerated, chicken soup.

- No antihistamine-containing medicines or other over-the-counter or prescription medications, which might be used when not pregnant, should be used without first checking with health care provider.

- Client is to contact provider if treatment approach not successful, or if symptoms become worse.

Follow-up

- Client to contact provider if signs/symptoms of secondary bacterial infection (e.g., URI symptoms beyond 10-14 days, persistent or rising fever after initial 2-3 days, nasal discharge or sputum become increasingly mucopurulent, sinuses become tender), other evidence of systemic disease develop, or if inadequate relief from discomfort obtained.

- If mild symptoms without complications, re-evaluate degree of symptoms and effectiveness of therapeutics on following visit.

- Document in progress notes and problem list if a significant ongoing problem.

URINARY FREQUENCY--PHYSIOLOGIC

Lucy Newmark Sammons

Abnormally frequent passage of urine is common in pregnancy, particularly in first and third trimesters. Bladder function is affected by vascular engorgement of the pelvis, progestational effects on smooth muscles, mechanical compression by the gravid uterus, and diuretic effects of pregnancy hormones.

Data Base

Subjective

- Complaints of increased frequency of urination coinciding with onset of pregnancy, particularly in first and third trimesters, <u>without</u> symptoms of UTI
- May complain of loss of urine when coughing or laughing
- Client not taking diuretic medication

Objective

- Afebrile, negative costovertebral angle tenderness (CVAT), lower abdominal exam and genitourinary exam within normal limits (WNL)
- Urinalysis (dipstick /microscopic) WNL, i.e., negative leukocyte esterase or nitrite; negative pyuria, bacteriuria, or hematuria
- Urine culture, if obtained, WNL

Assessment

- Urinary frequency--physiologic
- R/O UTI, asymptomatic bacteriuria
- R/O Diabetes mellitus, hypercalcemia, hypokalemia
- R/O Psychogenic origin, particularly if nocturia is absent (Seller, 1986)

Plan

Diagnostic Tests

- See laboratory tests under Objective Data.
- No specific diagnostics--a diagnosis by exclusion

Treatment/Management

- See Patient Education.

Consultation

- None required

Patient Education

- Explain multiple causes of changed bladder function during pregnancy, and expected reversion to previous function after delivery.

- Teach pelvic floor muscle exercises (Kegel's) to increase control over voluntary muscles.

- Instruct that while maintaining good hydration, reduce excessive fluid intake, especially late in evening, if nocturia is interfering with sleep.

- Reduce excessive intake of liquids containing alcohol and caffeine (e.g., coffee, cocoa, chocolate, and soft drinks).

- Use panty liner if desired.

- Advise to empty bladder frequently and fully to deter urinary stasis and infection.

- Explain the signs and symptoms of urinary tract infection that require further attention.

Follow-up

- Monitor degree of discomfort/dissatisfaction and effect of therapeutics at next regular prenatal visit.

- Document in progress notes and problem list if a significant ongoing problem.

VARICOSITIES

Lucy Newmark Sammons

Varicosities are veins that are enlarged, swollen, knotted or twisted. They are the most common vascular condition, occurring in 20% of the population (Ameli, 1986). In pregnancy, they are caused by proximal obstruction to return of venous blood caused by the gravid uterus, congenital and acquired weakness of vascular walls, increased venous stasis in legs due to the hemodynamics of pregnancy, inactivity and poor muscle tone, obesity, and decreased smooth muscle tone resulting from hormonal effects.

Diseases resulting from or potentially occurring with varicosities in pregnancy are rupture of the vein and deeper venous disease. Venous thrombosis with an inflammatory response is called thrombophlebitis; the term for thrombosis without inflammation is phlebothrombosis. The incidence of antepartum or postpartum thrombosis is between 1-7 per 1,000 (Cunningham, MacDonald, & Grant, 1989).

Data Base

Subjective

- Client describes prominent, enlarged blood vessels, which may feel painful, achy, or cause a feeling of heaviness, in the legs, feet, vulva, or anal area.

- Occurrence increases with following risk factors:

    - Family history of varicosities

    - Increased age

    - Greater gravidity

    - Obesity

    - Occupations requiring prolonged standing

Objective

- Pattern of purple or blue vessels, varying from flat and thin to raised and wide, visible superficially

- The following signs of thrombophlebitis are <u>absent</u>:

    - Inflammation, e.g., overlying skin is red and hot

    - Involved superficial veins feel firm, cord-like

    - Veins on dorsa of foot remain distended after elevation to 45o

    - Dependent cyanosis

    - Deep tenderness elicited on palpation

    - Positive Homan's sign--pain on abrupt ankle dorsiflexion

    - Louvel's sign--pain in calf upon sneezing or coughing, which disappears on digital compression proximal to obstruction

- Restlessness, fever, tachycardia
- Edema may be present.
- Peripheral pulses present and adequate

Assessment

- Varicosities of the _____
- R/O Thrombophlebitis
- R/O Edema--see Edema protocol

Plan

Diagnostic Tests

- No tests indicated

Treatment/Management

- See Patient Education.
- For hemorrhoids--see Hemorrhoids protocol

Consultation

- Medical consultation for severe/thrombosed varicosities

Patient Education

- Explain causes of varicosities and rationale for treatment approach.
- Advise modification of activities to allow rest and elevation of extremities.
  - Elevate legs at least 30 minutes twice a day.
  - Avoid prolonged standing.
  - Avoid sitting for more than one hour at a time without walking around.
- Advise use of supportive elastic stockings, placed prior to rising from bed.
- Explain that vulvar pad held snugly by belt or binder may give relief for vulvar varicosities; elevate hips with pillow when resting.
- Advise wearing loose, non-constrictive clothing, to avoid further impediment of circulation.
  - Avoid clothing such as knee-high socks or pants with constrictive bands.
  - Avoid crossing legs at the knee.
- Control weight gain and lose excess weight postpartally, as needed.
- Alert patient to possible complications and their prevention: orthostatic hypotension and faintness on standing, predisposition to postpartum thromboembolic disease, muscle aching, edema, or skin ulcers.
- Reassure women that visible veins are normal and require no treatment; early or primary varicose veins are benign and best dealt with conservatively with compression stockings, or by compression sclerotherapy; and if surgery or injection therapy is required, it is usually considered after all childbearing is completed.

Follow-up

- Re-evaluate discomfort/extent of varicosities and success of therapeutics on next regularly scheduled visit. If symptoms increase, are not responsive to treatment, or complications arise, see sooner.

- Document in progress notes and problem list if a significant ongoing problem.

Chapter 4

Obstetrical Complications

BACTERIURIA - ASYMPTOMATIC

Winifred L. Star

Asymptomatic bacteriuria is defined as the presence of actively multiplying bacteria in the urinary tract in a person without urinary tract symptomatology. Diagnosis is usually based upon isolation of >100,000 colony-forming units per milliliter (cfu/mL) on a freshly voided clean-catch midstream specimen. However, lower counts (especially of consistently cultured coliform organisms) may be significant. The pathogen responsible for 80-90% of asymptomatic infections is *Escherichia coli*. Other pathogens which may be isolated include: *Klebsiella pneumoniae, Proteus mirablis, Pseudomonas aeruginosa, Staphylococcus saphrophyticus, Enterococcus,* and *Group B beta-hemolytic Streptococcus* (Biswas & Perloff, 1987; McNeeley, 1988; Pauerstein, 1987).

The prevalence of asymptomatic bacteriuria in pregnancy ranges from 2-10%, similar to that in the non-pregnant population; thus, it is felt that pregnancy is **not** a predisposing factor. Forty percent of patients with untreated asymptomatic bacteriuria will progress to acute symptomatic infection including pyelonephritis (Davison & Lindheimer, 1989). Prompt treatment of asymptomatic infection, therefore, is warranted.

Pregnancy complications alleged to occur as a result of asymptomatic bacteriuria include low birthweight infants, fetal loss, preeclampsia, and maternal anemia. More recent studies do not support the occurrence of these factors (Davison & Lindheimer, 1989). The greatest concern is the risk of developing pyelonephritis and its complications of maternal sepsis and preterm labor (McNeeley, 1988).

Data Base

Subjective

- Lower socioeconomic status
- Increased age
- Increased parity
- Sickle cell trait/disease
- Diabetes
- Lifelong susceptibility to bacteriuria
- Reduced availability of medical care

Objective

- Urine dipstick may be leukocyte esterase, or nitrite positive.
- Microscopic urinalysis may reveal white blood cells, red blood cells, or bacteria.
- Urine culture reveals $>10^5$ cfu/ml of a single pathogenic bacteria.
- Urine culture may reveal $<10^5$ cfu/ml of a significant pathogen (particularly if specimen was not a first-void).

Assessment

- Asymptomatic bacteriuria
- R/O Vaginitis
- R/O Sexually transmitted disease(s)
- R/O Sickle cell trait
- R/O Obstetrical complication(s)
- Documentation of acute/chronic medical problem(s) as indicated

Plan

Diagnostic Tests

- Ideally, a complete urinalysis with culture and sensitivities (UA, C&S) on a clean-catch midstream specimen should be done on all patients at the first prenatal visit. Patients at risk for urinary tract infection should have a UA, C&S repeated at approximately 28 weeks.

- An acceptable cost-effective alternative to culture is the use of a urine dipstick evaluation for nitrites and leukocyte esterase activity (e.g., Chemstrip LN). It should be noted, however, that neither test alone is sensitive enough as a screening test for asymptomatic bacteriuria (Robertson & Duff, 1988).

- At times it may be necessary to obtain a sterile catheter specimen to assess bacteriuria in patients with repeated contaminated urine cultures from the vulvovaginal flora.

- Additional labs as indicated (e.g., cervical cultures, vaginal wet mounts)

Treatment/Management

- According to sensitivities on urine culture
- Commonly used antibiotic regimens include: (McNeeley, 1988)

  - Ampicillin 500 mg qid x 7-14 days

  - Nitrofurantoin (Macrodantin) 100 mg qid x 7-14 days

  - Sulfisoxazole (Gantrisin) 1 gram qid x 7-14 days

  - Cephalosporin (e.g., Velosef) 500 mg qid x 7-14 days

  NOTE: A seven day course is usually sufficient. Sulfa drugs and nitrofurantoin should not be prescribed to women with G6PD deficiency. Sulfa drugs should not be used in the weeks preceding delivery to avoid the risk of neonatal hyperbilirubinemia.

- Patients experiencing relapse (same pathogen) or reinfection (new pathogen) should be treated with a second course of antibiotic according to sensitivities.

- Long-term prophylaxis should be considered for those patients with persistent asymptomatic bacteriuria. This can be effected with a 100 mg daily dose of nitrofurantoin taken after dinner or at bedtime.

Consultation

- For prescription as necessary
- For repeated episodes of asymptomatic bacteriuria in pregnancy for which long-term suppression is being considered

104

Patient Education

- Discuss etiology of asymptomatic bacteriuria.

- Discuss normal anatomic changes of the urinary tract in pregnancy.

- Stress importance of completing medication despite absence of symptoms. Advise patient that untreated bacteriuria may lead to pyelonephritis. Alert patient to the signs and symptoms of acute cystitis and pyelonephritis--see Cystitis and Pylonephritis protocols.

- Teach or review personal hygiene techniques.

- Encourage liberal fluid intake throughout pregnancy and especially during treatment phase.

- Advise voiding following intercourse.

- Discuss preterm birth prevention routinely at about 20-22 weeks and as indicated--see Preterm Birth Prevention protocol.

Follow-up

- Patients treated for asymptomatic bacteriuria ideally should have a clean-catch midstream urine specimen assessed for protein, nitrites, and leukocyte esterase at each prenatal visit. Positive findings would warrant culture.

- Order UA, C&S upon completion of drug therapy and at regular intervals throughout the remainder of pregnancy. Some authorities recommend monthly cultures following treatment (Gilstrap & Cox, 1987; McNeeley, 1988).

- Patients on suppressive therapy should have monthly urine cultures.

- A UA, C&S should be ordered at the six-week postpartum appointment.

- Approximately 20% of women with bacteriuria have a minor abnormality of the urinary tract not clearly related to the infection. Postpartum intravenous pyelogram (IVP) is indicated for those patients with a history of acute recurrent symptomatic infections before or during pregnancy, in those whom bacteriuria is difficult to eradicate, and in those with postpartum recurrence (Davison & Lindheimer, 1989). Refer to urologist as indicated.

- Document in progress list and progress notes.

BATTERED WOMAN/PERINATAL DOMESTIC VIOLENCE

Lucy Newmark Sammons

A battered woman is defined as a woman over age 16 who has received physical abuse from an intimate male partner at least one time. A pattern of deliberate, severe physical abuse from the partner occurring three or more times is labelled the battered wife syndrome. Battering includes five types of interpersonal violence: physical, sexual, property, psychological, and social (Helton, 1987). Domestic violence, wife beating, and spousal abuse are other terms referring to violence between partners in an ongoing relationship. The abuse may also incorporate verbal and mental abuse, with variations in severity from verbal threats to life-threatening and fatal injury. Because of an interrelationship between suicidal and homicidal intent, suicidal threats by either the batterer or the victim may precede an actual homicide (Walker, 1984).

Since familial violence tends to be underreported, accurate incidence statistics are difficult to obtain. Estimates of spousal abuse range from 2-4 million women victims per year. Victims are found in all socioeconomic and racial groups. The incidence of battering during pregnancy is about 8-10%. The effect of pregnancy on the frequency of battering episodes varies, with reports of both increases and decreases (Hillard, 1985). The additional stresses on family dynamics of pregnancy, and later the care and demands of the newborn, may well precipitate violent episodes. The nature of the assault during pregnancy often includes sexual assault; blows to the abdomen, breasts, genitals, face and neck; choking; and broken bones. Potential risks to the fetus include miscarriage, low birthweight, and direct injury from abdominal blows.

Wife-battering is often found in an environment of family violence. Abusers often come from families where they themselves were victims of abuse. Furthermore, 53% of the men and 28% of the women in battering relationships report abusing their children (Walker, 1984).

Data Base

Subjective

- Client reports individual or repeated incidents of physical, mental, and/or verbal abuse by her partner.

- Client may deny or initially refuse to disclose abuse; report of how injuries occurred (e.g., "fell down") not consistent with nature of injuries.

- Client may report history of:

    - Abuse as a child or seeing own mother abused

    - Childhood in single-parent home

    - Marriage before age 20

    - Pregnancy before marriage

    - Drug or alcohol abuse/overdose; suicide attempt; depression

- Medical/health history may reveal:

    - Use of multiple caregivers/sites to maintain anonymity

- Frequent appointments for vague somatic complaints
- Noncompliance with medical recommendations, failure to keep appointed office visits
- Delay in seeking medical care for injuries
- Somatic complaints may include:
  - Headaches
  - Insomnia, violent nightmares, severe anxiety
  - Choking sensation
  - Hyperventilation
  - Gastrointestinal symptoms
  - Chest, back, or pelvic pain

Objective

- Physical examination may reveal signs of recent or past injury, particularly (Sammons, 1981):
  - Serious bleeding injuries
  - Broken bones, especially arms, legs, jaw, pelvis, skull or vertebrae
  - Burn injuries, as from cigarettes
  - Abdominal injury/bruising
- Multiple injuries may be present, from different time periods
- Behavioral manifestations may include:
  - Shyness, fright, embarrassment, evasiveness, jumpiness, passivity, depression, crying or sighing, anger or defensiveness
- Male partner may be resistant to leaving the client's presence throughout the health visit.

Assessment

- Domestic violence/battering
- R/O Concomitant child abuse/other family violence
- R/O Suicidal/homicidal intent

Plan

Diagnostic Tests

- No specific diagnostic test; reliant on disclosure by woman or other family member/reliable informant

Treatment/Management

- Directly ask all pregnant women if they are or have been injured/abused recently or in the past; repeat the question if circumstances warrant; interview woman privately if partner or children usually accompany her.

- Priority assessment of the pregnant woman who has experienced trauma includes checking for fetal heart rate, uterine contractions, vaginal bleeding, leakage of amniotic fluid, or other signs of progressing labor/imminent delivery (Bojanowski, Hill, & Martin, 1988).

- Where physical evidence will be collected for legal/forensic purposes, consent and specimen collection procedures should be in conformity with local requirements.

- Provide care in a non-judgmental manner, acknowledging the difficulty of disclosure, seeking assistance, leaving the batterer, or bringing legal action in a family violence situation.

- Assess the severity of the domestic situation, and offer realistic assessment of woman's safety to her own evaluation.

- Assist the woman in establishing contact with support services for battered women (shelters; financial, social, and legal support).

- Guide woman in development of an "exit plan" if she remains where violence may recur (Helton, 1986):

  - Pack essential clothing, toiletry articles, cash, and financial papers in a suitcase to be stored with a trusted friend.

  - Keep driver's license and necessary identification papers readily at hand for a rapid departure.

  - Predetermine a destination: friend, relative, or shelter if not injured; emergency room with assistance as needed by ambulance, police, or friend if she is injured.

Consultation

- Medical consultation required for all confirmed and highly suspicious cases of perinatal domestic violence

- Social services consultation for provision of, or referral to, specialized resources for domestic violence; emergency referral to protective services (legal, shelter, etc.) if woman in present danger

- Emergency mental health services consultation for suicidal/homicidal intent

- Police or social service agency notification required if evidence of child abuse has been provided

Patient Education

- Educate woman about cycle of violence: successive periods of increased tension, battering, and calm; signs of increasing physical danger include battering during pregnancy, involvement of weapons, extension of threats or assaults to other family members, observation of woman at her workplace, increased jealousy, forced sexual encounters, and decreased remorse in the calm phase (Helton, 1987).

- Convey that violence is not acceptable in family living; it is not appropriate for problem-solving or tension release; family violence is not a woman's fault because she "deserves it" for an act committed or ommitted.

- Provide written local battered women's resource contact numbers; the National Coalition Against Domestic Violence 24-hour hotline number is 1-800-333-SAFE.

- Battered women may particularly benefit from educational resources that increase knowledge of their legal rights and protections, provide job skills and facilitate re/entry into the market place, decrease social isolation, and increase self-esteem.

- Special educational needs if woman has opted to separate from her partner and is not settled in a permanent shelter/residence include:

  - Nutritional counseling emphasizing economic and convenient foods, possible application for food supplement programs

  - Need to maintain health care visits during pregnancy, despite potential chaotic and transient lifestyle; possible need to apply for medical financial assistance to continue prenatal care; need to maintain point of contact with provider, to follow-up on any abnormal laboratory results between office visits

- If woman stays with her partner, education prenatally addressed to the couple can include realistic expectations of the pregnant woman's needs and anticipatory guidance regarding neonatal care and family readjustments.

- Family planning counseling is important, since unplanned or unwanted pregnancy may precipitate spousal abuse.

- Advise against the use of alcohol or drugs as stress-reducing mechanisms, especially during pregnancy because of potential fetal effects.

Follow-up

- Follow the battered woman as a high-risk patient, with more frequent visits and interim telephone contact as needed.

- Contact pediatric care provider for appropriate follow-up of older children and neonate; contact intrapartum staff regarding battering situation, so they may provide additional support to family and be alert to any limitations/legal considerations regarding father of baby.

- Long-term care of woman and children often requires therapy program, with combination of group and individual approaches helpful; batterer may be involved in therapy on his own initiative or through legal requirement.

- Continue assessment of family dynamics into the postpartum period; the additional stresses of a new infant in the home and a fatigued mother unable to respond to the needs of all family members may precipitate violence.

- Encourage clinic/office administrative staff and other providers to tolerate non-appointed visits as scheduling permits during disorganized periods in battered woman's life.

- Document in progress notes, in accordance with legal evidenciary standards, and problem list.

BLEEDING: FIRST TRIMESTER BLEEDING

Maureen T. Shannon

Vaginal bleeding during the first trimester of pregnancy can be scant to extensive in amount; brown to bright red in color; and may or may not be accompanied by pain. Approximately 20% of pregnant women experience vaginal bleeding during the 1st trimester, with less than half of these women having a spontaneous abortion (SAB). There are multiple causes of first trimester bleeding, including the following: "implantation bleeding," threatened spontaneous abortion, inevitable spontaneous abortion, incomplete spontaneous abortion, complete spontaneous abortion, missed spontaneous abortion, ectopic pregnancy, gestational trophoblastic neoplasia (GTN), cervicitis, cervical polyps, cervical carcinoma, or normal hyperemia of the cervix.

Definitions

"Implantation bleeding": This usually occurs approximately 1-2 weeks after conception and is caused by blood escaping from blood vessels in the uterine epithelium that have been eroded by the implanting fertilized ovum. The bleeding is usually scant light pink, unaccompanied by pain, and lasts only for 1-2 days.

Threatened abortion: Vaginal bleeding with or without pelvic cramping and backache during the first trimester should signal the possibility of a threatened SAB. There are no cervical changes observed in a patient with this problem. Approximately 50% of threatened SABs do progress to complete SABs (Cunningham, MacDonald, & Gant, 1989; Willson, 1983b).

Inevitable spontaneous abortion: When vaginal bleeding increases, is accompanied by increasingly severe pelvic cramping, and there is evidence of cervical dilatation and/or effacement with or without the presence of fetal membranes or placenta at the cervical os, the term "inevitable spontaneous abortion" is used. At this point attempts to halt the progress of the SAB are useless (Cunningham et al., 1989; Willson, 1983b).

Incomplete spontaneous abortion: In the majority of SABs occurring during the 1st trimester some amount of placental tissue remains within the uterine cavity causing persistent vaginal bleeding, which can be profuse in some cases (Cunningham et al., 1989; Willson, 1983b). The patient usually reports the passage of tissue and clots with a history of vaginal bleeding and cramping. The bleeding and cramping will persist until all of the products of conception have been evacuated from the uterus.

Complete spontaneous abortion: A complete SAB occurs when the uterus spontaneously evacuates itself of all of the products of conception. This usually occurs before the 6th week and after the 14th week of pregnancy (Cunningham et al., 1989; Willson, 1983b).

Missed spontaneous abortion: This occurs when the products of conception are retained in the uterus after the embryo or fetus has died. Usually the patient will report the signs and symptoms of a threatened SAB which appears to resolve except for occasional brown spotting. Eventually the symptoms of pregnancy disappear, and the uterine size becomes smaller. The term "missed" SAB is usually applied to retention of a dead embryo or fetus for at least 4-8 weeks (Cunningham et al., 1989; Willson, 1983b).

Ectopic pregnancy: See the Ectopic Pregnancy protocol for the definition.

Gestational trophoblastic neoplasia (GTN) or Molar pregnancy: See the GTN protocol for definitions.

Cervicitis: See the Chlamydia and Gonorrhea protocols for definitions.

Cervical polyps: Painless bleeding, especially after coitus, which occurs early in gestation, may be caused by cervical polyps that usually increase in size during pregnancy (Pritchard, MacDonald, & Gant, 1985; Willson, 1983a). Cervical polyps usually appear as bright red pedunculated growths protruding from the cervical os (Neeson & Stockdale, 1981).

Cervical carcinoma: Painless vaginal bleeding, often after coitus, can be reported by women who have cervical carcinoma. However, patients with this disease have abnormal pap smear results.

Normal hyperemia of the cervix: Spontaneous light vaginal spotting or bleeding, which may or may not be related to coitus, can be caused by the increased vascularization of the cervix that normally occurs during pregnancy.

Data Base

Subjective

- Reports the symptoms of pregnancy.

- Reports vaginal bleeding that can be scant to profuse; brown, pink, or bright red in color.

- May have abdominal pain ranging from mild cramping to severe, sharp unilateral pain.

- May have passage of tissue, blood clots, or grape-like vesicles (in GTN).

- May report that the bleeding occurs at specific times (e.g., postcoitally) or that the bleeding is unrelated to activity.

- May report exposure to and symptoms of a sexually transmitted disease.

- May give a history of pelvic inflammatory disease, previous ectopic pregnancy, IUD use, infertility or adnexal surgery.

- May report disappearance of subjective signs and symptoms of pregnancy (in missed SABs).

Objective

- Beta HCG levels may be less than expected for gestational age--especially in threatened SABs and ectopic pregnancies.

- Uterine size may be normal for dates in threatened SABs; size less than dates in incomplete and missed SABs, and ectopic pregnancies (after 8 weeks); uterine size well contracted in complete SABs; and uterine size greater than dates in GTN (50% of GTN cases).

- Cervical dilitation and effacement in inevitable SABs

- Presence of products of conception at cervical os or in vaginal vault in incomplete SABs

- Nitrazine positive fluid in vaginal vault in some cases of inevitable and incomplete SABs

- Unilateral sausage-like enlargement of adnexa, usually accompanied by tenderness, is sometimes palpable in ectopic pregnancies.

- A bright red, pedunculated growth protruding from the cervical os may be observed if cervical polyp is causing the bleeding.

- Cervical inflammation, erythema, friability and leukorrhea may be seen in cervicitis.

- Absence of fetal heart tones (FHTs) when auscultating with Doppler at appropriate gestational age in missed SABs and GTN

- Sonogram may indicate the presence or absence of a fetal sac, fetal heart pulsations, or a "snow storm" pattern (in GTN).

Assessment

- IUP_____weeks with vaginal bleeding
- R/O Threatened SAB
- R/O Inevitable SAB
- R/O Incomplete SAB
- R/O Complete SAB
- R/O Missed SAB
- R/O Ectopic pregnancy
- R/O GTN
- R/O Cervicitis
- R/O Cervical polyp
- R/O Anemia

Plan

Diagnostic Tests

- Complete blood count (CBC) or Hemoglobin and Hematocrit (H/H)
- Beta HCG (may repeat serially in an asymptomatic patient with an uncertain diagnosis after consulting with an MD)
- Sonogram
- Type and Rh (if not already done)
- Cervical cultures for gonorrhea and chlamydia (if indicated)
- Coagulation studies in patients with missed SABs (since they may develop disseminated intravascular coagulation--especially if it has been 5 or more weeks since death of the embryo/fetus or 5 months after LMP)

Treatment/Management

- In threatened SAB the patient should be sent home and told to rest in bed until bleeding subsides. Pelvic rest is advised for at least 2 weeks after the bleeding has stopped.
- If a patient with a threatened SAB continues to have bleeding or if bleeding is accompanied by the passage of clots or tissue, then referral to MD is indicated.
- In patients with inevitable, incomplete, complete, or missed SABs, referral to MD care is indicated.
- If an ectopic pregnancy is suspected, referral to MD care is indicated.
- If a patient with a threatened SAB has resolution of her symptoms, continue routine prenatal care at two week intervals until normal uterine growth and fetal heart tones are confirmed.

- If anemia is present, then iron supplementation and high iron diet are prescribed--see Anemia protocol.

- If patient is Rh negative and she has a threatened SAB, incomplete or complete SAB, or an ectopic pregnancy, she should have an injection of RhoGam (if the pregnancy is 12 or more weeks gestational age) or Micro-Rhogam (if the pregnancy is between 8-12 weeks gestational age) within 72 hours after the completion of the SAB or termination of the ectopic pregnancy (Wible-Kant & Beer, 1983).

- If the patient has cervicitis, she should be treated with the appropriate medication.

- If cervical polyps are present, consultation/referral to MD for treatment is indicated.

- If the patient is diagnosed as having GTN, then referral to MD care is indicated.

Consultation

- Required in all patients with vaginal bleeding during the first trimester when a threatened, inevitable, incomplete, missed SAB, or ectopic pregnancy is suspected.

- Transfer to MD care all patients with vaginal bleeding during the first trimester when an inevitable, incomplete or missed SAB is suspected; or when GTN, ectopic pregnancy, or cervical polyps are suspected/diagnosed.

Patient Education

- Educate the patient about the diagnostic tests that are being ordered, and interpret the results for her.

- If an SAB has occurred it is important to help the patient and her partner work through any feelings of guilt and/or grief regarding their loss.

- If a threatened SAB is occurring, it may help the patient to know that she has a 50% chance of maintaining the pregnancy.

- Educate the patient regarding the importance of reporting the development of a fever, foul-smelling discharge, profuse or prolonged bleeding, passage of tissue or clots, or the development of abdominal or low-back pain.

- Educate the patient about the normal course of recovery from an SAB and the need to have follow-up evaluation of her physical (and psychological) recovery.

- If the patient is Rh negative and has had an SAB, then educate her about the need for RhoGam administration.

Follow-up

- If threatened SAB resolves, then the patient should return every two weeks for uterine growth assessment until normal growth and fetal heart tones are confirmed.

- Follow-up evaluations of patients who have experienced an inevitable, incomplete, complete, or missed SAB; or GTN, ectopic pregnancies or cervical polyps are per MD recommendation.

- Document in problem list and progress notes.

BLEEDING: SECOND AND THIRD TRIMESTER BLEEDING

Maureen T. Shannon

Vaginal bleeding during the latter half of pregnancy can be slight to severe; may or may not be accompanied by pain; and may be due to one of a number of problems including the following: placenta previa, abruptio placenta, gestational trophoblastic neoplasia (GTN), cervicitis, cervical intraepithelial neoplasia (CIN), cervical polyps, or postcoital bleeding due to increased vascularization of the cervix.

Definitions

Placenta previa: When the placenta implants very near or completely covers the internal cervical os. The incidence of this problem is approximately 1/150 - 1/200 births. There are 4 classifications of this abnormality:

1. Total placenta previa occurs when the placenta completely covers the cervical internal os (Cunningham, MacDonald, & Gant, 1989).

2. Partial placenta previa occurs when the cervical internal os is partially covered by the placenta (Cunningham et al., 1989).

3. Marginal placenta previa occurs when the edge of the placenta is at the very margin of the cervical internal os (Cunningham et al., 1989).

4. Low-lying placenta occurs when the edge of the placenta is located in the lower uterine segment in close proximity to, but not reaching, the cervical internal os (Cunningham et al., 1989).

Approximately 45% of all placentas are classified as "low-lying" during the 2nd trimester of pregnancy. However, at term only 1/150-1/200 pregnancies exhibit some form of placenta previa. This decrease in number of placenta previas is due to the progressive elongation of the upper uterine segment (Gottesfeld, 1983a). An increase risk of placenta previa has been noted in patients who are multiparous, 35 years or older, have had a previous c-section, have had a previous placenta previa (the recurrence risk is 4-8%), or have had GTN.

Abruptio placenta (placental abruption): When a normally attached placenta separates from either a portion or all of the uterine wall prior to the birth of the fetus (Cunningham et al., 1989; Gottesfeld, 1983b; Willson, 1983a). This complication occurs after the 20th week of pregnancy. The overall incidence of abruptio placenta has been noted to be between 1/85 and 1/200 births (Cunningham et al., 1989; Gottesfeld, 1983b). The wide variation in the incidence figures is due to the difficulty in diagnosing the milder degrees of this complication. There are two types of abruptio placenta:

1. External hemorrhage occurs when the blood which is escaping from beneath the placenta (close to the placental border) escapes between the membranes and uterine wall, and flows through the cervix (Cunningham et al., 1989).

2. Concealed hemorrhage (occult abruption) occurs when the bleeding is located in the central portion of the placenta and extends retroplacentally with extravasation of blood into

the myometrium (Couvelaire uterus). External bleeding may or may not be present. If vaginal bleeding is observed, it is usually less than would be expected from the severity of the signs and symptoms the woman may be exhibiting. Concealed hemorrhage has an associated increased incidence of DIC. Factors associated with an increased incidence of abruptio placenta are grand multiparity (gravida V or more), maternal hypertension, previous abruption, circumvallate placenta, sudden uterine decompression, short umbilical cords, and cocaine use (Cunningham et al., 1989; Gottesfeld, 1983b; Neeson & Stockdale, 1981; Willson, 1983a).

Gestational trophoblastic neoplasia (GTN)--see GTN protocol.

Cervical intraepithelial neoplasia (CIN)--see Abnormal Pap Smear protocol.

Cervical polyp and postcoital bleeding--see First Trimester Bleeding protocol.

Data Base

Subjective

Placenta previa

- Painless, bright red vaginal bleeding which begins in the late 2nd or the 3rd trimester. The amount of bleeding can vary from a slight amount to severe hemorrhage. Usually the first bleeding episode is mild.

- Approximately 7% of placentae previae are asymptomatic and are found on ultrasound exams being done for other problems (Gottesfeld, 1983a).

Abruptio placenta

- Vaginal bleeding occurring after the 20th week of pregnancy

- Abdominal pain that can be mild to severe

- Decreased fetal movements noted by mother

- May report fatigue, dizziness, or lightheadedness depending on the extent of the hemmorrhage.

- See specific protocols for subjective data for Cervicitis, GTN, Abnormal Pap Smear, First Trimester Bleeding.

Objective

Placenta previa: Do **not** do a speculum or bimanual examination unless an ultrasound done before the bleeding episode has determined that the placenta is in a normal location.

- Bright red vaginal bleeding may be observed when examining the external genitalia or a sanitary pad that the patient has used.

- Abdominal exam reveals a non-tender uterus which is soft.

- Fetal presenting part is usually not engaged and the fetus may be in an abnormal lie (e.g., transverse, oblique, or breech).

- Fetal heart tones (FHTs) are usually within normal limits unless the mother is in shock in which case the FHTs may be bradycardic or tachycardic.

- May exhibit signs of shock in severe hemorrhage (e.g., decreased BP; increased, thready pulse; pallor; etc.).

- Complete blood count (CBC) or Hemoglobin and Hematocrit (H/H) may reveal anemia.

- Sonogram will reveal abnormal location of the placenta.

Abruptio placenta: Do **not** do a speculum or bimanual examination unless an ultrasound done before the bleeding episode has determined that the placenta is in a normal location.

- Dark red vaginal bleeding varying in amount from slight to severe hemorrhage may be observed when examining the external genitalia.

- Uterine palpation will reveal uterine irritability ranging from minimal to extreme.

- Uterus will be minimally to extremely tender to palpation.

- Uterine resting tone will be normal in mild abruption increasing in severity until the uterus is hard, board-like and unrelaxing in severe abruptio.

- Uterine size will increase in severe concealed abruptions.

- FHTs will vary between a normal rate in mild abruptio to absent or faint bradycardic/tachycardic FHTs.

- Maternal vital signs will range from normal (in mild abruptio) to signs of shock (in severe abruptio).

- CBC or H/H may reveal mild to severe anemia depending on the amount of blood lost by the patient.

- Coagulation studies may reveal beginning disseminated intravascular coagulation (DIC) (e.g., decreased platelets, increased fibrin split products, etc.).

- Sonogram will reveal the absence of placenta previa and may indicate the degree of abruption. However, in posterior placentas the degree of abruption cannot be determined.

- See specific protocols for the objective data for Cervicitis, GTN, Abnormal Pap Smear, First Trimester Bleeding.

Assessment
- IUP_____weeks
- Vaginal bleeding
- R/O Placenta previa
- R/O Abruptio placenta
- R/O Anemia
- R/O Fetal distress
- R/O Cervicitis
- R/O GTN
- R/O CIN
- R/O Cervical polyps
- R/O "Bloody show"

116

Plan

Diagnostic Test

- CBC

- Sonogram to differentiate placenta previa from abruptio placenta

- Coagulation studies (as indicated)

- Type and cross match (as indicated)

Treatment/Management

- All patients with second and third trimester bleeding require consultation with an MD.

- If placenta previa or abruptio placenta is diagnosed, then transfer of care to MD management is warranted.

- If the patient is in shock or the fetus is in distress immediate MD management is warranted (i.e., to labor and delivery STAT).

- In Rh negative patients who experience second or third trimester bleeding, the administration of RhoGam is indicated (Wible-Kant & Beer, 1983).

- See specific protocols for the treatment/management of Cervicitis, GTN, Abnormal Pap Smear, First Trimester Bleeding.

Consultation

- See under Treatment/Management above.

Patient Education

- In mild cases of placenta previa or abruptio placenta a complete explanation of the problems, the diagnostic tests, and need for referral to MD can be given to the patient and her partner by NP/NM.

- In moderate to severe cases the patient and her partner should receive as complete an explanation as is possible (under the circumstances) regarding her immediate treatment and prognosis (this should be done by the MD treating the woman).

- Emotional and psychological support of the patient and her partner during the diagnosis and treatment of these problems should be available either through the NP/NM, social worker, clinical nurse specialist, or psych consults (when indicated).

- If a fetal demise occurs (there is a 10-25% chance in placenta previa and a 25-50% chance in an abruptio placenta), or if the fetus is premature or neurologically disabled, the patient and her family will need help working through the grieving process.

- The family with a neurologically disabled infant should be referred to the social worker for effective utilization of the community resources available to them.

Follow-up

- Follow-up of patients with placenta previa or abruptio placenta is by the MD treating these women.

- Document in progress notes and problem list.

BREAST MASS

Winifred L. Star

A breast mass may consist of normal glandular tissue or may be due to benign breast disease or cancer. During a woman's lifetime breast structure and composition varies because of endogenous hormonal fluctuations. Hypertrophy of glandular elements of breast tissue during pregnancy and lactation may impart increased nodularity to the breasts. Underlying parenchymal masses may be masked in pregnancy by normal breast enlargement (Borten, 1987).

Data Base

Subjective

- May complain of breast lump, mass, pain, tenderness, nipple discharge, burning, itching, swelling, skin changes.

- Diet may be high in methylxanthines (e.g., coffee, tea, sodas, chocolate).

- May be taking methylxanthine-containing medication (e.g., theophylline, phenothiazine).

- May have positive family history of benign breast disease or breast cancer.

Objective

- Inspection and palpation of breasts, supraclavicular areas and axillae (supine and sitting) may reveal: breast fullness/nodularity/ thickening/mass; nipple retraction/ulceration/ crusting/discharge; skin dimpling (peau d'orange), erythema, edema, induration; axillary or supraclavicular adenopathy.

- Carefully document findings using descriptive terms. Terms that may be applied to description of breast tissue include: thick, full, pronounced, prominent, soft, buoyant, fatty, ropey, granular, nodular, coarse, bumpy. Dominant masses should be described assuming a clock position, locating the mass in distance from the base of the nipple, the dimensions measured with a centimeter tape or ruler. The consistency, presence of tenderness, shape, and mobility of the mass should also be described. Skin changes of the breast should be noted. Diagrams are helpful.

Assessment

- Breast mass (with or without nipple or skin changes, discharge)
- Hypertrophy of normal breast tissue
- R/O Benign breast disease
- R/O Breast cancer
- R/O Cervical/dorsal radiculitis
- R/O Tietze's syndrome (costochondritis)

Plan

Diagnostic Tests

- Technologies for evaluating breast masses include:

    - mammography: most accurate for diagnosing early-stage cancers; generally avoided in pregnancy but safe to use during lactation (Feller, 1988)

    - ultrasonography: used as an adjunct to mammography to help distinguish solid from cystic masses but can not reliably detect microcalcifications or lesions <1 cm; can be safely used to evaluate breast masses in pregnancy (Ellerhorst-Ryan, Turba, & Stahl, 1988)

    - diaphanography (transillumination): currently under investigation as a screening procedure; used as an adjunct to mammography and physical exam

    - ductography or galactography: used to evaluate nipple discharge in a non-lactating breast; involves cannulating the involved duct and injecting a radiopaque dye, followed by xray evaluation; not likely to be used in pregnancy

    - CT scan and MRI: still under investigation

- Histologic evaluation of a biopsy specimen is the only definitive procedure that leads to the diagnosis of a breast mass and is indicated in the following instances (ACOG, 1983):

    - any dominant mass

    - bloody nipple discharge

    - eczema of the nipple

    - underlying induration

    - nipple retraction/elevation

    - skin dimpling/edema

    - unilateral persistent dominant thickening

    - suspicious axillary lymph nodes

    - suspicious lesions or microcalcifications found by other diagnostic aids despite normal physical exam

- Fine needle aspiration (FNA) is indicated for palpable cystic masses and may be used during pregnancy or lactation. Unresolved masses following aspiration require biopsy.

- Solid masses in a pregnant patient require excisional biopsy.

Treatment/Management

- Ask a second examiner to corroborate breast findings as indicated.

- Refer to breast specialist if a dominant breast mass is present.

- Elimination of caffeine substances has been suggested to reduce swelling in women with diffuse breast nodularity. Further research is needed to clarify the relationship of caffeine with symptomatic breast disorders.

- Vitamin E therapy has been reported to influence symptoms of breast pain and swelling. There are no studies on the use of vitamin E during pregnancy in women with breast complaints.

Consultation

- For suspicious mass

- MD management for dominant mass lesion is warranted.

Patient Education

- Teach/review breast self exam (BSE).

- Support/allay patient's concern for positive breast findings.

- Discuss changes of normal breast tissue during pregnancy.

Follow-up

- Encourage monthly BSE.

- Follow-up appointment for breast exam as indicated if patient has not been referred to breast specialist.

- Follow American Cancer Society's recommendations for routine mammogram in non-pregnant woman (American Cancer Society, 1988):

  - baseline at age 35-40

  - every year or two ages 40-49, depending on risk factors

  - yearly after age 50

  - women with a personal or family history of breast cancer may need more frequent mammograms; physician consultation should be sought.

- Document in progress notes and problem list.

CYSTITIS

Winifred L.Star

Acute cystitis occurs in about 1% of pregnant women, of whom 60% have had a negative urine culture on the initial screening (Davison & Lindheimer, 1989; McNeeley, 1988; Pauerstein, 1987). The urine culture in a patient with acute cystitis usually reveals >100,000 cfu/ml of a single pathogen, although lesser colony counts may exist in active infection (Davison & Lindheimer, 1989; McNeeley, 1988). In 75-90% of cases the infecting organism is *Escherichia coli*. Other organisms causing infection include: *Klebsiella, Proteus, coagulase-negative staphylococcus*, and *Pseudomonas* (Davison & Lindheimer, 1989).

Twenty five percent of women with untreated asymptomatic bacteriuria will eventually develop acute cystitis, which seems to occur more frequently in the second trimester (McNeeley, 1988). Pregnancy itself does not seem to predispose the woman to the development of lower urinary tract infection (Fowler, 1989). Normal pregnancy-related anatomic, physiologic, and hormonal changes may, however, predispose to the development of upper tract disease. Urinary tract symptoms normally present in a healthy pregnant woman may mimic those of acute cystitis.

The impact of maternal cystitis on the growing fetus has not been well-defined (Fowler, 1989). More is known regarding the impact of pyelonephritis during pregnancy. See the Pyelonephritis protocol.

Data Base

Subjective

- Predisposing factors may include:
    - inherent susceptibility to urinary tract infection
    - documented urinary tract infection in childhood
    - history of urinary tract infection as adult
    - recent new sexual partner
    - recent catheterization
    - diabetes
    - sickle cell trait
    - vaginal/cervical infection
- Symptoms may include:
    - urinary urgency, frequency
    - dysuria
    - nocturia
    - hesitancy, difficulty starting stream
    - incomplete emptying, dribbling
    - suprapubic discomfort

- tenesmus

- hematuria

- cloudy, malodorous urine

- vaginal discharge

- vulvar irritation

● Nausea, vomiting, fever, chills usually absent

Objective

● Vital signs usually within normal limits

● Abdominal exam may reveal tenderness in the suprapubic area.

● Pelvic exam may reveal findings consistent with vaginitis/cervicitis.

● Gross inspection of urine may reveal hematuria; urine may be cloudy and/or malodorous.

● Urine dipstick may be positive for nitrites, leukocyte esterase, protein, and/or blood.

● Microscopic urinalysis may reveal pyuria, bacteriuria, hematuria.

● Urine culture generally will reveal $\geq 10^5$ colonies of a single pathogenic organism. Lesser degrees of bacteriuria may be present.

● Wet mounts of vaginal discharge may be positive if vaginitis/cervicitis also present.

Assessment

● Acute cystitis

● R/O Asymptomatic bacteriuria

● R/O Pyelonephritis

● R/O Vaginitis/Cervicitis

Plan

Diagnostic Tests

● Routine urinalysis, culture and sensitivities on a clean-catch midstream specimen should be performed on all pregnant women at the initial prenatal visit. Repeat these tests each trimester in at risk patients.

● Complete urinalysis, culture and sensitivities on a clean-catch midstream urine specimen or sterile catheter specimen (although not usually necessary) to be performed when patient complaining of symptoms of acute cystitis, or if urine dipstick suggestive of infection.

● A "contaminated" urine culture will contain many mixed skin and/or vaginal flora and should be repeated in a symptomatic patient to ascertain the presence of a dominant pathogen.

● Dipstick for either nitrites or leukocyte esterase used alone is not sufficiently sensitive to detect bacteriuria but may provide a cost-effective alternative to culture if used in combination (Robertson & Duff, 1988).

Treatment/Management

● Ascertain drug allergy status of the patient.

- Ideally drug therapy is based upon sensitivities. However, in a patient with acute cystitis antibiotic therapy may be initiated immediately with change of drug as necessary.

- Drugs of choice in the pregnant population include:

  - Ampicillin 500 mg qid x 7-14 days

  - Nitrofurantoin (Macrodantin) 100 mg qid x 7-14 days

  - Sulfisoxazole (Gantrisin) 1 gram qid x 7-14 days

  - Cephalosporin (e.g., Velosef) 500 mg qid x 7-14 days

  NOTE: A seven day course is usually sufficient. Sulfa drugs and nitrofurantoin should not be prescribed to women with G6PD deficiency. Sulpha drugs should not be prescribed in the weeks preceding delivery to avoid the risk of neonatal hyperbilirubinemia.

- Suppressive antibiotic therapy for the remainder of pregnancy should be considered for patients with recurrent cystitis. A bedtime dose of nitrofurantoin 100 mg is usually prescribed.

Consultation

- For prescription as necessary

- For patients with repeated episodes of cystitis who are considered candidates for suppression with antibiotics during the remainder of pregnancy

- If acute pyelonephritis is suspected or diagnosed

Patient Education

- Discuss normal anatomical and hormonal changes of the urinary tract in pregnancy.

- Discuss etiology of acute cystitis.

- Encourage liberal fluid intake (minimum 8 cups of H_2O/day). Avoid caffeine. Recommend cranberry juice (home-made kind using fresh, smashed berries made into juice is the best!).

- Explain that symptoms should abate in 48 hours after initiation of drug therapy.

- Stress importance of finishing medication.

- Alert patient to signs and symptoms of pyelonephritis: fever, shaking chills, flank pain, nausea, vomiting, headache, malaise, anorexia, hematuria.

- Teach or review personal hygiene practices.

- Recommend urinating before and after intercourse.

Follow-up

- Order complete urinalysis, with culture and sensitivities after completion of drug therapy, at regularly scheduled routine OB visits (may be done monthly or once each trimester), and at 6-week postpartum visit.

- All patients should have a clean-catch midstream urine dipstick at each visit with follow-up culture if positive leukocyte esterase or nitrite noted on dipstick.

- Refer patient with repeated cystitis during pregnancy to urologist after third postpartum month to R/O renal anomalies.

- Document in progress notes and problem list. Note also on problem list the presence of Group B streptococcus in urine culture as indicated.

DEPRESSION--POSTPARTUM

Lucy Newmark Sammons

Mood disturbances occurring postpartum are commonly categorized into three classifications of increasing severity: "blues", depression, and psychosis. Excellent review articles of the growing literature describing postpartum depressions and their correlates (Affonso & Domino, 1984; O'Hara, 1987) support the following descriptions. Postpartum blues, with a prevalence of 39-85%, is a mild affective syndrome commonly occurring in the first week, but up to eight weeks, after birth. Symptoms last 1-10 days. Symptoms of the blues include depressed mood, crying spells, irritability, anxiety, mood swings, confusion, fatigue, insomnia, and appetite disturbances. Postpartum fatigue, increased burdens and responsibilities, and changing or absolute hormonal levels are implicated as causative factors, with reference to estrogens, progesterone, prolactin, cortisol, norepinephrine, and tryptophan. Consequences are generally benign, except when symptoms persist or increase to a more severe disorder.

Postpartum depression (PPD) occurs in 7-15% of women. It is characterized by lowered mood, some functional impairment, lack of affectional bonding between mother and infant, and symptoms associated with depression such as sleeping and eating changes, fatigue, psychomotor agitation or retardation, feelings of worthlessness, and loss of interest in usual activities. Inconsistencies have been found in attempts to associate PPD with age, parity, marital status, dysmenorrhea, previous pregnancy loss, obstetrical complications, hormonal disturbances, and other factors. Increased life stress, decreased social support, related personal and family psychopathology, and selected personality factors are more strongly associated with PPD. PPD may last for months. Consequences appear to include increased likelihood of additional depression for the woman and risk for emotional, cognitive, or social problems for her children.

Postpartum psychosis is characterized by severely impaired functional ability, often due to hallucinations, delusions, or severe mood depression or confusion. Suicidal or homicidal ideation may be present. The incidence of postpartum psychosis ranges from 1-4/1000. Most episodes occur in the first 2-4 weeks after birth, but may appear up to 90 days postpartum. Puerperal psychosis appears to be associated with first-time pregnancy, unmarried status, personal history of manic-depressive illness, and family history of psychopathology. Treatment may include psychotropic and electro-convulsive therapy, and hospitalization.

Data Base

Subjective

- Client or her family report sad, depressed, or lowered mood; mood swings; crying episodes; sleeping disturbances such as insomnia or excessive fatigue/hypersomnia; eating changes such as loss of appetite; confusion or inability to concentrate; inability to perform usual roles as mother, wife, or employee; loss of interest in usual sources of pleasure; feelings of worthlessness or inappropriate guilt; anger or hostility towards infant, other children, or partner.

- Possible pre-disposing factors include:

  - High levels of stressful life events in pregnancy and the puerperium

- Problematic interpersonal relationships, particularly poor partner relationship, or possibly poor relationship with own mother
- Inadequate social support from partner, family, and friends
- Personal history includes poor psychological adjustment before and during pregnancy; high levels of anxiety, neurotic behavior, depression/emotional distress
- Personal and/or family history of psychopathology

Objective

- May appear unkempt, personal grooming not maintained.
- Verbal/nonverbal responses may be inappropriate, e.g., flat affect or agitated.
- May demonstrate inappropriate weight loss or weight gain.

Assessment

- Postpartum blues, benign; or
- Postpartum depression
- R/O Postpartum psychosis or other psychopathology
- R/O Organic affective disorder, mood disorder secondary to underlying medical condition or as side effect of medication (Dreyfus, 1987)
- R/O Bereavement response
- R/O Substance abuse

Plan

Diagnostic Tests

- No specific diagnostic test

Treatment/Management

- Postpartum blues: a self-limited syndrome, no definitive treatment is required. Monitor woman for successful resolution.
- Postpartum depression: management under medical supervision. Treatment may include conventional chemotherapy (e.g., tricyclic antidepressants) or psychotherapy, with emphasis on inclusion of spouse/partner. Progesterone treatment is controversial.
- See also Patient Education.

Consultation

- Postpartum blues: no medical consultation necessary
- Postpartum depression, psychosis, or suspicion of other psychopathology: medical/psychiatric consultation required
- Presence of thoughts, dreams, or actions suggesting injury to self or others, particularly infant, require immediate consultation.

Patient Education

- Explain the causes and treatment approaches employed for the relevant level of postpartum depressed mood.

- Inform patient of feelings/behaviors that would require further health care assistance; assure woman of availability of continued routine or emergency services should they be needed.

- Involvement of family members and key support people is an integral aspect of prevention, identification, and management of postpartum mood disorders (Martell, 1990).

- Postpartum blues:

  - Reassure the woman that this mood alteration is self-limited, benign, and considered to be without future consequences for the woman or her family.

  - Assist woman and family in identifying and mobilizing resources to meet demands of infant and child care, family relationships, work, household maintenance, and social and leisure activities .

- Foster strategies to prevent postpartum emotional distress:

  - Avoid overload with non-essential tasks

  - Obtain plenty of rest and sleep

  - Maintain communication and share feelings with partner, family, and experienced friends.

  - Reduce responsibilities without eliminating social and recreational interests.

Follow-up

- Assure that patient/family have access to health care providers on 24-hour basis for crisis management, should need arise.

- Contact patient/family to reassess mood and functional status within one week. If symptoms are persisting or increasing in severity, further evaluation is required.

- Referrals to social services, financial services, mental health care professionals, public health nursing, community support groups, etc., as needed for assistance in coping and adjustment to demands of the puerperium

- Communication with pediatric providers required for appropriate follow-up of children in cases of severe depression or other psychopathology.

- No additional care required for resolved postpartum blues.

- For postpartum depression and severe psychopathology, document in progress notes and problem list.

ECTOPIC PREGNANCY

Maureen T. Shannon

The term "ectopic pregnancy" refers to the implantation of a fertilized ovum outside the endometrial cavity. Approximately 95% of ectopic pregnancies occur in the fallopian tubes (primarily in the ampulla or isthmus). Extratubal implantation sites include the cornua of the uterus (rudimentary horn), ovaries, cervix, broad ligaments, or abdominal cavity. Rarely can an ectopic pregnancy coexist with an intrauterine pregnancy. The incidence of ectopic pregnancy has been calculated to be 1.4/100 reported pregnancies (Dorfman, 1987) and is a leading cause of maternal mortality in the United States. Although maternal mortality due to ectopic pregnancy has decreased markedly during the past 15 years, the occurrence of this problem has continued to escalate, resulting in decreased fertility and an increased risk of recurrence of ectopic pregnancies in affected women (Dorfman, 1987).

Although the exact etiology is not known, mechanisms contributing to a woman's increased risk of experiencing an ectopic pregnancy include: 1) An alteration in the woman's tubal transport of a fertilized ovum, and 2) an alteration in the fertilization process itself (Russell, 1987; Sopelak & Bates, 1987). Treatment options currently available for the management of ectopic pregnancies include surgery, chemotherapy, and nonoperative expectant management. The treatment chosen is determined by several factors such as weeks of gestation, site of the ectopic, and ruptured or unruptured fallopian tube.

Data Base

Subjective

- Predisposing factors

    - History of a previous ectopic pregnancy

    - History of tubal surgery

    - History of pelvic inflammatory disease

    - History of infertility

    - Pregnant with an intrauterine device in utero

    - Pregnant while using low-dose progestins or postcoital estrogens for contraception

    - Pregnant after in-vitro fertilization

    - History of DES exposure

    - History of more than one therapeutic abortion (controversial)

- Symptomatology

    - Abdominal/pelvic pain--90-100% of patients will describe some type of abdominal/ pelvic pain varying from a vague ache to a sharp, colicky pain that may be diffuse or unilateral. Occasionally patients will report shoulder pain if there is blood in the peritoneum (Weckstein, 1987).

- Amenorrhea--40-95% of patients will report a lapsed menses (Rivlin, 1986; Weckstein, 1987).

- Irregular vaginal bleeding--usually described as light and intermittent, but can be profuse.

- Vertigo

- Syncope

- Nausea--10-25% of patients report this symptom (Weckstein, 1987).

- Breast tenderness--10-25% of patients report this symptom (Weckstein, 1987).

- May report passage of decidual tissue (rare).

Objective

- Blood pressure may be within normal limits (WNL), hypotensive, and/or demonstrate postural changes.

- Pulse may be WNL or tachycardic.

- Temperature (T) is usually WNL but 10% of patients will have a T> 38° C (Weckstein, 1987).

- Abdominal tenderness is present in 80-95% of patients (Weckstein, 1987).

- Rebound tenderness may be present.

- Uterine enlargement occurs in approximately 25% of patients (Rivlin, 1986), but uterine size is less than expected for weeks of gestation (Weckstein, 1987).

- Adnexal mass is present in 50-70% of patients (Rivlin, 1986; Weckstein, 1987).

- Vaginal bleeding may be observed.

Assessment

- Ectopic pregnancy
- R/O Intrauterine pregnancy with inaccurate dates
- R/O Incomplete or missed spontaneous abortion
- R/O Pelvic inflammatory disease
- R/O Appendicitis
- R/O Pelvic mass
- R/O Corpus luteum cyst
- R/O Endometriosis
- R/O Gestational trophoblastic neoplasia
- R/O Ureteral calculi

Plan

Diagnostic Tests

- CBC with differential--may reveal leukocytosis with a decreased hematocrit/hemoglobin depending upon the amount of blood lost.

128

- Type and Rh (if not already done).

- Serum Beta HCG--invariably positive but level is often less than expected for weeks of gestation. This test may be repeated serially in a stable patient with an uncertain diagnosis after consulting with an MD.

- Cervical cultures for chlamydia and gonorrhea (if indicated)

- Urine specimen--clean catch midstream urine for microscopic evaluation and culture

- Pelvic ultrasound--to evaluate for the presence or absence of an intrauterine or extrauterine pregnancy, or evidence of other pelvic pathology

Treatment/Management

- If an ectopic pregnancy is suspected, then consultation with an MD is mandatory.

- If an ectopic pregnancy is diagnosed, then transfer of care to MD management is warranted.

- If the patient is in shock, then immediate MD management is indicated. If the patient presents in shock in an outpatient setting that is geographically remote from a hospital, then procedures necessary to stabilize the patient should be initiated (e.g., insertion of an IV, oxygen therapy, etc.).

- In Rh negative women who experience an ectopic pregnancy, administration of Micro-RhoGam is indicated if the pregnancy is less than 12 weeks gestation, or RhoGam if the pregnancy is 12 or more weeks gestation (Wible-Kant & Beer, 1983).

Consultation

- Required in all patients suspected of having an ectopic pregnancy. Refer to MD care all patients diagnosed with an ectopic pregnancy.

Patient Education

- If the patient is stable, then a complete explanation of the possible problem(s), the diagnostic tests, and the need for consultation/referral to an MD can be given by the NP/NM.

- If the patient is exhibiting signs and symptoms of shock, then she (and her partner) should receive as complete an explanation as is possible regarding her immediate treatment and prognosis (this should be done by the MD managing her care).

- Emotional and psychological support of the patient and her partner should be available to help her/them work through the loss of a desired pregnancy and the implications this may have on future pregnancies.

- Educate the patient regarding her increased risk of having another ectopic pregnancy. Advise her that any time she may suspect that she is pregnant she should obtain medical evaluation due to her increased risk of a recurrence of this problem.

- Educate the patient about the signs and symptoms of possible complications following surgery for an ectopic pregnancy (e.g., infection, excessive bleeding, etc.). Ideally this should be done by the MD managing her care.

- Educate the Rh negative, antibody negative patient about the need for RhoGam administration after an ectopic pregnancy has been terminated.

Follow-up

- Follow-up evaluations of patients who have an ectopic pregnancy is per MD recommendation.

- Document in problem list and progress notes.

ENDOMETRITIS--POSTPARTUM

Lucy Newmark Sammons

Postpartum endometritis (PPE) is an inflammation of the inner lining of the uterus following childbirth. The phrases endomyometritis, endoparametritis, or metritis with pelvic cellulitis may be more accurate, since the decidua, myometrium, and parametrial tissues may be involved (Cunningham, MacDonald, & Gant, 1989). The conventional wisdom that fever during the puerperium must be regarded as resulting from genital tract infection until proven otherwise (Novy, 1987) continues to have merit. Postpartum endometritis is the most common infectious complication following childbirth (Soper, 1988). The incidence of PPE varies from 2-3% following vaginal birth to 10-95% following Cesarean delivery (Cox & Gilstrap, 1989).

Microbiologic studies have confirmed the polymicrobial character of perinatal genital tract infections. Common causative agents of PPE are mixtures of aerobic and anaerobic organisms indigenous to the lower genital tract, including anaerobic nonhemolytic *streptococci, coliform bacteria, staphylococci, chlamydiae, Mycoplasma hominis*, and *Bacteriodes* (Novy, 1987). Factors predisposing to postpartum endometritis or correlating with its occurrence are cesarean birth, prolonged labor, prolonged ruptured membranes, chorioamnionitis, midforceps delivery, size and number of incisions and lacerations, number of cervical examinations, and prolonged internal fetal monitoring (Cunningham et al., 1989; Gibbs, 1989). Extension of infection into the pelvic peritoneum can result in abscess formation, pelvic thrombophlebitis, generalized peritonitis, disseminated intravascular coagulation (DIC), septic shock, and infertility.

PPE may be categorized as either early-onset or late-onset (Soper, 1988). Early-onset endometritis generally occurs within 48 hours of birth, following operative delivery. Late-onset PPE usually occurs three days to six weeks after birth, often in women who delivered vaginally. These later infections tend to be clinically milder. Genital mycoplasmas and *chlamydiae trachomatis* are often the causative organisms in late PPE, while pathogenic anaerobic bacteria are not characteristic of late infections.

Data Base

Subjective

- Client complains of low back pain and low abdominal pain.
- Client may report:
  - Malodorous heavy vaginal discharge
  - Constipation
- History may include:
  - Cesarean delivery (especially surgery longer than 60 minutes, blood loss greater than 800 ml)
  - Premature rupture of membranes
  - Long labor
  - Temperature elevation in labor

- Instrumentation/other operative interference during current delivery

- Incomplete placental removal

- Perinatal hemorrhage/hematoma

- Indigent socio-economic status

- Low parity (Gibbs, 1989)

- Postpartum temperature elevation may be preceded by constitutional changes (malaise, anorexia, myalgia, diaphoresis, or chills).

Objective

- Temperature 38°C (100.4°F) or higher in any 2 of the first 10 days postpartum excluding the first 24 hours (Cunningham et al., 1989)

- Late onset fever (up to 7 weeks postpartum) may occur.

- Pulse rate may be normal or elevated.

- Blood count may reveal leukocytosis.

- Observable diaphoresis/chills if virulent infection

- Abdominal tenderness, possibly rigidity

- Abnormal (increased amount, dark red/brown, malodorous) discharge may be seen at external genitalia, vaginal vault, and cervix, although scant, odorless lochia is associated with beta-hemolytic streptococcal infection

- Cervical motion tenderness may be present.

- Uterus may be subinvoluted.

- Bimanual exam reveals swelling and/or tenderness in adnexa and pelvic peritoneum, as well as the uterus, with spread of infection.

- Macular rash and hypotension suggest postpartum toxic shock syndrome.

- Paralytic ileus may be concomitant problem; signs include abdominal distention, fecal vomiting, and constipation.

- Physical examination otherwise negative for signs of localized infection or systemic disease

Assessment

- Postpartum endometritis, early or late

- R/O Cystitis, pyelonephritis--see Cystitis and Pyelonephritis protocols

- R/O Mastitis, severe breast engorgement--see Mastitis protocol

- R/O Appendicitis

- R/O Mononucleosis or other viral disease

- R/O Septic ovarian vein thrombosis/peripheral ovarian vein syndrome--suggested by tender, linear, adnexal-lumbar mass and confirmed by computed tomography (CT scan)

- R/O Toxic Shock Syndrome (TSS)

- R/O Paralytic ileus

- R/O Respiratory complications, pulmonary atelectasis

- R/O Thrombophlebitis of lower extremities

Plan

Diagnostic Tests

- No specific diagnostic test used in clinical practice for mild cases, as treatment is empirical. Severe cases may warrant intrauterine and blood cultures.

- CBC, sedimentation rate

- Additional diagnostic tests as indicated by data base to exclude alternate assessments (e.g., urine culture)

Treatment/Management

- Antibiotics: varies by institution and early or late-onset pathophysiology. Severe cases require inpatient intravenous drug administration. Parenteral antibiotic regimens tending towards single agent second- and third-generation cephalosporins and newer semi-synthetic penicillins (Cox & Gilstrap, 1989). Sample outpatient regimens for milder cases:

  - Erythromycin 500 mg po qid x 7-10 days

  - Tetracycline 500 mg po qid x 7-10 days; effective against chlamydiae and mycoplasmas, but not recommended for lactating women (Briggs, Freeman, & Yaffe, 1986)

  - Ampicillin 500 mg po qid x 7-10 days

  - Cephalosporin, e.g., Keflex 500 mg po qid x 7-10 days

- Intravenous fluids for severe infection, nausea and vomiting

- Increased oral fluids, if tolerated

- Analgesics for pain relief--consider lactation status

- If subinvolution, treat per subinvolution protocol

- Prevention possibly enhanced by adequate diet and prevention/correction of anemia

- See also Patient Education.

Consultation

- Medical consultation required in all cases and for prescription as necessary

Patient Education

- Explain the causes and treatment approaches employed for endometritis.

- Advise bedrest in semi-Fowler position, providing concrete suggestions for realistic management of the newborn, self-care, household, and other family members.

- Maintain pelvic rest until infection is resolved.

- Obtain restorative diet and maintain good hydration.

Follow-up

- If symptoms worsen or fail to respond, reassess.

- If adequate symptom response and good patient compliance, reassess in 48-72 hours.

- Public health nurse/social services referral for woman with multiple children, demanding home situation, etc.

- Document in progress notes and problem list.

GESTATIONAL DIABETES MELLITUS

Winifred L. Star

The metabolic stress of pregnancy associated with fetal and placental growth results in various degrees of impairment of maternal carbohydrate tolerance. Both genetic and hormonal factors influence the development of gestational diabetes mellitus (GDM) in susceptible individuals.

In early normal pregnancy (0-20 weeks), estrogen/progesterone-induced metabolic alterations are reflected in hypertrophy of insulin secreting cells of the pancreas and increased insulin action at the level of muscle and adipose tissue. In the latter half of pregnancy (20-40 weeks), the increased level of human placental lactogen (HPL) and other placental hormones act as peripheral antagonists to the action of insulin. The sum of these hormonal changes results in a modest state of insulin resistance, increases in hepatic glucose production and mobilization of glycogen stores, and a stress on normal glucose tolerance (Nelson, 1984; Hollingsworth, 1985).

The majority of new onset diabetes diagnosed during pregnancy resolves postpartum. However, a significant number of women with GDM will develop overt diabetes mellitus in the ensuing 15-25 years.

Approximately 10% of pregnant women may have glucosuria without aberrations in blood glucose values. The increased GFR that occurs during pregnancy overcomes the renal threshold for resorbing glucose and results in renal glucosuria. This condition is more frequent in primiparas.

Worldwide, there is lack of uniform opinion regarding the definition or diagnostic criteria for GDM. The Second International Workshop - Conference on Gestational Diabetes Mellitus has defined GDM as..."carbohydrate intolerance of variable severity with onset of or first recognition during the present pregnancy. The definition applies irrespective of whether or not insulin is used for treatment or the condition persists after pregnancy. It does not exclude the possibility that the glucose intolerance may have antedated the pregnancy" (*Diabetes*, 1985, p. 123). In the U.S., the American College of Obstetricians and Gynecologists, the American Diabetes Association, and the National Diabetes Data Group (NDDG) support this definition. See Table 4.1, *Various Classifications of Diabetes in Use Today*, p. 141.

Depending upon the criteria used for diagnosis GDM occurs in approximately 1-5% of all U.S. pregnancies (Coustan & Carpenter, 1985). The majority of women with GDM can maintain normal glucose levels through diet alone. A sub-group of gestational diabetics (10-15%) will require insulin therapy to control fasting or postprandial hyperglycemia (Berry & Gabbe, 1986). These women face an increased risk of neonatal morbidity and mortality compared to their diet-controlled counterparts (Gabbe & Landon, 1987). Perinatal mortality of the gestational diabetic who is euglycemic may not be increased over the general population provided optimal obstetric care is maintained (Coustan & Carpenter, 1985; *Diabetes*, 1985; Gabbe & Landon, 1987).

The maternal/fetal risks associated with undetected GDM are significant and preventable. Perinatal mortality is a result of ketoacidosis, hypoxia, congenital anomalies, and respiratory distress syndrome. The most common neonatal complications include macrosomia, hyperbilirubinemia, and hypoglycemia. Maternal complications include spontaneous abortion, preterm labor and/or delivery, macrosomia, polyhydramnios, preeclampsia, and cesarean section (Kitzmiller et al., 1988; Reed,

1988). Advances in obstetrical care during the 1970s to 1980s have led to improvement in perinatal survival and decreased perinatal morbidity.

The management of the **insulin dependent** gestational diabetic is beyond the scope of this protocol and in many settings is primarily the responsibility of the MD. The reader is directed to an excellent monograph by Kitzmiller and associates, 1988 (see Bibliography section). Copies may be obtained from Year Book Medical Publishers, Inc., 200 N. La Salle St., Chicago, Ill. 60601 (customer service: 1-800-621-9262).

A program entitled "Sweet Success: Diabetes and Pregnancy Program" has established guidelines for care of women who have overt diabetes prior to pregnancy and who develop GDM. This protocol utilizes many of the guidelines of this program. The program is administered by the Maternal and Child Health Branch of the Department of Health Services. Their publication may be obtained through: Education Programs Associates, Center for Health Education Resources; 1 West Campbell Avenue, Campbell, CA 95008. Phone: (408) 374-1210.

Data Base

Subjective

- High Risk factors for the development of GDM include (Sweet Success, 1988):

    - previous obstetric history of gestational diabetes, macrosomic infant (>4000gm), unexplained stillbirth, malformed infant, polyhydramnios

    - obesity (>20% of IBW)

    - glucosuria (>2+)

    - family history of overt diabetes in first degree relative (i.e., parent, sibling, child)

    - age over 25 years

    NOTE: 50% of all patients with GDM fail to demonstrate the above risk factors

- Usually asymptomatic but may complain of polyuria, polydipsia, polyphagia (more common in uncontrolled overt diabetes predating pregnancy)

Objective

- Physical assessment of a well-controlled gestational diabetic should be within normal limits (WNL). Variations may include:

    - client that is obese and/or hypertensive

    - urine dipstick revealing glucosuria of> 1+ on >2 occasions or presence of ketones when GDM uncontrolled

    - evidence of bacteria on urinalysis or culture

    - uterine fundal height >2cm above that expected for dates in 2nd or 3rd trimester (suspect macrosomia or polyhydramnios)

- Macrosomia, polyhydramnios and/or presence of "thick placenta" may be evidenced by ultrasound in an uncontrolled gestational diabetic.

- Fetal movement should be in the normal range (10 moves within 2 hours) at 28 weeks and thereafter in an uncompromised pregnancy.

- If utilized NST should be reactive and CST negative in the absence of fetal distress at 34-36 weeks and thereafter. BPP should be 8-10 in an uncompromised pregnancy.

- In well-controlled gestational diabetes fasting blood sugar (FBS) should be <105 mg/dl, peak postprandial blood glucose <140mg/dl, and 2 hour postprandial <120mg/dl (Sweet Success, 1988).

Assessment

- Gestational diabetes mellitus (GDM)
- R/O Renal glucosuria
- R/O Asymptomatic bacteriuria
- R/O UTI
- R/O Hypertension/Preeclampsia
- R/O Macrosomia
- R/O Polyhydramnios
- R/O Fetal anomaly

Plan

Screening and Diagnostic Tests (See also Figure 4.1, *Screening and Diagnosis of Gestational Diabetes Mellitus,* p. 142)

- All pregnant women at 24-28 weeks to receive oral 50-gram glucose load followed 1 hour later with a venous plasma glucose measurement. Normal value= <140mg/dl. (O'Sullivan, Mahan, & Charles, 1973).
  NOTE: This test may performed at anytime of day without reference to the preceding meal. However, Coustan et al. (1986) recommends that if the 1 hour screen is administered to non-fasting women a value of 130mg/dl be used as the cut-off of normal. Capillary blood measurements using glucose oxidase-impregnated test strips are not sufficiently accurate for **diagnostic** purposes and are not to be used in this manner.

- A 1-hour glucose screen to be done earlier in pregnancy (~14-20 weeks) for the following categories (Sweet Success, 1988):

  - prior history of GDM
  - prior delivery of macrosomic infant
  - obesity
  - glucosuria of >2+
  - first degree relative with diabetes

- A 3-hour oral glucose tolerance test (GTT) to be done if the 1-hour glucose screen is 140-199mg/dl. This test is performed after an overnight fast of 8-14 hours. Some facilities require a 3-day diet preparation for the GTT which includes at least 150-g of carbohydrate/day. See Table 4.2, *Diet Preparation for Three-Hour Glucose Tolerance Test,* p. 143).

  Normal venous plasma values: fasting = <105mg/dl, 1 hour= <190 mg/dl, 2-hour= <165mg/dl, 3-hour= <145mg/dl (O'Sullivan & Mahan, 1964; NDDG, 1979). If two or more of the four values are met or exceeded a diagnosis of gestational diabetes can be made.

- If the 1-hour glucose screen is ≥200mg/dl order a FBS. If the FBS is ≥130mg/dl do **not** order a 3-hour GTT - patient to be managed as overt diabetic. If the FBS is <130mg/dl a 3-hour GTT may be performed (Sweet Success, 1988).

- If the 3-hour GTT is WNL at 24-28 weeks, consider retesting capillary blood glucose at 32-34 weeks under the following conditions (Sweet Success, 1988):

    - prior history of gestational diabetes

    - obesity

    - age >35

    - 1 value of 3-hour GTT abnormal

Treatment/Management

- See also Patient Education and Self-monitoring section. Ideally patient management should be coordinated closely with a multidisciplinary team including a nurse practitioner or nurse-midwife, physician, nutritionist clinical nurse specialist, and social worker. In some settings care of the gestational diabetic falls exclusively to the MD.

- Establish accurate dating in early first trimester (or as soon as possible).

- The following visit schedule is advised:

    - every two weeks from diagnosis to 36 weeks gestation

    - every week from 36 weeks gestation until delivery

    - more often as indicated

- Perform routine obstetrical evaluation at each prenatal visit with careful attention to serial McDonald's measurements; BP; weight; and urine for glucose, ketones, protein, leukocyte esterase, or nitrites.

- Routine OB lab studies should be ordered at the indicated times. See protocols on initial and return prenatal care.

- Urinalysis, culture, and sensitivities (UA, C&S) each trimester after diagnosis of GDM is advisable to R/O asymptomatic bacteriuria.

- Additional labs may include: thyroid, liver, renal function studies.

- Perform routine obstetrical ultrasound at 18-20 weeks to screen for fetal anomalies if GDM diagnosed early, if patient has past history of GDM, or if significant risk factors are present. Repeat as indicated to assess interval growth and perform prior to delivery to R/O macrosomia.

- Ideally refer patient to nutritionist for counseling regarding dietary controls. See Nutrition protocol. The goal is to achieve and maintain normal blood glucose levels throughout pregnancy (e.g., FBS <105 mg/dl, peak postprandial blood sugar <140 mg/dl, and 2-hour postprandial blood sugar <120 mg/dl) and to achieve a steady gradual pattern of weight gain (Sweet Success, 1988).

- Reassess nutritional status with a 24-hour dietary recall within one week of initial encounter, at monthly intervals, and prn if problems/complications develop.

- A psychosocial evaluation should be done on all patients preferably by a trained social worker. The assessment should include: review of diabetes history and social support systems, adjustment to pregnancy, and general emotional status. The goal of psychosocial services is to assist the patient in understanding and coping with the physical, emotional, and psychosocial stresses that may be encountered with GDM (Sweet Success, 1988).

- Patient to perform fasting and postprandial blood capillary glucose measurements if able to master finger stick procedure. It is recommended that patients perform these tests once a day, however, the frequency of testing should be individualized according to the clinical picture. Patient records should be maintained on flow sheets provided for this purpose. See Table 4.3, *Instructions and Flowsheet for Self-Blood Glucose Testing*, p. 144.

- Evaluate patient's glucose records carefully. If fasting and postprandial values are consistently elevated treatment with human insulin is required. Patient to be referred to MD.

- Fetal movement counts to be monitored by patient starting at 28 weeks.

- Standard antenatal fetal surveillance modalities such as the NST, CST, & BPP to be ordered at 34-36 weeks (and repeated weekly) for history of (Sweet Success, 1988):

    - prior stillbirth

    - hypertension

    - preeclampsia or PIH

- Induction of labor at 38-40 weeks with favorable cervix may be attempted to decrease the incidence of macrosomia and its associated complications. Fetal lung maturity should be documented for elective induction prior to 38 weeks.

- Spontaneous labor and vaginal delivery at term may be allowed unless complications arise (e.g., fetal distress, malpresentation, macrosomia, preeclampsia).

- If delivery has not occurred by 40 weeks routine postdate fetal surveillance with NSTs & amniotic fluid assessment should begin twice weekly. Follow-up with CSTs and/or BPPs as indicated. (Some facilities routinely order weekly NSTs after 34-36 weeks to follow uncomplicated gestational diabetes).

Consultation

- Patient may be referred to or comanaged with MD depending upon the practice setting. Ideal management utilizes a multidisciplinary approach.

- Ongoing consultation with an MD is strongly suggested if the NP/NM assumes primary care of the gestational diabetic.

- If the fasting or postprandial blood sugars are abnormal at any time, consult/refer to MD.

Patient Education and Self-Monitoring

- Engage in basic discussion of GDM and its obstetrical implications. Nutrition education ideally to be done by nutritionist. See Nutrition protocol.

- Discuss importance of careful and close follow-up, compliance with diet recommendations and blood glucose determinations.

- Explain the rationale and procedure for glucose testing:

    - First voided AM urine should be tested for ketones daily.

    - Fasting and postprandial capillary blood glucose should be performed by patient with the frequency of testing determined by MD. Assist patient in learning the proper technique for self finger-sticks and determining blood glucose readings with 'Chemstrip-bG'. The use of reflectance meters (e.g., Glucometer II, Glucoscan 3000, Accu-chek II) may also be utilized to determine capillary blood glucose.

    - Patient to keep accurate records on a flow sheet designed for gestational diabetes. See Table 4.3, *Instructions and Flowsheet for Self-Blood Glucose Testing*, p. 144.

- Recommend a 10-20 minute walk before or after meals to assist in lowering blood glucose (Sweet Success, 1985). Encourage continuation of regular daily exercise. The safe upper limit of exercise intensity is about 70% of maximum capacity (e.g., 220 - age x .70). Patients who regularly participate in aerobics may continue. "Vigorous" exercise programs should be discussed with the MD.

- Encourage postpartum follow-up of blood glucose as discussed in Follow-up Section below.

- Discuss long-term health maintenance measures, such as proper diet and exercise, to reduce the occurrence of nongestational diabetes mellitus.

- Address issues of parenting, sibling preparation, breast feeding, contraception and other perinatal issues as indicated by the individual patient.

Follow-up

- Consider postpartum follow-up with a 75 gram oral glucose tolerance test. This test should not be done during breastfeeding or prior to 6 weeks postdelivery. A venous plasma value at 2 hours of >200mg/dl is diagnostic of diabetes. Values between 140-199 are indicative of impaired glucose tolerance (Harris, Hadden, Knowler, & Bennett, 1985; NDDG, 1979).

- Alternately, a fasting blood sugar may also be ordered at 6 weeks postpartum. If the value is <115mg/dl overt diabetes is unlikely. Values ≥140 mg/dl indicate diabetes mellitus (Harris et al., 1985).

- Continue to support patient with psychosocial evaluation and referrals to appropriate systems or agencies.

- Continue to support long-term health maintenance (especially maintenance of normal weight) in order to prevent sequelae of diabetes.

- Assure that the patient has identified/established a safe and effective method of contraception.

- Document problem in problem list and progress notes.

Table 4.1

Various Classifications of Diabetes in Use Today

I. Modified White Classification

Pre-gestational Diabetes

Class	Age of Onset (year)		Duration (year)	Vascular Disease	Therapy
A	Any		Any	0	A-1, diet only A-2, insulin
B	>20		<10	0	insulin
C	10-19	or	10-19	0	insulin
D	10	or	20	Benign retinopathy	insulin
F	Any		Any	Nephropathy	insulin
R	Any		Any	Proliferative retinopathy	insulin
H	Any		Any	Heart disease	insulin

Gestational Diabetes

Class Level	Fasting Glucose Level		Postprandial Glucose
A-1	<105 mg/dl	and	<120 mg/dl
A-2	≥105 mg/dl	and/or	≥120 mg/dl

SOURCE:

American College of Obtetricians and Gynecologists (1986). *Management of diabetes mellitus in pregnancy* (Technical Bulletin No. 92). Washington, DC: Author. Reprinted with permission.

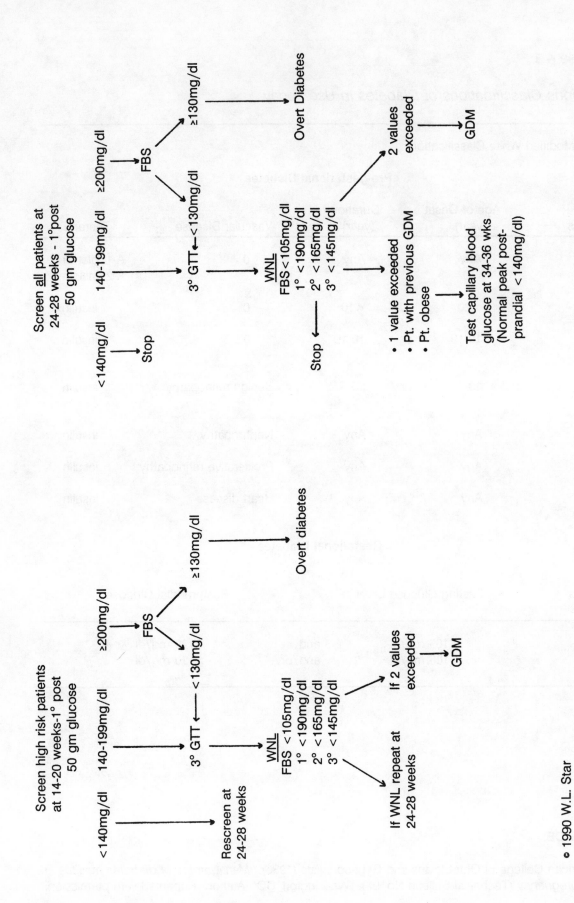

Figure 4.1. Screening and Diagnosis of Gestational Diabetes Mellitus (GDM)

© 1990 W.L. Star

142

Table 4.2

Diet Preparation for Three-Hour Glucose Tolerance Test

Your one-hour glucose screening test was abnormal. You will need to schedule a three-hour glucose tolerance test with the clinical laboratory. A glucose tolerance test checks how well your body responds to sugar. This test must be scheduled at a time that allows you to follow the special three-day diet. Please call the lab to schedule your appointment.

In order to decrease the chance of a falsely abnormal result follow the instructions below:

1. Continue to eat regular meals and all the foods you normally enjoy.

2. For three days before the test you must include extra carbohydrate (at least 150 grams or more) in your daily food intake. To make sure you are eating enough carbohydrate you must choose extra foods.

3. Choose <u>one</u> item from LIST 1 and <u>also one</u> item from LIST 2. Eat these foods in addition to the usual foods you eat for three days before the test.

LIST 1	LIST 2
2 slices of bread	
2/3 cup of cooked rice	8 tablespoons (4 oz) raisins
1 cup of cooked noodles	2 large apples
2 corn tortillas	2 small bananas
	16 oz orange or apple juice

4. <u>EXAMPLE</u>: Day 1 - extra 2 slices of bread
            10 oz of apple juice

          Day 2 - extra 1 cup of noodles
            16 oz orange juice

          Day 3 - extra 2 small bananas
            2 corn tortillas

- On the third day of your diet, eat nothing (not even toast), and drink nothing but sips of water <u>after 10:00 P.M.</u>, and until the test is over.

- Please arrive at the clinic lab no later than 8:30 A.M.

- First a fasting blood sample will be drawn, then you will be given a sugary liquid to drink.

- Each hour after the drink, blood will be drawn. This will be done three times. It is <u>important</u> that the blood is drawn at <u>exactly</u> one-hour intervals, so please be available at the indicated times.

- Please bring something to read, or do, while quietly sitting, until the test is over.

- Do not eat, smoke, or drink anything except water during the test. Sips of water should be taken only if you are very thirsty.

- After the last blood sample has been drawn, you may leave the laboratory and have your lunch.

- If you are unable to eat your usual diet, please inform your health care provider.

- Maintain your usual activity level on the days preceding the test.

Adapted from: University of California, San Francisco, OB Clinic

Table 4.3

Instructions and Flowsheet for Self-Blood Glucose Testing

Name: _____

1. Follow instructions on Chemstrip bG vial.

2. Check and record your blood sugar:
   ____ times a week before breakfast (fasting)
   ____ times a week 1 hour after breakfast
   ____ times a week 1 hour after lunch
   ____ times a week 1 hour after dinner

3. After you complete each test:
   a. Number the test strip with a test number
   b. Save used chemstrips in the vial, turning them in the opposite direction of the new Chemstrips
   c. Bring vial of chemstrips with the bar code to your next appointment.

4. Record your blood sugar value on the chart below with the test strip number. For example, if your blood sugar is 140 for test number 1, record "140 #1" in the appropriate box.

5. If your blood sugar is ever: 100 or more before breakfast or
                                   140 or more after meals
   call your health care provider at _____.

	Mon.	Tues.	Wed.	Thurs.	Fri.	Sat.	Sun.
Date							
Fasting Blood Glucose (BG)	#	#	#	#	#	#	#
Fasting Urine Ketones							
1 hr. after Breakfast BG	#	#	#	#	#	#	#
1 hr. after Lunch BG	#	#	#	#	#	#	#
1 hr. after Supper BG	#	#	#	#	#	#	#

	Mon.	Tues.	Wed.	Thurs.	Fri.	Sat.	Sun.
Date							
Fasting Blood Glucose (BG)	#	#	#	#	#	#	#
Fasting Urine Ketones							
1 hr. after Breakfast BG	#	#	#	#	#	#	#
1 hr. after Lunch BG	#	#	#	#	#	#	#
1 hr. after Supper BG	#	#	#	#	#	#	#

SOURCE:

Adapted from: Department of Ob/Gyn (1990). Kaiser Permanente Medical Center, San Francisco, CA.

144

GESTATIONAL TROPHOBLASTIC NEOPLASIA

Maureen T. Shannon

Gestational trophoblastic neoplasia (GTN) is a disease process caused by the abnormal development of the trophoblast which results in a benign or malignant tumor. The etiology of GTN is unknown; however, it is known that the chorionic villi become edematous grape-like vesicles which proliferate and eventually fill the uterus. The spectrum of this disease includes hydatidiform mole (partial or complete), invasive mole (chorioadenoma destruens), and choriocarcinoma (Celeste & Smith, 1986). The clinical classification of GTN is based on the location of the tumor, and the presence and extent of metastasis. The cure rate for persistent GTN of all severities is approximately 90%, with a cure rate of almost 100% being cited for low risk cases (Cunningham, MacDonald, & Gant, 1989). Early diagnosis of this disease is essential if successful treatment is to be attained. The overall incidence of GTN in the U.S. is 1/1,500 -1/2,000 pregnancies.

Data Base

Subjective

Predisposing factors

- Advanced maternal age (greater than 45 years old)

- History of previous mole (3.8% repeat molar pregnancy rate)

- Multiparity--a parity of 3 or more

- Geographic location--the highest incidences of GTN are in areas of Asia (1/125), the South Pacific (1/173-1/530) and in Mexico (1/500) (Celeste & Smith, 1986; Cunningham et al., 1989; Neeson & Stockdale, 1981).

Symptomatology

- Will report symptoms of pregnancy.

- Severe nausea and vomiting persisting after the 12th week of pregnancy

- Persistent dark-red or brownish vaginal bleeding which may be minimal or extensive

- Absence of fetal movement in pregnancies that continue through to the second trimester

- May be extremely fatigued due to increased loss of blood.

- May report passage of grape-like vesicles (usually this occurs before the 4th month of pregnancy).

Objective

- Uterine size not equal to dates--50% GTN will have uterine size greater than dates; 25% will have uterine size equal to dates; 25% will have uterine size less than dates.

- No fetal heart tones (FHTs) auscultated with Doppler by 12th week of pregnancy

- Signs of pre-eclampsia before the 24th week of pregnancy

- Ovarian mass due to theca-lutein cysts

- Decreased hematocrit/hemoglobin

- Increased thyroid functioning in about 2% of GTN cases

- Signs and symptoms of pulmonary embolism (e.g., cyanosis, tachypnea, tachycardia) secondary to the transportation of large amounts of the trophoblast to the lungs. Rarely is the volume of trophoblast transported to the lungs large enough to produce signs of pulmonary edema, although transport of small amounts of the trophoblast does occur and can result in lung metastasis (Cunningham et al., 1989).

- "Snow storm" pattern on sonogram

- Abnormally elevated Beta HCG levels 100 days or more after the woman's LMP

- Unexplained chest X-ray findings (e.g., "fungal" or "viral" pneumonias)

Assessment

- IUP _____ weeks

- R/O GTN

- R/O Anemia

- R/O Hyperemesis gravidarum

- R/O Threatened or missed spontaneous abortion

- R/O Hyperthyroidism

- R/O IUP with inaccurate dating

- R/O Pneumonia

Plan

Diagnostic Tests

- FHT auscultation--FHTs absent in GTN

- Beta HCG levels 100 days after LMP are persistently and abnormally elevated.

- Ultrasound exam reveals the "snow storm" pattern of molar pregnancy.

- Chest X-ray reveals unexplained findings (e.g., "viral" or "fungal" pneumonias), or evidence of pulmonary embolism.

- Complete blood count (CBC) or Hemoglobin and Hematocrit (H/H) reveals anemia.

- Thyroid studies may be elevated.

Treatment/Management

- In patients with suspected GTN order Beta HCG, sonogram and CBC.

- If GTN diagnosis is made, then immediate referral to MD care is warranted.

Consultation

- Required in all cases of suspected GTN.

- Transfer to MD care all patients with diagnosis of GTN.

Patient Education

- Explain the tests that are to be ordered and interpret the results for the patient.

- If GTN diagnosis is made, then the responsibility for educating the patient about this disease lies primarily with the treating physician, since the prognosis of the disease is based upon the extent of metastasis and duration of elevated Beta HCG levels. The cure rate is almost 100% in the majority of cases that are detected early and that do not have metastasis .

- Some patients will require help moving through the grieving process (grieving the loss of a "normal" pregnancy and working through the threat of a major disease).

Follow-up

- Follow-up of a patient diagnosed as having GTN is by the treating MD and includes:

    - Beta HCG levels every week until 3 consecutive negative results have been obtained after chemotherapy has been completed; then Beta HCG levels every month for six months; if negative, then Beta HCG levels every other month for one year.

    - Oral contraceptive use for one year after the HCG titers are negative.

    - Chemotherapy is started or restarted if a rise in the Beta HCG level occurs or if the level plateaus (does not drop).

- Patients who have been cured of GTN can become pregnant, but the recurrence rate for GTN is 3.8% for patients who have had one molar pregnancy and 28% for patients who have had two molar pregnancies (C. A. Braga, personal communication, 1986).

- Document in progress notes and problem list.

HYPERTENSIVE DISORDERS OF PREGNANCY

Maureen T. Shannon

Hypertensive disorders of pregnancy encompass a spectrum of hypertensive vascular diseases that includes the following: pregnancy-induced hypertension (PIH) without proteinuria and gross edema; PIH with proteinuria and edema (pre-eclampsia); PIH with tonic-clonic convulsions (eclampsia); chronic hypertension preceding pregnancy; chronic hypertension with superimposed pre-eclampsia or eclampsia; and the HELLP syndrome. See definitions below.

PIH is the most common hypertensive complication of pregnancy affecting up to 12% of all pregnancies (Ales, Norton, & Druzin, 1989). It is a leading cause of both perinatal and maternal morbidity and mortality, and is responsible for the majority of maternal deaths occurring at term (Gavette & Roberts, 1987). The delineation of subcategories of PIH is an attempt to differentiate them based upon their clinical signs, symptoms, and severity. However, the pathophysiology of these disorders is believed to be the same and involves the following components: 1) Generalized vasospasm resulting in an increased peripheral vascular resistance with a subsequent decreased perfusion to vital organs (e.g., brain, liver, kidneys, placenta); 2) the development of vascular lesions in several organ systems (e.g., placenta, liver); 3) stimulation of coagulation mechanisms; and 4) an alteration in the production and destruction of the prostacyclin-thromboxane mechanisms resulting in hemolysis and thrombocytopenia (Sibai & Moretti, 1988). The recognition of predisposing factors and subtle clinical signs and symptoms that a woman may exhibit during the early stages of PIH is paramount in preventing or significantly reducing the severity of the adverse maternal and fetal outcomes associated with this disorder.

Definitions

Hypertension induced by Pregnancy (PIH): This condition is characterized by the development of an elevation of a patient's blood pressure during the latter half of pregnancy. PIH is categorized as follows:

A. PIH without proteinuria and gross edema:
The occurrence of two blood pressure recordings done at least 6 hours apart that are equal to or greater than 140/90, or a rise in the systolic pressure of at least 30 mm/Hg or in the diastolic pressure of at least 15/mm Hg without proteinuria or edema (ACOG, 1986).

B. PIH with proteinuria and gross edema (Pre-eclampsia)

1. Mild Pre-eclampsia: The development of an elevation in BP as described under section A above with the additional development of the following: proteinuria equal to or greater than 1+ on a clean catch midstream urine; non-dependent edema of equal to or greater than 1+; and rapid, excessive weight gain equal to or greater than 2 lb/week or 6 lb/month (ACOG, 1986).

2. Severe Pre-eclampsia: The diagnosis of severe pre-eclampsia is made if one or more of the following signs occur in addition to those listed under mild pre-eclampsia: two blood pressure recordings greater than 160/110 taken at bed rest at least 6 hours apart; proteinuria equal to or greater than 3+ using a clean catch midstream urine, or equal to or greater than 5gm/24 hour urine collection; oliguria; pulmonary edema; thrombocytopenia (platelets less than 100,000); impaired liver function; epigastric or right upper quadrant pain; and cerebral or visual disturbances (ACOG, 1986).

a. <u>HELLP Syndrome</u>: The acronym "HELLP" reflects the clinical hallmarks of a PIH syndrome that include hypertension and hemolysis (H), elevated liver enzymes (EL), and low platelets (LP) (Abrams, 1989; Kirshon & Cotton, 1989; Sibai, 1988). It is observed in 4-12% of severe pre-eclamptic and/or eclamptic patients and is associated with poor maternal and fetal outcomes (Sibai et al., 1986). Reported perinatal mortality rates for this disorder have been as high as 33% (Sibai, 1988). There is an increased incidence of HELLP syndrome observed in patients with a delayed diagnosis of pre-eclampsia (Sibai, 1986), with as much as 20% of the cases first manifesting signs and/or symptoms of the syndrome during the early postpartum period (Weinstein, 1986). The most common symptoms reported by these patients are fatigue, nausea and/or vomiting, epigastric or right upper quadrant pain, and edema (Abrams, 1989; Weinstein, 1986). Early recognition of the signs and symptoms of this disorder is essential, since prompt, aggressive management is necessary to reduce the likelihood of significant maternal and perinatal morbidity and mortality.

C. Eclampsia: Eclampsia occurs when a pre-eclamptic patients develops tonic-clonic convulsions that are not related to a pre-existing neurologic condition such as epilepsy.

<u>Chronic Hypertension Preceding Pregnancy</u>: The diagnosis of chronic hypertension preceding pregnancy can be made when persistent hypertension, due to any etiology, is present before the 20th week of pregnancy and is not a result of gestational trophoblastic neoplasia (GTN); or when hypertension continues beyond 6 weeks postpartum (ACOG, 1986).

<u>Chronic Hypertension with Superimposed PIH</u>: The diagnosis of chronic hypertension with superimposed PIH (Either pre-eclampsia or eclampsia is made when a patient with chronic hypertension or renal disease develops the signs and symptoms of pre-eclampsia or eclampsia (ACOG, 1986).

Data Base

Subjective

<u>Predisposing Factors</u>

- Parity--it occurs primarily in primigravidas
- Maternal age--more common in teenagers (16 years or younger) and women greater than 35 years of age
- Lower socioeconomic status
- Family history of pre-eclampsia
- Severe malnutrition
- Women with vascular diseases--essential hypertension, diabetes mellitus, renal disease, systemic lupus erythematosus
- Gestational trophoblastic neoplasia (GTN)
- Multiple gestation
- History of pre-eclampsia with previous pregnancy

<u>Symptomatology/History</u>

PIH WITHOUT PROTEINURIA AND EDEMA

- Usually no physical complaints

PIH with Proteinuria and Gross Edema (Pre-eclampsia)

- Mild Pre-eclampsia

  - Usually no physical complaints except for edema of fingers (e.g., tightness of rings) and/or face (e.g., "puffy looking")

- Severe Pre-eclampsia

  - May complain of edema of fingers and/or face

  - May experience severe headaches (often in the frontal or occipital areas)

  - May report blurred vision, "flashes of light," "spots before eyes," or blindness (due to retinal detachment)

  - May complain of nausea and vomiting

  - May complain of epigastric or right upper quadrant pain

  - May complain of fatigue and "generally not feeling well"

  - May report decreased fetal movement

- HELLP Syndrome

  - See also subjective section under severe pre-eclampsia and eclampsia.

  - May complain of fatigue (50% of patients) (Weinstein, 1986)

  - May complain of nausea and/or vomiting (approximately 50% of patients) (Weinstein, 1986)

  - May complain of epigastric or right upper quadrant pain (approximately 50% of patients) (Weinstein, 1986)

  - May complain of edema (approximately 40% of patients) (Weinstein, 1986)

  - May report jaundice (up to 40% of patients with significant hemolysis) (Weinstein, 1986)

Eclampsia

- Reports loss of consciousness with drowsiness or coma following (relative or friend may describe patients having had a seizure or "fit")

- May report having experienced severe dyspnea and/or shortness of breath (due to pulmonary edema)

Chronic Hypertension

- May report history of hypertension prior to pregnancy

Chronic Hypertension with Superimposed PIH

- See subjective section under pre-eclampsia and eclampsia.

- May report history of hypertension prior to pregnancy.

Objective

PIH without Proteinuria and Edema

- BP equal to or greater than 140/90, or a rise in systolic pressure equal to or greater than 30 mm Hg, or the diastolic pressure equal to or greater than 15 mm Hg after the 20th week gestation measured on 2 separate occasions 6 hours apart

- Absence of significant proteinuria (equal to or less than 1+) and gross, generalized edema

- Lab tests (e.g., BUN, serum creatinine, etc.) are within normal limits (WNL).

- Reflexes WNL

- Usually no evidence of intrauterine growth retardation (IUGR)

- Woman is normotensive after delivery.

PIH with Proteinuria and Edema (ACOG, 1986)

- Mild Pre-eclampsia

  - Two blood pressure recordings (at least 6 hours apart) equal to or greater than 140/90, or an increase in the systolic pressure equal to or greater than 30 mm Hg, or the diastolic pressure equal to or greater than 15 mm Hg over a baseline reading.
    NOTE: in mild pre-eclampsia the diastolic pressure is usually less than 100 mm Hg).

  - Rapid, excessive weight gain equal to or greater than 2 lbs/week or 6 lbs/month (usually this increase in weight will precede evidence of non-dependent edema)

  - Proteinuria equal to or greater than 1+ on a clean catch midstream urine sample on 2 separate occasions (at least 6 hours apart), or greater than 300 mg protein in a 24-hour urine collection

  - Non-dependent edema (e.g., orbital, fingers, sacral) and/or pretibial edema equal to or greater than 1+

  - Reflexes are usually normal.

- Severe Pre-eclampsia

  - Two blood pressure recordings (at least 6 hours apart) greater than 160/110 mm Hg

  - Persistent proteinuria equal to or greater than 3+ using a clean-catch midstream specimen, or equal to or greater than 5 gm/24-hour urine collection

  - Generalized non-dependent edema, pretibial edema equal to or greater than 3-4+

  - Urinary output equal to or less than 400-500 ml/24 hours (oliguria)

  - Uterine size less than dates (evidence of IUGR)

  - Cyanosis (if pulmonary edema present)

  - Tachypnea, dyspnea (if pulmonary edema present)

  - Retinal changes (e.g., arteriolar spasm, papillary edema, ischemia, retinal detachment--rare) may be present

  - Hyperreflexia (3+-4+) with or without clonus may be present

  - Jaundice may be present

- HELLP Syndrome

  - See also objective section under severe preeclampsia and eclampsia.

  - Tenderness to palpation in epigastric or right upper quadrant area

- Enlarged, firm liver

- Ascites may be evident.

- Jaundice--approximately 40% of patients will develop jaundice (Weinstein, 1986).

- Adult respiratory distress syndrome (ARDS) may be evident with cyanosis, dyspnea, tachypnea.

Eclampsia

- Tonic-clonic seizure(s) with coma following for varying lengths of time

- May be anuric

- Jaundice (approximately 10% of eclamptic women)

- Cyanosis and tachypnea may be present (due to pulmonary edema).

- Excessive bleeding from I.V. sites (if woman develops disseminated intravascular coagulation [DIC])

- Absence of fetal movement & fetal heart tones if fetal demise

Chronic Hypertension

- BP equal to or greater than 140/90, or a rise in systolic pressure equal to or greater than 30 mm/Hg, or in diastolic pressure equal to or greater than 15 mm/Hg before the 20th week of gestation (without evidence of GTN) on two separate occasions

- Absence of significant proteinuria (less than 1+)

- Absence of gross, generalized edema

- Lab tests usually WNL unless severe hypertension

- Reflexes WNL

- Hypertension will persist after 6 weeks postpartum if not treated.

Chronic Hypertension with Superimposed PIH

- See objective section for PIH with and without proteinuria and edema.

- Hypertension will persist after 6 weeks postpartum if not treated.

Assessment

- PIH without proteinuria and edema

- Pre-eclampsia--mild or severe

- Pre-eclampsia or eclampsia with HELLP syndrome

- Eclampsia (R/O convulsive disorder)

- R/O Chronic hypertension

- R/O Chronic hypertension with superimposed pre-eclampsia

- R/O Gestational proteinuria

- R/O GTN (if clinical features of pre-eclampsia occur before 24th week of pregnancy)

- R/O Chronic renal disease

- R/O Endocrine disorders (e.g., Pheochromocytoma)

- R/O Connective tissue disorders (e.g., Lupus erythematosus)

- R/O Intrauterine growth retardation (IUGR)

- R/O Liver disease (e.g., hepatitis)

- R/O Cholelithiasis

- R/O Pyelonephritis

- R/O Idiopathic thrombocytopenia purpura (ITP)

Plan

Diagnostic Tests

PIH without Proteinuria and Edema

- Urine dipstick for protein will be negative or trace.

- Kidney function studies will usually be WNL.

- Hematologic, coagulation & hepatic studies (if ordered) will usually be WNL.

- Ultrasonography--if any clinical evidence of IUGR

- Sequential non-stress tests (NSTs) with fluid check, contraction stress tests (CSTs), or biophysical profile (BPP) of the fetus ordered in late pregnancy (34-36 weeks) or earlier if other problems (e.g., IUGR) are suspected.

PIH with Proteinuria and Edema (Pre-eclampsia)

- Mild Pre-eclampsia

  - CBC--hemoconcentration is a common finding in severe pre-eclampsia; a low platelet count may also be present.

  - SGOT, serum creatinine, uric acid--often elevated with worsening pre-eclampsia

  - Ultrasonography--if any clinical evidence of IUGR

  - Sequential (NSTs) with fluid check, CSTs, and/or BPPs of fetus beginning when the diagnosis is made.

  - 24-hour urine for protein and creatinine clearance to be followed serially $\downarrow Ca^{++}$

- Severe Pre-eclampsia--All of the diagnostic tests listed under mild pre-eclampsia as well as:

  - Liver function studies (e.g., LDH & SGOT) may be elevated.

  - Coagulation studies--decreased clotting factors and platelets and increased fibrin split products in severe pre-eclampsia with developing DIC or HELLP syndrome

- HELLP Syndrome

  - See also components listed under severe pre-eclampsia.

  - CBC--initially hemoconcentration is usually observed; however, in 60% of patients there will be a rapid, significant decrease in hematocrit observed after delivery that is not consistent with the patient's blood loss (Abrams, 1989; Weinstein, 1986).

  - Peripheral blood smear--will reveal shistocytes and/or Burr cells

- Platelets--usually significantly decreased (less than 100,000/mm^2, often less than 50,000/mm^2)

- PT and PTT--WNL

- Fibrinogen--WNL

- Serum glucose--can be significantly decreased in some patients (Weinstein, 1986)

- SGOT and SGPT--elevated

- BUN and creatinine--elevated

- Uric acid--elevated

Eclampsia

- See components listed under severe pre-eclampsia.

Chronic Hypertension

- Urine dipstick for protein will be negative or trace.

- Kidney function studies may be altered depending on the severity of hypertension and any renal damage associated with it.

- Hematologic, coagulation, and hepatic studies (if ordered) will usually be WNL.

- Ultrasonography--if any clinical evidence of IUGR

- Sequential NSTs with fluid checks, BPP of fetus, or CSTs beginning at 34-36 weeks or earlier if other problems (e.g., IUGR) are suspected.

Chronic Hypertension with Superimposed PIH

- See diagnostic tests for mild and severe pre-eclampsia.

Treatment/Management

Mild PIH without Proteinuria and Edema/Mild Pre-eclampsia

- Bed rest at home in left lateral recumbent position to enhance placental perfusion--hospitalization if BP does not respond to rest

- Weekly visits for BP, urine, weight, and uterine growth checks; every other week client to see MD

- Observation and questioning for development of signs and symptoms of pre-eclampsia

- Nutritional counseling for bed rest diet; increased protein; avoidance of excessive salt intake; increased fluids. See Nutrition protocol.

- Fetal movement counts beginning the 28th week

- Weekly NSTs/CSTs beginning at 34-36 weeks gestation (or earlier if indicated). Attempt to schedule these tests on the same day as the office visit.

- Fetal monitoring during labor and delivery

Severe Pre-eclampsia/Eclampsia

- Managed by MD in hospital

- HELLP Syndrome

-   Managed by MD in hospital

Chronic Hypertension

-   Managed by MD

Chronic Hypertension with Superimposed PIH

-   Managed by MD

Consultation

-   Required in all cases of hypertensive disorders of pregnancy

-   Co-management with MD of mild PIH without proteinuria or mild pre-eclampsia is possible in reliable, compliant patients.

-   Refer to MD care all severely pre-eclamptic patients, all non-compliant patients, and all patients with chronic hypertension.

Patient Education

-   Explanation regarding the problem and the plan of care

-   Explanation of tests and interpretation of results

-   Teach the woman how to count fetal movements and when she should notify NP/NM or MD regarding a decrease in these.

-   Advise the woman about the necessity of maintaining bed rest (in left lateral recumbent position)--the benefits to her and her baby.

-   Discuss and help with child care arrangements if woman has other children.

-   Nutrition counseling--high protein, bed rest diet; increased fluids; avoidance of excessive salt intake (see Nutrition protocol)

-   Explain the importance of recognizing and reporting signs and symptoms of progressing pre-eclampsia and of other possible complications (e.g., obstetrical bleeding, pre-term labor, etc.).

-   Teach the woman breathing techniques for labor and birth (since it is unlikely she will be able to attend a formal childbirth class if she maintains strict bed rest); provide anticipatory guidance regarding labor and birth; direct her to available books and/or video tapes on labor and birth, childcare, and breastfeeding.

-   Review procedures involved in labor and birth (e.g., analgesia, anesthesia, episiotomy, etc.).

-   Advise that continuous fetal monitoring during labor and delivery will be indicated.

-   Consider home health visits, if available, for noncompliant patients.

-   Provide instruction on taking BPs at home if cuff available.

Follow-up

-   If signs and symptoms of PIH are resolved after birth of infant, then schedule woman for 2 and 6-week postpartum office visits.

-   If PIH persisted after delivery of infant (e.g., 24-48 hrs) then schedule the office visit one week after birth (if no follow-up by MD scheduled). Refer to MD if persistent hypertension occurs postpartum.

- If the infant is small for gestational age then a public health nurse home visit should be scheduled for 1-2 weeks after birth.

- Make sure mother has scheduled pediatric visits for the infant at 2 and 6-8 weeks after birth.

- Document in progress notes and problem list.

INTRAUTERINE GROWTH RETARDATION/
SMALL FOR GESTATIONAL AGE

Lisa L. Lommel

Intrauterine growth retardation (IUGR) affects 5% to 10% of all pregnancies (Hobbins, Berkowitz, Manning, & Medearis, 1988). It has been found that one-third of infants with birthweights less than 2,500 grams are not premature but are term infants whose birthweight is the result of impaired uterine growth. The impact of this problem is evident by the significantly higher perinatal morbidity and mortality rates compared to infants who grow normally. The perinatal mortality is four to ten times higher in growth retarded neonates than those with normal growth patterns (Chiswick, 1985; Simpson & Creasy, 1984). Although the majority of full-term infants with IUGR demonstrate normal intelligence, the risk for long-term neurologic and developmental disorders is substantially increased.

A newborn is classified as growth retarded, or small for gestational age (SGA), when birthweight falls below the 10th percentile for gestational age. Birthweight below the third percentile, birthweight more than two standard deviations below the mean for gestational age, and a ponderal index below the 10th percentile for gestational age have also been used to designate intrauterine growth retardation (Chiswick, 1985; Mintz & Landon, 1988). Although growth retardation is usually defined in terms of weight for gestational age, there are variables that must be considered when measuring weight and age alone. These include accurateness of determined gestational age, ethnicity, genetic factors, altitude, and parameters such as body size and length. Sonographic evaluation of IUGR includes the measurement of several fetal parameters. Measurements include: biparietal diameter (BPD), femur length (FL), abdominal circumference (AC), estimated fetal weight (EFW) (calculated from BPD or FL and AC), total intrauterine volume (TIUV), and amniotic fluid volume (AFV). The ratios most commonly used to identify growth disturbances are the head to abdominal circumference and femur to abdominal circumference. Most studies have shown the abdominal circumference to be the best indicator for IUGR (Mintz & Landon, 1988).

Two types of abnormal growth patterns have been recognized by sonography in the IUGR fetus. These types of IUGR reflect differences in parameters of body length and size (Table 4.4, *Clinical Classification of IUGR*, p. 162).

- Symmetrical IUGR: This type of IUGR occurs when the fetus has experienced an early and prolonged deprivation resulting from chronic maternal malnutrition, intrauterine infection, congenital malformation, fetal chromosomal anomaly, substance abuse, placental insufficiency, or multiple gestation. Fetal cell size is normal but is generally deficient throughout the body. The neonate's body and head are proportional but small (proportional growth retardation). Head circumference falls below the 10th percentile, brain size is diminished, and permanent mental retardation may result.

- Asymmetrical IUGR: This type of IUGR results from nutritional deficits and placental deficiency in late pregnancy caused by a variety of maternal disorders including chronic hypertension and pregnancy induced hypertension. Diminished cell size results from atrophy of pre-existing cells, without reduction in the number of cells. Head size of the neonate appears disproportionately large in relation to the body (disproportional growth retardation). The body contains little subcutaneous fat and appears long and emaciated. Generalized muscle wasting, poor skin tugor, sparse hair, wrinkled abdomen, and widely separated sutures are all indicative of asymmetrical IUGR. Postnatal growth and development of the infant is rapid, and potential for normal intellectual growth is excellent.

There are a variety of socioeconomic, nutritional, and clinical factors that have been found to predict IUGR (see Data Base). When IUGR is suspected in a pregnancy, however, the cause is identified in only a minority of cases. Even after birth, a cause for growth retardation in the SGA infant can be found in fewer than one-half of the cases.

Data Base

Subjective

- Socioeconomic status
  - low socioeconomic status
  - lack of access to medical care
  - exposure to occupational hazards
  - substance abuse (tobacco, alcohol, drugs) (strong correlation with IUGR)
- Nutrition
  - low prepregnancy weight (strong correlation with IUGR)
  - inadequate weight gain during pregnancy
  - lack of access to food
  - vegetarian, food fetishes
- Medical conditions
  - chronic hypertension (strong correlation with IUGR)
  - diabetes
  - renal disease
  - autoimmune disease
  - hemoglobinopathies
  - severe anemia
  - congenital heart condition
- Maternal infections
  - viral: rubella, cytomegalovirus, herpes simplex, varicella zoster
  - bacterial: listeriosis, tuberculosis, poliomyelitis
  - spirochete: syphilis
  - protozoa: toxoplasmosis, malaria, trypanosomiasis
- Obstetrical history
  - previous SGA infant (recurrence risk 25%)
  - previous stillborn
  - unsure dates/late entry for prenatal care
  - maternal age (extremes of youth or increased age)
- Pregnancy complications
  - pre-eclampsia (strong correlation with IUGR)

- third trimester bleeding
- prolonged pregnancy
- extrauterine pregnancy
- placental/cord abnormalities
- multiple gestation
- poor uterine fundal growth
- Fetal chromosomal abnormalities
  - trisomies 13, 18, 21
  - Turner's syndrome
  - neural tube defects
  - congenital heart defects

Objective

- Maternal weight gain less than expected
- Fundal height measurement less than expected for gestational age
- Nutrition recall deficient in expected caloric intake for weight, maternal age, and gestational age
- Urine dipstick may be positive for ketones
- Sonographic evidence of estimated fetal weight less than the 10th percentile for gestational age
- Presence of clinical indicators for conditions that have been associated with IUGR (i.e., increased blood pressure in chronic hypertension, positive TORCH titer, congenital malformation detected by ultrasound)

Assessment

- Intrauterine growth retardation: estimated fetal weight below 10th percentile for gestational age
- R/O Inaccurate dating of pregnancy
- R/O Inaccurate fundal height measurement/estimation of fetal weight
- R/O Oligohydramnios
- R/O Transverse lie
- R/O Small but normal fetus
- Presence of condition(s) known to be associated with IUGR

Plan

Diagnostic Tests

- Accurate dating of gestational age should be performed as early as possible in the pregnancy including LMP, pelvic exam, doptone and fetoscope auscultation of fetal heart tones, and quickening.
- Sonogram before 20 weeks' gestation to confirm dates in patients at risk for IUGR.
- Assessment/measurement of uterine fundus at every prenatal visit preferably by the same examiner.

- Maternal weight

- Second trimester sonogram to evaluate fetal growth and assess fetal anatomy and function. Second trimester fetal measurements include BPD, HC, AC, and FL. Ratio relationships of HC to AC, FL to AC, and estimated fetal weight are used to estimate fetal growth.

- Serial sonograms approximately 3 weeks apart will estimate the interval fetal growth and percentile rank of fetal weight for gestational age.

- Sonogram to assess the amount of amniotic fluid. Amniotic fluid is frequently reduced with placental insufficiency. Oligohydramnios is recognized as a feature of IUGR. The finding of a single amniotic fluid pocket of 1 cm or less is associated with a 90% chance of IUGR.

- Sonogram evaluation of the placenta for maturation.

- Doppler ultrasound to evaluate the blood flow of the fetoplacental unit and uterine arteries. It has been found that growth-retarded fetuses with abnormal flow patterns are at higher risk for adverse perinatal outcome (Hobbins et al., 1988).

Treatment/Management

- Cessation of maternal smoking and/or drug use

- Nutritional counseling and referral to supplemental food program as indicated--see Nutritional protocol).

- Financial assistance when appropriate

- Bed rest on left side to enhance placental perfusion

- Initiate fetal movement counts at 28 weeks--see Antepartum Fetal Surveillance protocol.

- Weekly (or more often as indicated) non-stress test and bio-physical profile--see Antepartum Fetal Surveillance protocol.

- Management/treatment of conditions known to be associated with IUGR

- Amniocentesis to determine fetal lung maturity as appropriate

- Early delivery when maternal illness is aggravated by the pregnancy (i.e., pre-eclampsia/eclampsia), when fetal growth is poor or absent, oligohydramnios develops or evidence of fetal distress with non-reassuring fetal function test

- Fetal monitoring during labor and delivery

Consultation

- Required for suspected IUGR

- Referral to MD when IUGR is diagnosed

Patient Education

- Avoid using the term intrauterine growth retardation when talking with patients. Use the terms slow fetal growth or small for gestational age

- Discuss the plan of care with the patient including an explanation of tests and interpretation of results.

- Explain that a small fetus does not always mean there is a problem.

- Explain how to obtain fetal movement counts.

- Encourage a well-balanced, high-caloric, high-protein diet.

- Advise the patient to rest as much as possible in the left lateral recumbent position.

Follow-up

- Refer to nutritionist for diet counseling.
- Refer to social worker for assistance with socioeconomic problems.
- Refer to public health nurse as appropriate.
- Document in progress notes and problem list.

Table 4.4

Clinical Classification of IUGR

	Type I: Symmetrical	Type II: Asymmetrical
Incidence	25%	75%
Causes	"Intrinsic" genetic anomalies, "Extrinsic," TORCH teratogens, severe malnutrition (?), drugs, smoking, alcohol	"Extrinsic" utero placental insufficiency i.e., maternal disorders
Timing of insult	< 28 weeks gestation	> 28 weeks gestation
Cell number	Decreased (hypoplastic)	Normal
Cell size	Normal	Decreased (hypotrophic)
Head size	Microcephalic	Usually normal
Brain size	Decreased	Usually normal
Liver, thymus size	Decreased	Decreased
Brain/liver weight ratio (NL 3:1)	Normal	Increased > 6:1
Placental growth	Frequently normal though cell number decreased	Decreased
Congenital anomalies	Frequent	Rare
Ponderal index	Normal	Decreased
Ultrasound evaluation		
BPD	Small	Early-Normal Late-Small
AC	Small	Small
HC:AC ratio	Normal	Early-Increased Late-Normal
Doppler		
Umbilical and aortic resistance index	Increased	Increased
Carotid resistance index	Increased "no brain spairing"	Decreased "brain spairing"
Postnatal catch-up growth	Poor	Good

SOURCE:

Brar, H. S., & Rutherford, S. E. (1988). Classification of intrauterine growth retardation. *Seminars in Perinatology, 12* (1), 2-10. Reprinted with permission.

KETONURIA

Lisa L. Lommel

Ketonuria is defined by the presence of ketones excreted in the urine as metabolic end-products of fatty acid metabolism. Fats are used when glucose is unavailable to the body's cells. The three ketone bodies in the urine are acetone, acetoacetic acid, and beta-hydroxybutyric acid. Clinically available strips and tablets test for the presence of acetone and acetoacetic acid.

The unavailability of glucose as an energy source is usually due to glucose not being transported to the cells, as in diabetes, or because insufficient amounts of glucose exist in the body. Since insulin is necessary for transport of glucose to the cells, ketonuria in the pregnant, diabetic patient indicates an insulin/glucose imbalance. Testing the urine for the presence of ketones is often used for monitoring diabetes in pregnancy (Corbett, 1987). Ketonuria due to insufficient amounts of glucose in the body may be the result of fasting, heavy exercise, or when the pregnant woman cannot maintain food intake because of nausea and vomiting (Varney, 1987).

Data Base

Subjective

- History of diabetes

- Dieting, fasting, pica

- Nausea and vomiting

- Hyperemesis gravidarum

- Excessive exercise

Objective

- Ketonuria 1-4+ as identified by dipstick

- Weight loss

- Failure to gain weight

- Signs of dehydration: decreased skin turgor, dry mucous membranes, ketones on breath, increased pulse rate and temperature

- Document type, amount, and frequency of exercise

Assessment

- Ketonuria 1-4+

- R/O Diabetes

- R/O Hyperemesis gravidarum

- R/O Dieting/Pica

- R/O Excessive exercise

Plan

Diagnostic tests

- Perform a urine dipstick for ketones and glucose.

- Obtain patient weight.

- Collect a twenty-four hour diet recall.

- Serum acetone may be ordered in presence of significant ketonuria.

- Routine screening of all patients for diabetes at 24-28 weeks as indicated

Treatment/Management

- Prescribe an adequate diet.

- Provide an antiemetic for severe nausea and vomiting.

- Decrease the amount of exercise when excessive.

- Refer to labor and delivery unit for IV hydration if severe hyperemesis.

- Refer to Pica, Nausea/Vomiting, and Gestational Diabetes protocols.

Consultation

- In cases of excessive, prolonged nausea and vomiting

- With persistent significant ketonuria

Patient Education

- Ensure that the patient knows that ketonuria is of concern during pregnancy.

- Discuss the value of adequate exercise; emphasize the problems that may be associated with excessive and/or prolonged exercise.

- Explain the importance of adequate nutritional intake and the problems of dieting or fasting during pregnancy.

- Patients practicing pica will require an understanding of its meaning during pregnancy.

Follow-up

- Adjust clinical visits as necessary for non-compliant patients.

- Refer to nutritionist for dietary counseling. See Nutrition protocol.

- Offer psychological counseling for the hyperemesis gravidarum patient as indicated.

- Document in problem list and progress notes.

MALPRESENTATION OF THE FETUS

Maureen T. Shannon

Malpresentation of the fetus occurs whenever the presenting fetal part is other than vertex. There are several different types of malpresentations with many factors contributing to their development (e.g., placenta previa, contracted pelvis, fetal malformations, etc.). Often, a fetal malpresentation will not become apparent until labor has started (e.g., brow presentation, face presentation). However, some malpresentations are evident during the antepartum period, and include the following:

Breech Presentation: The fetus is in a longitudinal lie with the fetal buttocks, knees or feet as the presenting part, and the fetal sacrum is the denominator (Whitley, 1985). Breech presentations are more common during the second trimester than at term, when the incidence is approximately 2-4% (Cunningham, MacDonald, & Gant, 1989; Whitley, 1985). There are four types of breech presentations:

1. Complete breech presentation occurs when the fetal thighs and knees are flexed. The fetus appears to be in a tailor-sitting position (Whitley, 1985).
2. Frank breech presentation occurs when the fetal thighs are flexed and the knees are extended. About 2/3 of breech presentations are frank breeches (Cunningham et al., 1989; Whitley, 1985).
3. Footling breech presentation can be single or double and occurs when the fetal thigh(s) and knee(s) is/are extended, and one foot or both feet present(s).
4. Kneeling breech presentation occurs when the fetal thighs are extended, the knees are flexed, and the knees are the presenting part. A kneeling breech can be single or double.

Transverse Lie: This fetal position occurs when the long axis of the fetus is perpendicular to the mother's body. Often the fetal shoulder is over the pelvic inlet and the term "shoulder presentation" (or acromion presentation) is used.

Oblique Lie: An oblique lie occurs when the fetal head or breech is in the maternal iliac fossa. This is usually a transitory presentation which will evolve into either a transverse or longitudinal lie (e.g., a cephalic or breech presentation) when labor begins (Cunningham et al., 1989).

Data Base

Subjective

Breech Presentations

- May feel fetal movements in the lower abdomen, and may complain of painful "kicking" in her cervical or rectal areas.

- May not feel the fetus "drop" before the onset of labor.

Transverse or Oblique Lie

- May feel fetal movements in right or left side.

- Will not feel the fetus "drop" before the onset of labor unless the oblique lie converts to a cephalic or breech presentation.

Objective

Breech Presentation

- Leopold's maneuvers will reveal the fetal head (harder and more globular than the buttocks, ballotable) in the fundus, and a soft, irregular, non-ballotable mass lying over the pelvis. The presenting part often is not engaged.

- Fetal heart tones (FHTs) are usually heard loudest above the umbilicus.

- Bimanual examination will usually reveal that the presenting part is not engaged and is soft without suture lines or fontanelles. The anal orifice or a foot of the fetus may be felt.

- Ultrasound examination will confirm the presence of a suspected breech presentation.

Transverse or Oblique Lie

- Leopold's maneuvers will reveal that neither the fetal head nor the buttocks are palpable in the uterine fundus or over the pelvis. The fetal head will be felt in one of the mother's sides with the fetal buttocks palpated in the opposite side.

- The appearance of the abdomen is asymmetrical and wider than usual.

- Measurement of the uterine fundus will usually reveal that it is lower than expected for the weeks of gestation.

- The FHTs are usually heard below the umbilicus.

- Bimanual examination (done only if no history of second or third trimester bleeding or if previous sonographic evaluation has R/O the possibility of a placenta previa) will reveal that neither the fetal head nor buttocks can be felt by the examiner, and that the presenting part is not engaged. Occassionally, an examiner may feel a fetal shoulder, back, hand, or rib cage.

- Ultrasound examination will confirm the presence of a suspected transverse or oblique lie.

Assessment

- IUP ___ weeks
- R/O Breech presentation
- R/O Transverse lie
- R/O Oblique lie

Plan

Diagnostic Tests

- Whenever a fetal malpresentation is suspected during the last 5 weeks of pregnancy, an ultrasound should be ordered.

- If a spontaneous conversion of a malpresentation to a cephalic presentation is suspected 5 weeks before term, then an ultrasound should be ordered to confirm this.

Treatment/Management

● The incidence of breech presentations decreases weekly from approximately 30% at 27 weeks gestation to between 2-4% at term. If a breech presentation, transverse lie or oblique lie is present at 35-36 weeks gestation, then an ultrasound should be ordered to confirm the malpresentation. Prior to this time, an ultrasound may not be warranted due to the increased occurrence of spontaneous conversion of both breech presentations and transverse lies.

● In recent years, several studies have reported the successful conversion of breech presentations to cephalic presentations by external version under tocolysis after 36-37 weeks gestation (Dyson, Ferguson, & Hensleigh, 1986; Morrison et al., 1986). Therefore, referral of a patient with a breech presentation or transverse lie to an MD who is qualified and experienced in this technique should occur as soon as the malpresentation is confirmed by sonogram after 35 weeks.

● Postural exercises can be done in an attempt to facilitate the conversion of a breech presentation to a cephalic presentation. These exercises consist of pelvic rocking on the patient's hands and knees; and having the patient elevate her hips on pillows in the supine position so that her hips are approximately 9-12 inches higher than her head for 10 minutes twice a day. This latter exercise should be started at 30 weeks of gestation and should continue for 4-6 weeks or until the conversion occurs (Whitley, 1985).

Consultation

● Required in all malpresentations which occur from 35-36 weeks gestation and are confirmed by sonography. MD evaluation and education of a patient with a malpresentation is essential so that she can explore all of the options available to her (e.g., external version, if not contraindicated; the need for a cesarean section if indicated; etc.).

Patient Education

● Reassure patients who have a breech presentation or a transverse or oblique lie early in the third trimester that most of these presentations spontaneously convert to a cephalic presentation as the pregnancy progresses.

● Educate the patient about the need for a sonogram if a malpresentation is suspected at 35-36 weeks gestation.

● Educate the patient regarding the need for an MD referral if a malpresentation is confirmed by sonography after 35 weeks gestation.

● Education of the patient regarding her options (e.g., external version, cesarean section, vaginal birth) should be done by the MD evaluating the patient who has a malpresentation occurring after 35 weeks gestation.

● Postural exercises which may facilitate the spontaneous conversion of a breech presentation or a transverse lie to a cephalic presentation should be taught to patients who present with these malpresentations at 30 weeks gestation.

Follow-up

● Routine prenatal follow-up of patients with malpresentations which have spontaneously converted to a cephalic presentation, or in women who have had successful external versions for malpresentations.

● Co-management with an MD those patients whose malpresentation cannot be corrected by external version, or patients who do not want this procedure attempted. It is necessary that these patients establish rapport with the MD who will be attending their births.

● Document problem in progress notes and problem list.

MASTITIS

Lucy Newmark Sammons

Mastitis is an inflammation of the breast. Nonpuerperal mastitis usually is associated with a ductal abnormality or local manifestation of a systemic process. Puerperal mastitis occurs in association with lactogenesis and lactation following childbirth. The term "congestive mastitis" may be used to refer to non-infectious breast engorgement. Simple early breast engorgement is treated by suppression of lactation with binding and mild analgesia, if lactation is not desired, or by thorough breast emptying if lactation is being established. This discussion of mastitis, however, focuses on sporadic puerperal mastitis, which is a nonepidemic breast infection during the puerperium.

The incidence of puerperal mastitis is about 5% of lactating women, with reported ranges of 2.5-26% (Neifert & Seacat, 1986; Ogle & Davis, 1988). Of these women, 5-10% will go on to develop a breast abscess. The responsible pathogen may enter the breast at the site of nipple injury, such as cracking or abrasion. Milk stasis or a clogged milk duct predisposes to a noninfectious inflammation that can develop into infectious mastitis. Hence, infection is commonly seen at the time of weaning or with incomplete breast emptying. Mastitis is generally differentiated from a clogged duct by suddeness of onset, fever, systemic symptoms, and local findings (Ogle & Davis, 1988). Characteristic flu-like symptoms have led to the traditional warning that flu in the nursing mother is mastitis until proven otherwise. Recurrence of mild mastitis suggests the presence of a predisposing factor such as inadequate draining of the breast due to poorly emptying lobules or ducts, poor letdown, breast constriction from clothing or feeding technique, poor infant positioning, ineffectual infant sucking, missed feedings, mother-baby separation, or maternal fatigue or stress (Ogle & Davis, 1988). Recurrent severe mastitis suggests ductal abnormalities or persistent lobular problem, chronic nipple fissures or cracks, or inadequate antibiotic therapy (Lawrence, 1985).

The most common organism causing mastitis is *Staphylococcus aureus*. Other common skin inhabitants, including *micrococcus dyogenes, streptococci*, and *hemophilus species*, or occasionally *Escherichia coli*, may also be responsible. The offending bacteria usually are from the infant's nose and throat, but may be from nursery/hospital personnel, or the mother's hands or circulating blood. In suppurative mastitis, the bacteria forms pus, which leads to abscess formation. A frank abscess requires incision and drainage.

Data Base

Subjective

- Client complains of flu-like aching, fatigue, chills, and fever.

- Breast: tender, painful area or lump; often outer quadrant of breast, persisting through and between feeding periods; may be hard, warm and reddened; pain may be aggravated when infant nurses; usually unilateral

- More common occurrence:

  - Primiparous women (Kapernick, 1987)

  - Caucasian women (Cunningham, MacDonald, & Gant, 1989)

  - First two months postpartum, peaking in incidence between second and fourth weeks; rarely occurs before fifth postpartum day

- History of weaning, interruption of regular nursing, or failure to empty breasts adequately

Objective

- Fever, often high

- Tachycardia, common

- Breast examination:

    - Affected area(s) usually demonstrate increased warmth, redness, tenderness, swelling; erythematous lobule often outer quadrant, often wedge-shaped area

    - Crack or abrasion of nipple common

    - May be distended with milk, indurated

    - Absence of pitting edema and fluctuation (wavy impulse felt on palpation produced by vibration of underlying fluid, which would indicate abscess formation)

- Blood count, if done, shows leukocytosis.

- Remainder of physical exam within normal limits

Assessment

- Mastitis, infectious puerperal

- R/O Clogged duct, milk stasis, non-infectious inflammation

- R/O Breast abscess

- R/O Other breast disease, inflammatory carcinoma--see Breast Mass protocol

- R/O Viral syndrome

- R/O Other sites of infection, e.g., endometritis, cystitis

- R/O Toxic Shock Syndrome

Plan

Diagnostic Tests

- Microscopic and microbiologic laboratory analysis of secreted milk for bacterial count and leukocyte count is possible, and may contribute to differential diagnosis, but is rarely employed; infectious mastitis milk corresponds to greater than 10^3 bacterial colonies/ml and greater than 10^6 WBC's (Thomsen, Espersen, & Maigaard, 1984)

- Culture and sensitivity of breast milk from affected breast may identify the causative organism.

- Perform other tests as needed to rule out alternate pathology.

Treatment/Management

- Continue emptying breasts--nursing or with pump.

- Apply moist heat.

- Rest

- Increased fluids by mouth

(handwritten in left margin: + 14 day)

- Antibiotics: Dicloxacillin sodium (Dynapen, Dycill, Pathocil) 250 mg, 500 mg caps. <u>Sig</u>: cap i po qid x 7-10 days. Consider alternate drugs if patient penicillin-sensitive or infection not responsive: <u>clindamycin 150 mg qid</u>, or a <u>cephalosporin or erythromycin</u> for 7-10 days

- Over-the-counter analgesic/antipyretic. Acetaminophen is preferred over aspirin/acetyl-salicylic acid if the woman is still breastfeeding, because breakdown products from aspirin compete for bilirubin binding sites, putting the infant at risk for kernicterus. Neonates handle acetaminophen well (Lawrence, 1985).

- See also Patient Education.

Consultation

- Physician consultation for prescription as necessary

- Medical consultation for suspected abscess or other breast pathology

- Referral to lactation consultant/specialist if indicated, for assistance with techniques and expanded education

Patient Education

- Explain cause of mastitis and rationale for therapeutics employed.

- Interruption of nursing during antibiotic treatment usually unnecessary; emptying by nursing or use of breast pump prevents milk stasis; initially, frequent nursing (every 1-2 hours) will promote good drainage; deferral of weaning, if planned, may be suggested to reduce chance of abscess formation

- Comfort measures to reduce discomfort while nursing from sore breast include immersion of breast in warm water before nursing.

- Advise woman to continue taking full course of antibiotics, although symptom relief may occur within a few days.

- Woman should be alert to signs of infection in the infant, e.g., umbilical cord.

- Preventive measures include good breast hygiene; prevention, early detection, and care of nipple fissures, milk stasis, or clogged ducts; use of variety of positions to enhance emptying; avoidance of constrictive clothing (especially bras); avoidance of prolonged intervals between nursing and unrelieved engorgement; regular handwashing practices; and gradual weaning.

- Subsequent to antibiotic treatment, problems with sore nipples or breast pain may indicate candida albicans infection, which would require re-evaluation by provider.

- Explore rest-promoting and stress-reduction strategies, particularly around infant-feeding periods.

- Encourage liberal po fluids, especially water.

Follow-up

- Patient is to contact provider if she does not experience symptom relief in 24-36 hours. Failure to achieve relief may indicate the infectious organism is not sensitive to the prescribed antibiotic, or abscess formation may have occurred.

- Document problem in progress notes and problem list.

MITRAL VALVE PROLAPSE

Maureen T. Shannon

Mitral valve prolapse (MVP) is the protrusion of the mitral leaflets into the left atrium during ventricular contraction. It is the most common congenital cardiac lesion affecting between 5-10% of the general population, with the diagnosis often occurring in women of childbearing age (Abrams, 1989; Arias, 1988; Rivlin, 1986). In the vast majority of cases, mitral valve prolapse is asymptomatic and benign; however, in some instances it has been associated with complications such as mitral insufficiency, infective endocarditis, ruptured chordae tendineae, transient ischemic attacks, arrhythmias, and, rarely, sudden death (Jeresaty, 1985). Asymptomatic, benign MVP is not associated with an increase in maternal or perinatal morbidity or mortality. The use of prophylactic antibiotics for normal labors and vaginal births remains controversial, but is recommended for any complicated deliveries and for patients with a systolic click and evidence of MVP on echocardiogram.

Data Base

Subjective

- May report a history of MVP diagnosis
- Usually asymptomatic
- May complain of fatigue, palpitations, anxiety, lightheadedness
- May complain of retrosternal chest pain of varying severity that is unrelated to exercise

Objective

- Heart-rate--usually normal but may be tachycardic with occasional ectopic beats
- Auscultation of heart may reveal a midsystolic click (a high-pitched, crisp sound) that increases in intensity when patient is sitting or in a left lateral decubitus position. A late systolic or pansystolic murmur may also be evident.

Assessment

- Probable mitral valve prolapse
- R/O Mitral regurgitation
- R/O Hemic murmur of pregnancy
- R/O Marfan's syndrome

Plan

Diagnostic Tests

- EKG--may reveal low or inverted T waves in the inferior leads with or without S-T depression (Gottlieb, 1987; Jeresaty, 1985).
- Echocardiogram--will confirm MVP diagnosis in 80% of patients (Gottlieb, 1987; Jeresaty, 1985).

- Holter monitoring is recommended in patients with tachyarrhythmias and/or syncopal episodes (Gottlieb, 1987; Jeresaty, 1985).

Treatment/Management

- Consultation with an MD is warranted in all patients being evaluated for MVP. Transfer to MD care all patients with MVP who are symptomatic.

- Use of antiarrhythmic medications (if indicated) and/or prophylactic antibiotics (during labor and delivery) is determined and prescribed by an MD consultant.

Consultation

- Required in all patients who are suspected of having MVP.

Patient Education

- Education of the patient diagnosed with MVP should include information about MVP, the diagnostic tests ordered and their results, and the fact that there are no adverse maternal or fetal effects known to occur in patients with asymptomatic MVP.

- In patients with symptomatic MVP, explain the reasons for transferring their care to an MD.

- Reassure asymptomatic MVP patients about their diagnosis, emphasizing that between 5-10% of the population have this condition and the majority of these people do not develop any significant problems.

- Educate the patients regarding signs and symptoms that should be reported to an NP/NM/MD for further evaluation (e.g., palpitations, ectopic or "skipped" beats, excessive fatigue, etc.).

- Discuss the familial tendency of MVP and recommend screening of other family members for this condition.

Follow-up

- Follow-up evaluations of patients with MVP who are symptomatic is determined by the MD managing their care.

- Follow-up care of patients with asymptomatic MVP involves only routine prenatal visits unless symptoms develop that require more immediate evaluation.

- Document in problem list and progress notes.

MULTIPLE GESTATION

Lucy Newmark Sammons

Twins are the most commonly occurring multiple gestations, with an incidence of about 1 in 80 pregnancies in the United States. Twins developing from two separately released and fertilized ova are labelled dizygotic, double-ovum, or fraternal twins. Rates of dizygotic twinning are higher in women with a personal or familial history of multiple ovulation/dizygotic twinning, higher in blacks, higher with increasing age and parity, higher in larger and taller women, higher in drug-induced ovarian hyperstimulation (e.g., clomiphene citrate [Clomid] or human gonadotropins [Pergonal and HCG]), and possibly increased when stopping oral contraceptives or with seasonal exposure to increased light (Hollenbach & Hickok, 1990; Scerbo, Rattan, & Drukker, 1986). Dizygotic twinning is less common in Asians and during periods of malnourishment. Twins developing from a single fertilized ovum are labelled monozygotic, single-ovum, or identical twins. They account for a third of all United States-born twins, and have a world-wide incidence of about 1/250 pregnancies, unaffected by known risk factors.

Combinations of dizygotic and monozygotic processes may be involved in higher order multifetal pregnancies. The incidence of triplets is between 1/1,696 and 1/7,925 live births, with population differences, diagnostic inconsistencies, and increased use of ovulation-inducing drugs and infertility treatments accounting for the wide range (Alvarez & Berkowitz, 1990). Pregnancies with four or more embryos are labelled grand multifetal pregnancies.

Certain maternal and fetal risks are increased with multiple gestation. Twin transfusion syndrome results from unequal fetal circulations due to vascular anastamoses between placentas. The recipient twin is usually larger, polycythemic, and edematous, with cardiac and renal hypertrophy. The donor is usually smaller, hypoglycemic, hypovolemic, and anemic. An acute bood shifting emergency may occur at birth when arterial connections exist. Other fetal risks in multiple gestation pregnancies are increased spontaneous abortions, often with reabsorption of one fetus and continued viability of the other/s; increased incidence of congenital anomalies; possibly placenta previa and abruptio; cord accidents; and increased morbidity and mortality secondary to prematurity, intrauterine growth retardation, birth trauma, and maternal anemia. Maternal risks are increased for anemia (iron deficiency, folate deficiency, acute blood loss), hypertension, hydramnios, premature rupture of the membranes, abnormal fetal presentation, operative delivery, and antepartum and postpartum hemorrhage (Cunningham, MacDonald, & Gant, 1989; Jones, Sbarra, & Cetrulo, 1990; Scerbo et al., 1986).

The greatest cause of the increased morbidity in multigestational offspring is related to prematurity and associated complications. The emphasis in care of multifetal pregnancies is early detection, so that these potential complications can be either prevented or detected early and minimized if possible.

Data Base

Subjective

- Client may have following risk factors:
    - Use of drugs causing ovarian hyperstimulation or infertility technology involving transfer of multiple fertilized ova

- Personal or familial history of dizygotic twins
- Black racial background
- Increased age or parity
- Recent cessation of oral contraceptives
- Client may report:
    - Exagerrated or prolonged nausea and vomiting
    - Sensations of excessive fetal movement
    - Sensation of feeling larger than expectation for gestational age

Objective

- Fundal height measurements greater than expected for gestational date, particularly discrepancy of 4 cms or more in second and third trimester
- Palpation of multiple fetal parts or more than two fetal poles
- Simultaneous auscultation of more than one distinct fetal heart sound
- Client may demonstrate:
    - Rapid weight gain pattern
    - Anemia, due to additional fetal demands
    - Elevated blood pressure, especially suspicious if before 20 weeks gestation
- Maternal alpha-fetoprotein (AFP) results higher than expected for singleton pregnancy. Human placental lactogen (HPL), Beta-HCG, estriol, and pregnanediol levels may all be elevated, but these are less indicative of multiple gestation.
- If ultrasound has been performed for routine screening or other indication, multiple gestation is confirmed.

Assessment

- Multiple gestation
- R/O Size-date discrepancy due to inaccurate dating, hydramnios, uterine myomas, or adnexal mass--see Size/Dates Discrepancy protocol
- R/O Discordant twin syndrome--seen as disparity in fetal abdominal circumference and biparietal diameter measurements on ultrasound
- R/O Intrauterine growth retardation
- R/O Hydatidiform mole--may co-exist with normal fetus
- R/O Maternal complications: Anemia, hypertension, polyhydramnios
- R/O Preterm labor

Plan

Diagnostic Tests

- Ultrasound examination to determine multiple gestation and assess fetal status

Treatment/Management

- Initiate preterm labor prevention program, consider use of ambulatory monitor--see Preterm Birth Prevention protocol

- Initiate fetal assessment program, which may include weekly nonstress testing (NST) in third trimester and biophysical profiles for discordant or nonreactive NSTs; continuous wave Doppler ultrasound may be used in assessing intrauterine growth retardation; serial ultrasound examinations (every 3-4 weeks starting at 24-26 weeks) are necessary to monitor fetal growth and detect potential malpresentation at birth, as well as part of biophysical profile; daily fetal movement counts important from 28 weeks on, but may be difficult to attribute to an individual fetus--see Fetal Surveillance protocol

- Activity reduction/bedrest as indicated; site-specific routines vary regarding this controversial aspect of management

- Nutritional support:

  - An addition of at least 300 kcal/day above singleton pregnancy recommendations

  - Prenatal vitamin and mineral supplementation daily, including 2 mg folic acid

  - Iron supplement of 60-100 mg/day, modified by individual hematologic status, nutritional stores, and dietary patterns

  - Weight gain goal of 40-60 pounds; optimal level not known. See Nutrition protocol.

- Fetal pulmonary lung maturation may be difficult to assess: Lecithin-sphingomyelin ratios may normally exceed "2" by 32 weeks (vs 36 weeks in singleton pregnancies), and values may vary among fetuses; corticosteroids may be used to stimulate lung maturity.

- Routine prophylactic tocolytic agents, elective cerclage, and in-hospital bedrest do not appear to be justified for twin pregnancy (Jones et al., 1990).

- When systemic tocolytics are required for premature labor in multiple gestations, monitor more carefully, since risk of complications (e.g., pulmonary edema) appears higher than in singleton pregnancy; magnesium sulfate may be preferred over beta-adrenergics (Nageotte, 1990).

- Cervical and vaginal cultures at 28 weeks to aide in amniotic infection control may be performed (Halfar, 1987).

- See also Patient Education.

Consultation

- Medical consultation required for management of multiple gestation pregnancy in Special Care/High Risk clinic

- Pediatric provider to be alerted when labor imminent for optimal neonatal care

Patient Education

- Explain the work-up and diagnosis for multiple gestation pregnancy. When diagnosis is confirmed, assure that woman understands the implications for herself and her baby in terms of potential complications, their early detection, and their management.

- Reinforce preterm birth prevention strategies.

- Continuation of sexual intercourse to term may be permissible (Neilson & Mutambira, 1989).

- Reinforce activity restrictions, which may be imposed from 26-34 weeks; clarify extent of restriction (bedrest, modified bedrest, minimum 10 hours rest at night and 2 hours in day, or frequent resting with avoidance of exertional activity, etc). Assist in planning for household maintenance emphasizing nutritious meal preparation, disability income if outside employment stopped, child care, childbirth and homecoming preparation.

- Emphasize cessation of tobacco use.

- Postpartal care of the infants, especially feeding and scheduling, and household maintenance, especially cleaning and cooking, may well be problematic the first three months (Neifert & Thorpe, 1990). Plans for assistance should be made well before delivery.

- Explore family reactions to potential multiple additions to family life; work with family to develop their own resources and contact additional financial, social, and community resources as may be needed prenatally and postpartally. In addition to institutional and local services, assistance may be obtained by contacting:

  - Twin Line, P.O. Box 10066, Berkeley, CA 94709, (415) 524-0863

  - National Organization of Mothers of Twins Clubs, Inc., 12404 Princess Jeanne NE, Albuquerque, NM 87112 (505) 275-0955

  - The Triplet Connection, P.O. Box 99571, Stockton, CA 95209, (209) 474-0885

- Provide symptom specific education for discomforts of pregnancy, which may be increased with multiple gestation, e.g., nausea and vomiting, increased esophageal reflux, fatigue and insomnia, shortness of breath, varicosities--see separate protocols.

- Support breastfeeding if selected. Discuss scheduling patterns (simultaneous, individual complete demand, modified demand, alternating or same-side breast), desireability of piston electric breast pump use after feedings to establish adequate milk supply, positioning, maternal nutritional needs (Neifert & Thorpe, 1990; Sollid, Evans, McClowry, & Garrett, 1989); referral to lactation support group or lactation specialist may be valuable.

Follow-up

- Patient to be followed in Special Care/High Risk Obstetrics Clinic by multi-disciplinary team; visits every 2 weeks to 28 weeks, then weekly, or as needed

- Referrals to social services, public health nursing, specialty support groups and other services prenatally and postpartally as needed

- Document in progress notes and problem list.

OLIGOHYDRAMNIOS

Lisa L. Lommel

Oligohydramnios is defined as abnormally low amniotic fluid volume: less than 200 ml (Beischer & MacKay, 1986). Since the amount of amniotic fluid is difficult to quantitate, sonographic criteria such as no pockets of amniotic fluid with vertical dimensions >2 cm (Chamberlain et al., 1984) or the four quadrant Amniotic Fluid Index (Rutherford, Phelan, Smith, & Jacobs, 1987) have been proposed.

The incidence of oligohydramnios is difficult to establish since clinical features and the effect on the mother are often unremarkable. Often it is diagnosed as an incidental finding on ultrasound.

There is no significant etiologic factor for oligohydramnios in 40-60% of patients with this condition. Of the known causes, oligohydramnios is associated with intrauterine growth retardation in the majority of cases. Fetal malformations including renal agenesis or obstruction of the lower urinary tract are also responsible since urination *in utero* is important in maintaining the amniotic fluid volume. A chronic leak from a defect in the amniotic membrane may reduce the amniotic fluid appreciably. In this case, labor usually begins.

When oligohydramnios occurs in early pregnancy, adhesions between the amnion and part of the fetus may occur, causing serious deformities including musculoskeletal malformation or amputation. Pulmonary hypoplasia due to compression of the fetal thorax by the uterus, which prevents chest wall excursion and lung expansion, is also a consequence of oligohydramnios in early pregnancy. In late pregnancy, the incidence of cord compression and fetal distress is increased in the presence of small fluid volume. In most cases of oligohydramnios the skin of the fetus appears dry, leathery, and wrinkled.

Perinatal mortality is significantly increased if oligohydramnios presents early in pregnancy, in severe oligohydramnios, and when accompanied by fetal malformations. Many cases of oligohydramnios are associated with chronic fetal hypoxia, and the finding of oligohydramnios in the third trimester always warrants intensive antenatal surveillance.

Data Base

Subjective

- Small uterine size

- Previous growth-retarded pregnancy or risk factor for intrauterine growth retardation (IUGR)

- Postdate pregnancy

- Continuous, slow fluid leakage from vagina

- Uterine contractions

Objective

- Data review to rule out inaccurate dating

- Uterine size small for gestational age

- Fetal outline easily felt through the abdominal wall
- Incidental finding on ultrasound
- Vaginal fluid ph 7.0-7.5 (positive nitrazine test)
- Positive fern test
- Position, dilatation, effacement, and consistency of the cervix

Assessment

- Size less than dates
- R/O Oligohydramnios
- R/O IUGR
- R/O Fetal anomaly
- R/O Preterm labor
- R/O Rupture of membranes
- R/O Inaccurate dating

Plan

Diagnostic Tests

- Monitor weight gain.
- Compare changes in fundal height.
- Obtain ultrasound to:
  - assess amniotic fluid volume
  - assess fetal growth
  - rule out presence of fetal malformation
- Clinical diagnosis by uterine palpation
- Nitrazine and Fern Test to rule out rupture of membranes

Treatment/Management

- Antenatal surveillance (e.g., NST, CST, biophysical profile) weekly or twice weekly at 34-36 weeks or as soon as oligohydramnios is diagnosed
- Rest in left lateral recumbent position.
- For preterm labor see Preterm Birth Prevention protocol.
- Initiate fetal movement counts at 28 weeks. See Fetal Movement Count protocol.

Consultation

- Refer to MD.

Patient Education

- Discuss need for close prenatal surveillance and tests that will be used.
- Provide information regarding etiology of the condition.

- Provide anticipatory guidance and counseling when fetal anomaly has been identified by sonography.

- Educate regarding sign and symptoms of preterm labor and rupture of membranes with emphasis on prompt reporting by the patient.

- Explain how to record fetal movement counts.

Follow-up

- Document in problem list and progress notes.

PAP SMEAR--ABNORMAL

Maureen T. Shannon

A Class II-V Pap smear is considered atypical (Class II) or abnormal (Classes III-V) and warrants further evaluation (see chart below for classifications of Pap smears).

Class I Normal smear No abnormal cells	
Class II Atypical cells present below the level of cervical neoplasia.	
Class III Smear contains abnormal cells consistent with dysplasia.	Mild dysplasia = CIN 1 Moderate dysplasia = CIN 2
Class IV Smear contains abnormal cells consistent with carcinoma *in situ*.	Severe dysplasia and = CIN 3 Carcinoma *in situ*
Class V Smear contains abnormal cells consistent with invasive carcinoma of squamous cell origin.	

SOURCE:

Nelson, J. H., Averette, H. E., & Richart, R. M. (1984). Dysplasia, carcinoma in situ, and early invasive cervical carcinoma. *CA-A Cancer Journal for Clinicians, 34*(6), 307. Reprinted with permission.

Recently, a newly devised method to classify Pap smear results, called the Bethesda System, has been developed. This system gives a detailed analysis of Pap smear findings so that clinicians will have more comprehensive information regarding the results and the possible need for further evaluation. The Bethesda System attempts to provide the following information for the clinician: 1) Determines whether or not the specimen is adequate for interpretation, and if it is not, gives specific reasons for the unsatisfactory nature of the specimen; 2) determines if the specimen is within normal limits; and 3) provides a detailed descriptive diagnosis of any pathology that is identified (e.g., infections, reactive and reparative changes, epithelial cell abnormalities, nonepithelial malignant neoplasm) (National Cancer Institute Workshop, 1989).

Additionally, the Bethesda System utilizes the term "squamous intraepithelial lesion" (SIL) to describe the cervical changes that are currently classified as cervical intraepithelial neoplasia (CIN). According to the Bethesda System, "low grade SIL" findings would encompass cellular changes associated with human papilloma virus (HPV) and CIN 1, while "high grade SIL" would describe lesions encompassing changes seen in CIN II through CIN III (carcinoma in situ). These results would also include a detailed description of the actual cell analysis.

Data Base

Subjective

- May be asymptomatic.

- May report having previously abnormal Pap smear.

- May report having had condylomata in past.

- May complain of painless spotting or bleeding after coitus, and/or intermenstrually.

- May complain of a thin, watery vaginal discharge.

- Usually no complaints of problems or discomfort until the latter stages of carcinoma of the cervix

- May report one or more of the epidemiologic factors associated with an increased incidence of cervical intraepithelial neoplasia (CIN): lower socioeonomic status, multiple sexual partners, early age of first coitus, pregnancy before age 20, smoking, DES daughter (still controversial).

- May have complaints associated with cervicitis (e.g., increased leukorrhea).

- Complaints of weight loss and painful vaginal bleeding occur only in the latter stages of carcinoma of the cervix.

Objective

- Cervix may appear normal.

- Cervix may be erythematous, friable and/or ulcerated.

- Failure of abnormal epithelium to stain with iodine (Schiller Test)

- Bimanual palpation of cervix can reveal hard, enlarged mass (in latter stages of carcinoma of cervix).

- Condylomata of vagina and cervix may be visualized.

- Cervical cultures for herpes, chlamydia or gonorrhea may be positive if concomitant vaginal/cervical infection.

- No effect on clinical parameters of pregnancy unless in latter stages of carcinoma (e.g., weight loss with subsequent intrauterine growth retardation)

Assessment

- Class (I-V) Pap smear

- Bethesda System Classification--specific to findings

- Cervicitis--if culture for specific organism is positive, then document (e.g., chlamydial cervicitis).

- Condylomata--if present

Plan

Diagnostic Tests

- Class II--cervical cultures to R/O infections (e.g., chlamydia, gonorrhea, etc.)
- Repeat Pap smear (3 months after treatment of infection causing class II result)
- Colposcopy for persistent Class II result or for Class III-V Pap smear result
- Biopsy of lesion

Treatment/Management

- Class I: Routine follow-up for Pap smears (annual Paps)
- Class II: Culture and treat any inflammation/infection and repeat Pap smear in 3 months. If repeat Pap smear after treatment is WNL, then Pap smears annually. If repeat Pap smear after treatment is still Class II, then refer for colposcopy.
- Class III: Refer for colposcopy, MD evaluation, and management.
  NOTE: In some settings, Class III Pap smear result are managed by NP/NMs who are trained in colposcopy. Management generally undertaken with physician consultation.
- Class IV: Refer for colposcopy, MD evaluation, and management.
- Class V: Refer for colposcopy, MD evaluation, and management.
- The use of cryo and laser therapy in treatment of CIN is deferred until postpartum recovery is completed. Pregnant patients with CIN may be followed with serial colposcopy (every 3 months) and directed biopsy as indicated.

Consultation

- Required for all Class II-V Pap smear results.
- Refer to MD all clients with Class III-V Pap smear results.

Patient Education

- Explain laboratory tests and interpret results for the client. Discuss the importance of having follow-up testing (when indicated).
- If a sexually transmitted disease (STD) is present, discuss with client the importance of partner evaluation and treatment, and methods to prevent re-infection (e.g., condom use in condylomata even with treatment--see specific STD protocols for patient evaluation, treatment and education).
- Reassure client regarding the outcome of her pregnancy (i.e., abnormal Pap smear results will not adversely affect her baby).

Follow-up

- Class I Pap result--annual Pap smear
- Class II result that reverts to Class I after treatment for infection--annual Pap smears
- Pap smear that remains Class II after treatment for inflammation/infection--refer for colposcopy by appropriate health care provider.
- Class III-V results--colposcopy performed by appropriate health care provider

- Serial colposcopic evaluation with directed biopsy as indicated for pregnant patients with CIN

- Clients with condylomata (with or without abnormal Pap smear result) require Pap smears every 6 months.

- Clients treated for chlamydial or gonococcal cervicitis need test of cure cultures--see specific protocols for test of cure schedules.

- Repeat Pap smears on all clients at the 6 week postpartum visit.

- Document Pap results in lab section of chart; if abnormal, then record in progress notes and problem list.

POLYHYDRAMNIOS

Lisa L. Lommel

Polyhydramnios is defined as the excessive quantity of amniotic fluid in the amniotic sac. Normally the volume of amniotic fluid increases to about 1,000 ml by 36 weeks gestation and then decreases at a rate of about 150 ml/week. Amniotic fluid in excess of 2,000 ml is considered to be polyhydramnios. Acute polyhydramnios is the very sudden increase of amniotic fluid over the course of a few days occurring, before the 24th week of gestation. Chronic polyhydramnios is the gradual increase of amniotic fluid and is more commonly diagnosed than acute polyhydramnios.

Polyhydramnios (chronic) occurs in 0.20 to 1.6% of all pregnancies (Cardwell, 1987). The incidence varies because of the difficulty of complete collection of the amniotic fluid making the diagnosis dependent on clinical impression or sonographic estimation.

Polyhydramnios is often associated with fetal malformation (20% incidence) and maternal disease. However, one-third of individuals with polyhydramnios have no significant etiologic factor (Beischer & MacKay, 1986). Fetal malformations associated with polyhydramnios include gastrointestinal obstructions (esophageal or duodenal atresia) and central nervous system abnormalities (50% of congenital anomalies presenting with polyhydramnios). Central nervous system malformations associated with increased fluid from the exposed meninges into the amniotic cavity are anacephaly, spina bifida, and hydrocephaly. Down's syndrome, congenital heart disease, and twin pregnancy (monozygotic more often than dizygotic) are other fetal factors associated with polyhydramnios. Maternal factors include diabetes, isoimmunization, and syphilis.

Perinatal mortality is higher in the more severe cases of polyhydramnios, especially if accompanied by a fetal malformation. Premature labor and delivery, caused by overdistention of the uterus and premature rupture of membranes, further increase perinatal mortality. Malpresentation and prolapse of the cord are also common in polyhydramnios. The most frequent maternal complications are discomfort from the distended uterus, placental abruption, uterine dysfunction, and postpartum hemorrhage.

Data Base

Subjective

- Multiple pregnancy

- Maternal diabetes mellitus

- Dyspnea, generalized edema

- Rapid enlargement of the abdomen

- Maternal discomfort from distended uterus, and/or possible decreased mobility

- Regular/irregular uterine contractions

- Most commonly occurs about seven months gestation

Objective

- Data review to rule out inaccurate dating
- Uterine size large for dates
- Palpation of excessive fluid in the uterus
- Difficulty in palpating fetal parts and position
- Difficulty in palpating any part of the fetus in severe polyhydramnios
- Difficulty in hearing fetal heart tones
- Ultrasound shows increased volume of amniotic fluid
- Uterine contractions felt with abdominal palpation
- Position, dilation, consistency, and effacement of the cervix

Assessment

- Size greater than dates
- R/O Polyhydramnios
- R/O Diabetes mellitus
- R/O Multiple pregnancy
- R/O Inaccurate dating
- R/O Macrosomia
- R/O Fetal anomaly
- R/O Irregular antibody
- R/O Preterm labor

Plan

Diagnostic Tests

- Monitor weight gain.
- Compare changes in fundal height.
- Ballot for fetal parts.
- Screen for irregular antibodies by indirect Coombs test.
- Screen for syphilis.
- Order 1-hour glucose screen to rule out diabetes mellitus.
- Obtain an ultrasound to:
  - demonstrate increased amniotic fluid status
  - rule out presence of malformation, multiple fetuses, macrosomia, or malpresentation
- Order fetal echocardiogram to rule out congestive heart failure.

Treatment/Management

- Management of idiopathic polyhydramnios is conservative and includes:

- maintenance of the pregnancy until 37 weeks or when the L/S ratio indicates fetal lung maturity

- maintenance of partial bed rest and high protein diet

- Management of severe polyhydramnios when the women is experiencing respiratory distress or marked uterine irritability includes:

    - amniocentesis to withdraw excessive amniotic fluid; as much as 1,500-2,000 ml fluid may be withdrawn at the rate of 50 ml per hour (this will rapidly reaccumulate).

- Observe the patient for signs of congestive heart failure.

- Sedation may be indicated.

- Initiate fetal movement counts at 28 weeks. See Fetal Movement Count protocol.

- Sterile pelvic exam if membranes ruptured to rule out cord prolapse

- For preterm labor see Preterm Birth Prevention protocol.

Consultation

- MD management

Patient Education

- Discuss the need for close prenatal surveillance and the tests that will be used.

- Provide information regarding etiology of the condition.

- Provide sensitive emotional support to the mother and her partner when an antenatal diagnosis of fetal anomaly has been made.

- Educate regarding signs and symptoms of preterm labor and rupture of membranes with emphasis on prompt reporting by the patient.

- Explain how to record fetal movement counts.

Follow-up

- Document in problem list and progress notes.

POSTDATE PREGNANCY

Lisa L. Lommel

There are various terms that describe pregnancy that continues past the estimated date of delivery. Postdate pregnancy is used to describe pregnancy that exceeds 42 weeks (294 days) from the onset of the last normal menstrual period. This term includes patients with uncertain dates. Prolonged pregnancy is used to describe pregnancy that is well documented by ovulation or conception to have exceeded 294 days (Freeman, 1986; Lagrew & Freeman, 1986). The terms postterm and postmature are most often used to describe the maturity of the neonate which cannot be assessed until after birth (Lagrew & Freeman, 1986; Nichols, 1985).

The incidence of postdate pregnancy is reported to be 3.5 to 14% of all pregnancies (Hendricksen, 1985). Inaccurate dating of pregnancies and irregularity of ovulation accounts for the variation in incidence of postdate pregnancy. Seventy percent of postdate pregnancies are misdiagnosed term pregnancies (Nichols, 1985). Early and accurate evaluation of the patient is important in determining the estimated date of delivery. The known date of the last menstrual period (LMP) is considered to be the best clinical predictor of date of delivery. If the last menstrual period is unknown, additional clinical and physical parameters should be collected to aid in the determination of this date.

The risk of mortality and morbidity is increased in the postdate pregnancy. Pregnancy of greater than 300 days accounts for 15% of all perinatal mortality (Hendricksen, 1985). Mortality rates are lowest in deliveries before 42 weeks gestation. The leading causes of perinatal mortality in the postdate pregnancy are congenital malformations, including anencephaly and adrenal hypoplasia, and asphyxia from impaired uretoplacental perfusion.

Postmaturity syndrome is evident in less than 20% of postdate pregnancies. The infant with this syndrome will show signs of uretoplacental insufficiency and increased maturity. Indications of postmature syndrome include oligohydramnios, decreased subcutaneous fat, respiratory distress, loss of vernix, malnourishment, and meconium staining (Eden, 1989). Low apgar scores at one and five minutes and increase in the number of illnesses experienced during the first three years of life have also been associated with this syndrome (Nichols, 1985).

Maternal morbidity can be significantly affected by the postdate pregnancy. The incidence of cesarean section is increased from 13.6% at term to 25.6% in postdate pregnancies (Lagrew, 1986). In addition, if fetal growth continues normally, macrosomia in the fetus may contribute to dysfunctional labor, shoulder dystocia, and traumatic delivery.

Management of postdate pregnancy has focused on assessment of fetal well-being and induction, either elective or because of signs of fetal compromise.

Data Base

Subjective

Maternal factors associated with postdate pregnancy (Hendricksen, 1985):

- LMP induced by oral contraceptives

- Uncertain dating of pregnancy
- History of postdate pregnancy
- Symptoms may include decreased fetal movement.

Objective
- Maternal weight loss
- Decreasing fundal height secondary to oligohydramnios and fetal wastage
- Decreasing abdominal girth secondary to reduced amounts of amniotic fluid
- Data review including:
  - accuracy of LMP including history of regular/irregular menses
  - predicted ovulation by temperature and/or coital records
  - oral contraceptive use
  - positive pregnancy test 5-6 weeks after LMP
  - ultrasound before 20 weeks gestation that agrees with LMP
  - first visit estimation of uterine size in relation to LMP
  - date of fetal heart tones first heard with the electronic doppler
  - date of fetal heart tones first heard with the fetoscope
  - date of first fetal movement
  - anatomic location of uterus at 20 weeks past LMP
- Result of:
  - ultrasound, non-stress test (NST), contraction stress test (CST) or biophysical profile (BPP)
- Position, dilatation, effacement, and consistency of the cervix
- Station of the presenting part

Assessment
- Intrauterine pregnancy greater than 42 weeks
- Size equal dates
- Size greater than dates
- Size less than dates
- R/O Oligohydramnios
- R/O Fetal anomaly

Plan

Diagnostic Tests
- Obtain ultrasound to:
  - determine placental senescence
  - assess amniotic fluid volume

189

- rule out congenital anomaly

- NST to evaluate fetal well-being. See NST protocol.

- CST is used if the NST is non-reactive. The nipple stimulation stress test (NSCST) is more commonly used than the oxytocin challenge test (OCT). See CST protocol.

- BPP to evaluate fetal heart reactivity, fetal breathing movements, fetal muscular tone, fetal body movements, and amniotic fluid volume. See BPP protocol.

- Amniocentesis may be conducted by a MD to assess amniotic fluid color and the lecithin/sphingomyelin (L/S) ratio.

Treatment/Management

- Initiate fetal movements counts at 28 weeks on all patients. See Fetal Movement Count protocol.

- Weekly cervical assessments beginning at approximately 40 weeks

- Semi-weekly NST and/or weekly CST and/or BPP (or more often as indicated) starting at 41 weeks until delivery

- Labor induction as appropriate

- Vaginal delivery when there is no evidence of fetal distress, labor dystocia, or fetal macrosomia

Consultation

- Referral to MD after 41 weeks gestation

Patient Education

- Discuss postdate pregnancy and its implications.

- Explain how to obtain Fetal Movement Counts.

- Counsel patient regarding the tests that will be performed and their use in fetal surveillance.

- Reassure patient that the majority of infants (approximately 80%) experience no problems after postdate gestation.

Follow-up

- Routine postpartum follow-up for mother and infant at appropriate intervals

- Document in progress notes and problem list.

PREMATURE RUPTURE OF MEMBRANES

Winifred L. Star

Premature rupture of membranes (PROM) is defined as loss or leakage of amnionic fluid prior to the onset of labor. Preterm PROM indicates membrane rupture prior to 37 weeks gestation. Prolonged rupture of membranes refers to rupture that occurs more than 24 hours prior to the onset of labor. The latent period is defined as the interval from rupture of membranes to the time labor ensues.

Spontaneous onset of labor following PROM occurs within 24 hours in 80-90% of term pregnancies. An inverse relationship exists between gestational age at the time of membrane rupture and the duration of the latent period (i.e., latent periods tend to be longer in preterm pregnancies with PROM) (ACOG, 1988). The reported incidence of PROM is 3-18.5% of all deliveries. The incidence is significantly higher in preterm deliveries (Gibbs & Sweet, 1989).

The etiology of PROM is not well-understood. Factors predisposing to PROM may include decreasing collagen content of the amnion and inflammatory weakening of the membranes via subclinical infection with Group B streptococcus, gonococcus, chlamydia, or anaerobic organisms (Pauerstein, 1987).

The major complications of PROM are infection (amnionitis, endometritis) and prematurity. The incidence of infection in mother and fetus at term increases with the duration of PROM. In the preterm pregnancy the greater concern is respiratory distress syndrome (RDS) which occurs in 10-40% of neonates. Controversy exists regarding whether a longer duration of ruptured membranes (i.e., 16-48 hours) will accelerate fetal lung maturity (ACOG, 1988). Asphyxia is the most common complication among very low birth weight infants. Other complications of PROM (especially preterm) include malpresentation, cord prolapse, fetal distress from cord compression, fetal deformation syndrome, intraventricular hemorrhage, pulmonary hypoplasia, and congenital anomalies. (ACOG, 1988; Pauerstein, 1987).

The management of PROM is still controversial with respect to aggressive versus expectant management and the use of technologies such as tocolytics, corticosteroids, and prophylactic antibiotics. This protocol will utilize management modalities supported by the American College of Obstetricians and Gynecologists (ACOG, 1988).

Data Base

Subjective

Associated variables may include:

- Cervical incompetance
- Cervical surgery/lacerations
- Multiple pregnancies
- Amniocentesis
- Polyhydramnios

191

- Antepartum hemorrhage (abruptio placenta)
- Cervical/vaginal infection
- Smoking (heavy)
- Lower socioeconomic status
- Adolescence
- Recent coitus/douching
- Low ascorbic acid levels
- Low collagen content

Symptomatology may include:

- Gush or leakage of fluid from the vagina: fluid may be clear, yellow brown, or red-brown and may or may not have an odor. (Provider to establish time of rupture or onset of leaking; timing of last coital/douching event.)
- No awareness of fluid leakage
- Associated normal or abnormal vaginal discharge
- Fever, chills, increased pulse rate (especially with increased duration of PROM)

Objective

- See Plan section.

Assessment

- R/O PROM
- R/O Physiologic leukorrhea
- R/O Urinary Incontinence
- R/O Recent coital/douching event
- R/O Umbilical cord prolapse
- R/O Amnionitis
- R/O Oligohydramnios
- R/O Preterm labor
- R/O Fetal demise

Plan

Diagnostic Tests

- Confirm gestational age with review of history, prenatal records, previous ultrasound etc.
- Perform Leopold's maneuvers and McDonald's measurements to assess fetal position, estimated size and gestational age of the fetus.
- Palpate uterus for contractions/tenderness to R/O labor/amnionitis.
- Perform a sterile speculum examination:
  - Observe for prolapse of umbilical cord in vagina.

- Observe for presence of amnionic fluid; note its color and odor. Ask the patient to bear down (Valsalva's maneuver) or cough if no fluid is readily seen and observe for a gush or leaking from the cervical os. Observation of a pool of fluid ("pooling") in the posterior vaginal fornix or visualization of fluid from the cervical os strongly suggests ROM. (If pooling of fluid is noted, draw-up the fluid in a syringe; it may be sent for phosphatidylglycerol analysis later).

- Touch a sterile cotton swab to the posterior vaginal pool then rub onto Nitrazine paper. A blue color change (pH >7.0) indicates amnionic fluid.
  NOTE: Accuracy 74-97%; false positive readings may result from urine, blood, vaginal discharge, cervical mucus, or antiseptic solution.

- Place a sample of fluid from the posterior fornix onto a glass slide and allow to air dry. Under a microscope observe for presence of a ferning pattern.
  NOTE: Accuracy 75-98%. False positives may result if a cervical mucus sample is obtained or from fingerprints on the glass slide. False negatives occur with blood, meconium, cervical/vaginal infections.

- If first exam negative repeat in 30 minutes to 1 hour using Valsalva's maneuver and fundal pressure.

- Do not perform a bimanual examination if PROM confirmed by sterile speculum exam. Consider sterile bimanual exam to evaluate baseline cervical status in a term pregnancy in which the patient is geographically remote from hospitalization or MD evaluation.

- Utilize ultrasound to assess amnionic fluid, fetal position, gestational age, and fetal anomalies.
  NOTE: Ultrasound to assess oligohydramnios not sufficiently sensitive; do not use as primary means of diagnosis as other causes of oligohydramnios may be involved.

- Assess BP, temperature, heart rate (maternal and fetal), and respirations to R/O amnionitis. Objective signs of amnionitis include: maternal/fetal tachycardia (>100/180 beats/min respectively), maternal fever (>38 degrees C or 99.4 degrees F), leukocytosis with left shift (i.e., increased number of bands), purulent and malodorous amnionic fluid from the vagina, uterine tenderness.

- Assess fetal maturity via lecithin/sphingomyelin (L/S) ratio and phosphatidylglycerol (PG) measurements:

  - Aspirate fluid from the vaginal pool or cervical os for the presence of PG. Fluid from a sanitary pad may also be used for this purpose (Golde, 1983).
    NOTE: False positive results may occur in the presence of semen.

  - Amniocentesis for determination of L/S ratio may be attempted to determine fetal lung maturity.

- Cervical cultures for chlamydia and gonococcus and rectal/introital cultures for Group B streptococcus should be obtained.

- Other diagnostic tests may include:

  - injection of dye (indigo carmine) into amnionic cavity (rarely used)

Treatment/Management

- Patients with suspected or confirmed PROM should be managed by an MD.

- There are many controversial aspects regarding medical management of patients with PROM; care needs to be individualized. ACOG (1988) guidelines will be utilized in the management plans below.

Term (36 weeks and beyond)

- Labor generally ensues spontaneously.

- Patients in active labor without infection should be allowed to progress and should be managed routinely.

- Patients not in labor should be evaluated for infection and fetal distress (via clinical signs; amniocentesis specimen for gram stain/culture; WBC; serum C-reactive protein, non-stress test [NST]/biophysical profile [BPP]).

- If labor has not started within a reasonable amount of time, induction may be attempted (in the absence of infection prolonged expectant management is also an option).

    . Induce labor with oxytocin or effect delivery with cesarean section (for malpresentation, fetal distress, failure to progress in labor, cephalopelvic disproportion [CPD])

    . Obtain cervical and blood cultures, amniocentesis specimen for gram stain/culture.

    . Begin antibiotic therapy if clinical signs of infection.

Preterm (34-36 weeks)

Management goals are to prolong gestation if patient not in labor, not infected, and has no evidence of fetal distress.

- patient usually in hospital setting but in rare cases may be managed at home (e.g., reliable woman, cephalic presentation, home environment conducive to maternal/fetal assessment)

- patient on bedrest with bathroom/meal privileges

- digital exams to be avoided

- external FHT monitoring at frequent intervals or continuously

- careful monitoring for evidence of infection:

    . cervical cultures for gonococcus, chlamydia, Group B streptococcus

    . vital signs q 4 hours

    . laboratory tests including WBC q 12-24 hours, and possibly C-reactive protein

    . amniocentesis for gram stain/culture (optional)

    . ultrasound at periodic intervals to detect oligohydramnios

    . BPP at least every other day to evaluate fetal signs

- prophylactic antibiotics usually not administered; antibiotics may be given to women with positive genital cultures

- tocolytics may be employed if in preterm labor

- corticosteroids may be given to accelerate fetal lung maturity

- delivery indicated for infection, fetal distress, or preterm labor

- alternate approach to expectant management at less than 36 weeks is to evaluate fetal lung maturity (via amniocentesis or vaginal fluid collection for L/S ratio or PG determination) and deliver once lungs are mature

Consultation

- Required in all cases of suspected or confirmend PROM

- Management directed by medical consultant

Patient Education

- Discuss diagnostic tests to be utilized.

- Educate regarding signs of infection (e.g., fever, chills, foul smelling discharge) if patient being managed at home.

- Explain PROM and discuss implications for mom and baby.

- Medical management plans ideally should be discussed with the patient by the MD managing her care.

Follow-up

- To be determined by MD or high risk team according to clinical presentation

- Refer to social services as indicated. Patient may need assistance with child care arrangements if on bedrest.

- If patient to be managed at home make referral to public health nurse or home care team.

- Ongoing psychosocial support is important for patients with PROM or those who may be anticipating a preterm delivery.

- NP/NM may resume care of patient in postpartum period as indicated by patient's condition and her preference of provider.

- Document problem in problem list and progress notes.

PRETERM BIRTH PREVENTION

Winifred L. Star

Over the last several decades there has been no consistent decrease in the incidence of low birth weight and preterm infants. Preterm delivery is the single most important problem facing obstetrics today, and its incidence must be decreased in order to significantly improve perinatal mortality (Creasy, 1989; Iams & Creasy, 1988).

Preterm labor is defined as labor occurring between 20-37 completed weeks of pregnancy (114-259 days of gestation). A preterm birth is any delivery that occurs prior to 37 completed weeks of pregnancy (less than 259 days from the last menstrual period [LMP]). The true incidence of preterm delivery is not well documented and depends upon the population studied; estimates lie between 5-10% of all births in developed countries (Creasy, 1989). Preterm births are responsible for the majority of perinatal deaths in newborns without anomalies. Respiratory distress syndrome and intercranial bleeding are the primary neonatal complications (Arias, 1984; Creasy, 1989).

Multiple factors are antecedent to preterm labor and delivery many of which are poorly understood. It appears that equal numbers of preterm births are caused by preterm labor (PTL), preterm premature rupture of membranes (PPROM), or maternal/fetal complications (Main, 1988). There is growing evidence to indicate that cervicovaginal microbial colonization is associated with preterm labor and delivery (McGregor, 1987; Romero & Mazor, 1988). Individual risk factors are presented in the Subjective section. It should be kept in mind that the predictive value of any of these is relatively low, most being <30% (Iams & Creasy, 1988).

Several risk scoring systems for preterm labor are in existence today. Risk scoring helps identify patients at risk for preterm labor/delivery, however the systems currently available are not discriminating enough to identify approximately 50% of patients who have spontaneous preterm deliveries (Creasy, 1989). As well, the systems cannot be reliably transferred from one population to another without prospective testing (Iams & Creasy, 1988). Additional means of identifying high-risk patients (e.g., biochemical/biophysical) need to be developed (Creasy, 1989).

The various components of preterm birth prevention programs include: a) identification and close observation of patients at risk for preterm labor, b) patient education regarding the signs and symptoms of preterm labor and self-detection of uterine contractions, c) use of ambulatory home monitoring via tocodynamometry, d) education of staff regarding the problem of preterm labor, signs and symptoms, and e) prompt treatment with tocolysis once the diagnosis is made. Although many suggestions have been made, there is no **proven** method for the prevention of PTL.

Data Base

Subjective: Risk Factors

<u>Demographic Factors</u>

- Age <17 or >35
- Black race
- Single status

- Low socioeconomic/educational status

Behavioral Factors

- Smoking
- Substance use/abuse
- Poor nutrition
- Underweight status
- Inadequate weight gain in pregnancy
- Lack of/inadequate prenatal care
- Excessive physical activity
- Psychological stress

Medical/Obstetrical Factors

- Prior preterm labor or delivery (recurrence risk 17-30%)
- Prior second trimester pregnancy loss
- Uterine anomaly
- Cervical incompetence (congenital, iatrogenic)
- DES exposure (especially if associated cervical/uterine anomaly)
- Cone biopsy
- Multiple induced abortions with dilatation >8 mm
- Multiple gestation
- Leiomyomata (multiple, large)
- Uterine bleeding after 12 weeks
- Vaginal/cervical/intrauterine infection
- Uterine irritability
- Cervical effacement or dilatation
- Premature rupture of membranes
- Placenta previa
- Abruptio placenta
- Poly/oligohydramnios
- Abdominal surgery in second or third trimester
- Renal disease
- Bacteriuria
- Pyelonephritis
- Pregnancy induced hypertension
- Systemic infection
- Diabetes (complicated by polyhydramnios)
- Asthma ?

- Hyperthyroidism ?
- Heart disease ?
- Obstetric cholestasis ?
- Hepatitis ?
- Anemia (<9 gm/100 ml) ?

Fetal Factors

- Polyhydramnios
- Renal agenesis
- Multiple congenital anomalies
- Central nervous system anomalies

Subjective: Signs and Symptoms

- Menstrual-like cramps
- Low, dull backache (intermittent or constant)
- Rhythmic pelvic pressure
- Abdominal cramping
- Diarrhea
- "Balling-up" of uterus (i.e., uterus rises up and hardens, then softens)
- Change in vaginal discharge (more pasty, sticky, or bloody)
- Fluid leaking from vagina
- Vaginal bleeding or spotting
- Overall sense of feeling unwell
- Fever may be present if patient has systemic illness.

Objective

- Identify maternal risk factors through comprehensive history taking and use of Preterm Labor Screen. Complete PTL screen at initial visit and rescreen at 20 weeks. See Figure 4.2, *Preterm Labor Screen*, p. 203).
- Document baseline cervical status at initial OB examination. Record position, consistency, length (preferably in centimeters), degree of dilatation of external and internal os.
- Assess routine OB clinical parameters at each visit.
- Routinely question patient regarding signs and symptoms of preterm labor and document in prenatal chart. This should be done at every prenatal visit especially after 20 weeks.
- Identify presence or absence of uterine contractions by palpation of the uterus and/or with use of maternal uterine contractility monitor as indicated.
- Identify presence or absence of cervical change by gentle digital cervical examination as indicated. Comment on position, consistency, length, and status of the external/internal os. Serial cervical exams should be done by the same examiner whenever possible.

NOTE: Digital exams should be avoided in the presence of ruptured membranes. A sterile speculum exam may be performed in this instance to assess amniotic fluid leakage along with careful visual inspection of the cervix.

- Additional physical exam components as indicated by patient complaints and concerns

Assessment

- R/O Preterm labor
- R/O Normal fetal activity
- R/O Gastrointestinal activity
- R/O Irritable uterus
- R/O Dehydration
- R/O PROM
- R/O Asymptomatic bacteriuria
- R/O Cystitis
- R/O Pyelonephritis
- R/O Chorioamnionitis
- R/O Vaginitis/cervicitis
- Identify any abnormal physical and/or laboratory findings.
- Identify any maternal or fetal pathologic condition.

Plan

Diagnostic Tests

- Sterile speculum exam with testing for rupture of membranes as indicated. See PROM protocol.
- If ROM is ruled out gentle digital cervical examination may be undertaken to assess position, consistency, length, and status of the external/internal os.
- Maternal uterine contractility monitor may be employed to assess presence/absence of contractions.
- Ultrasound to confirm/establish gestational age, and to assess presence of abnormalities of the uterus, cervix, fetus, placenta
- Cervical cultures for *neisseria gonorrhea, chlamydia trachomatis, group B streptococcus, gardnerella vaginalis*, and *listeria monocytogenes* may be done to R/O vaginal/cervical infection.
- Amniocentesis for diagnosis of fetal maturity as indicated (assessment of L/S ratio, phosphatidylglycerol). Bacteriologic studies of amniotic fluid may be done to R/O chorioamnionitis.
- Maternal serum alphafetoprotein elevations (not explained by fetal anomalies) (Hamilton Abdalla, & Whitfield, 1985)
- Lupus anticoagulant (associated with recurrent pregnancy loss, preterm delivery, and abruption) (Lubbe & Wiggins, 1985)
- Serum collagenase or C-reactive protein elevations (not routinely used)

- Other labs as indicated by history or physical findings (e.g., CBC, urinalysis, urine culture & sensitivity, cervical cultures, clotting studies)

Treatment/Management

- Ideally preterm labor prevention begins preconceptually attempting to correct for maternal risk factors.

- Routine prenatal care with special attention to:

  - regular prenatal visits

  - avoidance of overexertion

  - stress reduction

  - avoidance of smoking/substance use

  - good nutrition

  - identification and treatment of bacteriuria, vaginal/cervical infections

  - prompt evaluation of febrile illness

  - careful evaluation/treatment of all medical complications

  - patient education regarding PTL

- Complete Preterm Labor Screen at initial OB visit and rescreen at 20 weeks. If 1 major or 2 minor factors identified, begin preterm labor surveillance and education. Patient may be seen every two weeks (or more often as indicated) until 36 weeks and then weekly until delivery. A careful history and gentle digital cervical exam should be undertaken at each visit.

- In identified at risk patients or in patients with irritable uteri restriction of physical and sexual activity is recommended. Ideally patient should be on modified bedrest (bathroom privileges, up for meals & shower) until 36 weeks or until signs/symptoms of PTL abate completely. Alternatives to intercourse/orgasm to be suggested. Avoidance of breast stimulation is also warranted.

- Serial ultrasound exam of cervical length and dilatation may be performed in the early second trimester in women with prior second trimester pregnancy loss or with a history suggestive of cervical incompetence (Parisi, 1988).

- Cervical cerclage should be reserved for patients with cervical incompetence (identified by a history of rapid, painless cervical effacement and dilatation resulting in second trimester pregnancy loss; or in women who have sufficient cervical change without uterine activity in the current pregnancy (Iams & Creasy, 1988; Parisi, 1988).

- Ambulatory home monitoring of uterine activity with the use of a tocodynamometer has been utilized in several ways (Katz & Scheerer, 1988):

  - screening of low risk women for preterm labor

  - making the early diagnosis of preterm labor in at risk women

  - improving tocolytic therapy once the diagnosis of preterm labor is made

The utilization of this modality is site-specific and depends upon availability of equipment and support services. The monitor is worn for one hour in the morning and evening and the tracing is transmitted through a telephone to a receiving unit. Trained nurses evaluate the monitor strips daily and are available on a twenty-four hour basis to respond to emergencies. A sudden increase in uterine contractility in the 24 hours prior to diagnosis

200

of PTL may be identified via the use of the tocodynamometer (Katz, Gill, & Newman, 1986). Iams, Johnson, and O'Shaughnessy (1988) believe that the success reported in reducing the incidence of prematurity via home uterine activity monitoring is most likely the result of daily nurse-patient contact regarding attention to the early symptoms of preterm labor.

- Hospital admission is indicated for rupture of membranes, vaginal bleeding, diagnosis of preterm labor with cervical change, or strong suspicion of preterm labor. Inpatient management is beyond the scope of this protocol.

- Tocolytic therapy may be initiated provided the following criteria are met (Pernoll, 1987):

    - gestational age 20-34 weeks

    - membranes intact

    - cervical dilatation <4 cm, effacement <80%

    - fetus not in distress

- If intravenous tocolysis was instituted the patient will usually be started on oral doses while in the hospital and if stable will be discharged on oral maintenance therapy (as well as bedrest) until 36 weeks of pregnancy. Betamimetic agents are the most commonly used oral tocolytics and their dose is tailored to the individual patient based on maternal heart rate, uterine activity, and undesirable side effects. The resting pulse rate should be <120 beats/minute. Sustained increased pulse rate, uterine contractions not controlled by medication, and/or poor compliance with medication or bedrest regimen warrants re-evaluation and possible re-admission to the hospital.
NOTE: Side effects and adverse reactions of beta-adrenergic tocolytic agents include: tachycardia, nervousness, anxiety, tremor, palpitations, nausea, vomiting, diaphoresis, headache, chest pain, dyspnea, hypotension, cardiac arrythmias, myocardial ischemia, pulmonary edema.

- Patients admitted for suspected PTL that do not demonstrate cervical change and whose contractions cease may be discharged from the hospital to be further evaluated with regular frequent OB visits as described above.

Consultation

- Mandatory if preterm labor suspected or confirmed, or if PROM evidenced

- May refer to special care or high risk OB team if available, or to MD for primary management.

- Co-management with MD is also feasible.

Patient Education

- Encourage good care of self during pregnancy paying attention to adequate nutrition and fluid intake, avoidance of extreme physical activity and fatigue, minimization of psychological stress, regular prenatal visits, and prompt reporting of problems.

- Pregnant women/couples should be educated regarding the risk factors for premature delivery and encouraged to make necessary lifestyle changes in an attempt to prevent this outcome.

- Intensive education/counseling is mandatory for patients at risk for or with suspected PTL. At many facilities patient education materials are available on the subject of preterm birth prevention.

- Educate the patient regarding the signs and symptoms of preterm labor as described in the Subjective section. Be sure the patient understands these.

- Teach self-detection and timing of uterine contractions.

- Establish criteria for notification of the health care provider:

    - regular uterine contractions: 10 minutes apart or closer, or more than 4-5 contractions in one hour

    - vaginal bleeding or leaking of fluid

    - other signs/symptoms of preterm labor

- Stress importance of compliance with bedrest and the reporting of signs and symptoms of PTL.

- Offer suggestions for meal planning if on bedrest. See Nutrition protocol.

- Review danger signs of pregnancy relative to spontaneous abortion, preeclampsia, placenta previa/abruption.

- Provide Labor & Delivery, emergency, and health care provider phone numbers.

Follow-up

- Assess presence or absence of signs/symptoms of preterm labor at each visit. Assess compliance with tocolytic medication as indicated. Use of a Preterm Labor Monitoring Log may assist in patient evaluation. See Table 4.5, *Preterm Labor Monitoring Log*, p. 204).

- Perform gentle serial cervical exams at each prenatal visit and as indicated in patients at risk for or with signs/symptoms of PTL.

- Review with patient at each visit signs and symptoms of preterm labor, self-detection and timing of uterine contractions, and criteria for notification of health care provider. Have patient verbalize understanding.

- Assess activity level and compliance with bedrest regimen.

- Support need for sexual expression exclusive of breast stimulation, intercourse, and orgasm.

- Advance activity slowly as indicated by history and cervical exam.

- Assess social situation and support systems. Refer to social services or public health nurse as indicated. Assist with child care arrangements as necessary if patient on bedrest.

- Patient to be referred to Labor & Delivery if preterm labor suspected or confirmed, or in cases of PROM.

- Preterm delivery may precipitate an emotional crisis for the patient and family. Support for the normal responses of grief, guilt, and anxiety should be demonstrated.

- The mother should be aware that one preterm delivery places her at risk for another; therefore in future pregnancies early, comprehensive prenatal care should be sought.

- Document in progress notes and problem list.

Preterm Labor Screen	1st Visit	Rescreen
MAJOR FACTORS		
Previous preterm labor with or without preterm delivery		
DES daughter		
Cone biopsy		
2nd trimester abortions, 2 or more		
Uterine anomalies		
Current pregnancy		
Multiple gestation		
Effaced and/or dilated cervix (<1 cm long or 1 cm dil. int. os)		
Uterine irritability		
Abdominal surgery after 18 weeks		
Hydramnios		
Cerclage		
MINOR FACTORS		
Fibroids		
2nd trimester abortion, 1		
1st trimester abortion, 3 or more		
Current pregnancy		
Bleeding after 12 weeks		
Febrile illness (including pyelonephritis)		
Cigarette smoking (10 or more a day)		
ANY MAJOR AND/OR 2 MINOR FACTORS PRETERM LABOR SURVEILLANCE/EDUCATION INDICATED		

SOURCE:

Laros, R. (1988). University of California, San Francisco. Reprinted with permission.

Figure 4.2. Preterm Labor Screen

Table 4.5

Preterm Labor Monitoring Log

Name

To assist your health care team to take the best care of you and your baby, your help is needed. Please record information about your condition throughout the day and night. Be sure you understand what you are to record before you leave the hospital. Bring this form with you to your visits.

Date	Time	Preterm Labor Symptoms-- contractions, cramps, tightening, pelvic pressure, low backache that comes and goes, intestinal cramps or diarrhea, vaginal discharge changes. Call your provider if contractions occur 4 or more times/hour.	Pulse Take for 30 sec. & multiply by 2, or 15 sec. & multiply by 4	Medication--Do not take if pulse greater than 120/minute, you have shortness of breath or chest pain. Call your provider if these occur.

Adapted with permission from Kaiser Permanente Medical Center, San Francisco, CA. *Preterm labor monitoring log* (1988).

PROTEINURIA

Lisa L.Lommel

Protein is excreted in the urine (proteinuria) when the renal system is stressed by disease or infection. Protein is normally not present in the urine. However, small amounts (traces) may be found in a specimen contaminated by vaginal secretions or blood. Large amounts of protein (1-4+) is a common characteristic of renal dysfunction. In the pregnant client, proteinuria may indicate a kidney or bladder infection, a sign of pre-eclampsia, or chronic/acute renal disease.

Albumin is the primary protein of clinical significance excreted in all of these conditions (Corbett, 1987). The dipstick method is used most often to monitor for proteinuria in the pregnant client. Prenatal clients should have their urine evaluated for protein at every prenatal visit.

Data Base

Subjective

- Usually asymptomatic

- Pain or burning on urination, urgency, frequency, fever and/or chills

- Flank or suprapubic pain

- Headache, visual disturbances, epigastric pain, decreased urinary output, generalized edema

- Vaginal discharge, accompanying signs and symptoms of vaginitis

- History of chronic renal disease

Objective

- Amount of protein recorded on dipstick

- Elevated temperature, rapid pulse

- CVA or suprapubic tenderness

- Positive leukocyte esterase and/or hemoglobin on dipstick

- Positive urine culture

- Elevated blood pressure

- Sudden weight gain

- Edema of hands, feet, and/or face

- Hyperreflexia

- Positive wet mount/culture for vaginitis

Assessment

- Proteinuria

- R/O Urinary tract infection (UTI) or pyelonephritis

- R/O Pre-eclampsia
- R/O Vaginal contamination/infection
- R/O Chronic renal disease

Plan

Diagnostic Tests

- Obtain urine specimen and dipstick
- If initial dipstick is positive for protein ($\geq 1+$), obtain clean-catch urine specimen and repeat dipstick.
- If unable to obtain clean-catch urine in presence of subjective and/or objective signs and symptoms, obtain catheterized urine specimen and dipstick.
- If repeat dipstick is positive for protein ($\geq 1+$), obtain complete urinalysis and urine culture with sensitivities.
- Assess for pre-eclampsia (see Hypertensive Disorders of Pregnancy protocol).
- Obtain wet mounts and cultures as indicated.
- For persistent proteinuria of $1-4+$ order:
    - serum creatinine and uric acid
    - 24-hour urine for total protein, creatinine, and creatinine clearance

Treatment/Management

- If repeat dipstick contains no protein, initiate routine follow-up as indicated.
- See Bacteriuria, Cystitis, and Pyelonephritis protocols.
- See Hypertensive Disorders of Pregnancy protocol.
- See Vaginitis protocol.

Consultation

- Consult with MD when there is persistent proteinuria, recurrent UTI, or possible pre-eclampsia.
- Refer to MD when pre-eclampsia is diagnosed or the patient has a past history of recurrent UTI or pyelonephritis.

Patient Education

- Explain the need for a clean-catch urine specimen and the method of collection.
- Stress the importance of perineal hygiene to prevent UTI.
- See Patient Education of Bacteriuria, Cystitis, Pyelonephritis, and Vaginitis protocols.

Follow-up

- Evaluate the patient's urine for proteinuria at each visit.
- Document in progress notes and problem list if a significant, on-going problem.

PYELONEPHRITIS

Winifred L. Star

Acute pyelonephritis is one of the most common complications affecting pregnancy, with an incidence of 1-2.5%. *Escherichia coli* causes about 70% of infections. Other common pathogens include *Proteus mirablis* and *Klebsiella pneumoniae* (Pauerstein, 1987). The presence of asymptomatic bacteriuria is a major risk factor for the development of pyelonephritis; twenty to forty percent of untreated women with asymptomatic bacteriuria will go on to develop this complication (Gibbs & Sweet, 1989; Pauerstein, 1987). Early detection and treatment of bacteriuria will reduce the incidence of pyelonephritis by 70-80% (Gibbs & Sweet, 1989). Recurrence rates of pyelonephritis in pregnancy are 10-18% (Gibbs & Sweet, 1989; Pauerstein, 1987).

Several pregnancy-related factors predispose to the development of acute pyelonephritis. Anatomical and hormonal changes encourage dilatation and relaxation of the collecting system of the kidney leading to stasis of urine and facilitation of bacterial migration. Glycosuria, common in pregnancy, favors bacterial overgrowth. Estrogen may enhance growth of *E. coli.* The cumulative effects of these physiological changes is an increased risk that infection, which may begin in the bladder, will ascend to the kidneys (Gibbs & Sweet, 1989).

The most significant complication of pyelonephritis is preterm labor and delivery. Other reported complications include anemia, thrombocytopenia, hypertension, adult respiratory distress syndrome, transient renal dysfunction, and intrauterine death. Maternal sepsis may develop in 10% of cases of pyelonephritis; septic shock may ensue in these women (McNeeley, 1988; Pauerstein, 1987).

Data Base

Subjective

- Risk factors may include:

    - physiologic changes of pregnancy

    - asymptomatic bacteriuria

    - cystitis

    - recent catheterization

    - history of renal anomaly/calculi

- Symptoms may include:

    - urinary frequency, urgency

    - dysuria

    - shaking chills

    - fever

    - flank pain

    - nausea, vomiting, anorexia

    - headache

- lower abdominal pain

Objective

- Fever (universal sign)
- Tachycardia may be present.
- Hypotension may occur.
- Costovertebral angle tenderness (CVAT), usually on the right
- Lower abdominal tenderness may be present.
- Signs of dehydration may be present.
- Urine dipstick may be positive for nitrites, leukocyte esterase, protein.
- Urinalysis reveals presence of pyuria, bacteriuria, and/or white blood cell casts.
- Urine culture shows >100,000 colonies of a significant pathogen.
- Urine immunofluorescence test (if done) may be positive for antibody-coated bacteria.
- Perform pelvic exam as indicated.

Assessment

- Pyelonephritis
- R/O Acute hydronephrosis/hydroureter
- R/O Urinary tract calculus
- R/P Perinephric abscess
- R/O Sepsis
- R/O Spontaneous rupture of renal pelvis secondary to obstruction (rare)
- R/O Preterm labor
- R/O Vaginitis/Cervicitis

Plan

Diagnostic tests

- Complete urinalysis, urine culture and sensitivities on a clean-catch midstream urine specimen
- Additional labs may include: CBC, sedimentation rate, urine immunofluorescence, renal function studies, blood cultures

Treatment /Management

- Inpatient hospitalization required.
- Therapeutic interventions include: broad spectrum intravenous antibiotics (ampicillin, cephalosporins, and aminoglycosides may be employed), hydration, lowering of temperature, monitoring of renal function, intake and output assessment, observation for shock. The details of inpatient management is beyond the scope of this protocol.
- Treat vaginitis/cervicitis as indicated.

Consultation

- Required

Patient Education

- Discuss the etiology of pyelonephritis and need for hospitalization.

- Discuss the importance of antibiotic therapy and compliance with medication regimen.

- Educate regarding health maintenance and prevention measures for urinary tract infection. See Cystitis protocol.

- Discuss preterm labor signs and symptoms. See Preterm Birth Prevention protocol.

Follow-up

- Patients with pyelonephritis are usually given suppressive antibiotic therapy for the duration of pregnancy. Nitrofurantoin 100 mg q hs is usually prescribed. Sulfonamides or ampicillin are alternate drugs that may be employed.

- An alternative to suppressive therapy is evaluation of urine cultures q 2-4 weeks for the remainder of pregnancy, with antibiotic treatment if bacteriuria identified.

- A complete urine culture should be done at the 6 week postpartum visit and on an annual basis.

- Patients with repeated urinary tract infection/pyelonephritis in pregnancy should be referred to a urologist to R/O renal abnormalities. An intravenous pyelogram at three months postpartum may be considered.

- Document in progress notes and problem list.

RADIATION EXPOSURE

Lisa L. Lommel

High-energy ionizing radiation (x-ray) has the capacity to damage chromosomes within the nuclei of cells. After ionization of a cell, the resulting chemical injury to the DNA may lead to cell death or replication of the abnormal cell. Although most often, the cell repairs itself before it divides. Effects of radiation are dependent on a variety of factors including the amount of exposure and susceptibility of the recipient.

Exposure of the fetus/embryo to radiation is not uncommon and is often unavoidable. Radiation exposure from the atmosphere, building materials, the ground, and naturally occurring radioisotopes account for approximately 0.075 to 0.1 rem during gestation (NCRP, 1977a). A routine chest x-ray accounts for <.05 rems of exposure to the fetus (Drugan & Evans, 1988). The majority of diagnostic examinations expose the fetus to less than 5 rems (Table 4.6, *Exposure to Fetus from X-ray Studies*, p. 213). It has been determined that exposure of 5 rems or less presents a low risk of pregnancy loss, congenital anomalies, mental defectiveness, and growth retardation. Some studies have shown that the threshold for radiation effects in the embryo occur in the 15-20 rem range. At levels of 5 rems or less, the risk for a fetus is not increased substantially above general risks of pregnancy loss (30% to 50%) and malformations (2.75%). At these levels, termination of the pregnancy is not recommended.

Exposure to radiation above 50 rems during the first 10 to 14 days of human development is unlikely to produce congenital malformations but there is a substantial risk of pregnancy loss. Exposure to these levels during the period of organogenesis (two to nine weeks) places the embryo at risk for major anatomical malformation including mental retardation, microcephaly, and ocular abnormalities (Jankowski, 1986). During the second and third trimester, central nervous system anomalies and ophthalmic defects may occur at high doses. Although not well substantiated, it has been reported that diagnostic levels (up to 5 rems) of *in utero* exposure increase the risk of childhood cancer (Jankowski, 1986).

The physical and biological characteristics of microwave and ultrasound energy are different than that of ionizing radiation (x-rays). The embryo is not at risk of mutagenic or carcinogenic effects from microwave radiation (Jankowski, 1986). Properly constructed microwave ovens do not represent a hazard during pregnancy (Brent, 1980b).

Ultrasonography uses sound waves to study anatomical features of the fetus. This procedure has greatly reduced the need for fetal exposure to x-rays. There has been no identifiable adverse effects to the fetus from diagnostic ultrasound. It is currently considered to be safe during pregnancy (Maulik, 1989).

Video display terminals are of minimal risk to the fetus. A woman sitting at a VDT console for 30 hours a week would accumulate a maximum dose of 0.006 rads during the first trimester. As gestation of the pregnancy increases there is protection from the increased amount of amniotic fluid surrounding the fetus. It has been found that the video display terminal offers no radiation hazard (Jankowski, 1986).

Data Base

Subjective

- No symptoms related to exposure
- Women who may be pregnant and need diagnostic evaluation with x-rays
- Women with unknown pregnancy who were exposed to ionizing radiation
- Women at occupational risk are health care personnel who work with patients receiving x-rays, those who handle radioactive material and workers exposed to nuclear material on the job.

Objective

- No signs of exposure
- Number or rems accumulated as determined by use of film or thermoluminescent dosimeter (TLD) badge
- Type, date, and number of radiation exposures
- Use of protective clothing (lead equivalent) equipment
- Stage of pregnancy when radiation exposure occurred
- Calculation of embryonic exposure

Assessment

- Patient exposure to ionizing radiation

Plan

Diagnostic Tests

- Diagnostic x-rays that are essential for optimal medical care of the mother and evaluation of medical problems should be performed.
- Elective tests need not be performed on a pregnant woman even though the risk to the embryo is small.
- Ultrasound to determine possible fetal anomalies
- Ultrasound at 28-34 weeks gestation to rule out intrauterine growth retardation (IUGR)

Treatment/Management

- Patient support and education
- It is the position of the American College of Radiology that termination of pregnancy is not justified secondary to exposure of the fetus to a diagnostic x-ray exam (Medical News, 1976).

Consultation

- MD consultation to evaluate level of embryonic exposure and need for genetic risk counseling

Patient Education

- Advise non-pregnant women working with or in the presence of radiation (occupational exposure) that it is required they be:

  - eighteen years of age or older and

  - monitored for radiation exposure by film or thermoluminescent dosimeter (TLD) badge if there is a possibility of receiving more than a quarter of the recommended limit of 1.25 rems. (The numbers of workers who actually receive an annual dose that approaches 5 rems is minimal) (Jankowski, 1986).

- Advise pregnant women who are occupationally exposed to radiation that the exposure to the embryo/fetus should not exceed a maximum dose of 0.5 rems. This is equivalent to 1.5 rems to the pregnant women because absorption of radiation by the abdominal wall usually reduces the fetal dose to 0.5 rems or less. Women working in areas of radiation exposure whose fetus could receive 0.5 rems or more before birth should seek ways to reduce their exposure within their present job or:

  - request reassignment to an area of less exposure

  - delay childbearing until they change jobs

  - continue working in their present position with the awareness that there is a small risk to the unborn child

- Advise women radiologists who are pregnant to limit radiation dose to 0.5 rems by the use of an 0.5 mm lead-equivalent wrap-around apron and avoidance of the radiation beam.

- Educate the patient that no special shielding precautions need to be taken during x-ray of a part away from the maternal pelvis (e.g., dental films). Shielding of the pregnant woman's abdomen is routinely done however, in most cases. Reassure the patient that if she has been unshielded, radiation dose to the fetus is minuscule.

- Agencies employing workers exposed to radiation are responsible to provide employees with specific instructions concerning the risks of radiation and in-utero radiation which include:

  - shielding for x-rays

  - wearing protective clothing when working with radioactive chemicals

  - wearing long-sleeved protective uniforms

  - using protective lead-lined aprons and gloves, and protective eye wear

  - wearing personal radiation monitoring devices, which monitor individual cumulative radiation exposure, at all times during work hours

  - avoiding all unnecessary exposure to radiation sources

Follow-up

- Routine postpartum follow-up

- Document exposure in progress notes and problem list.

Table 4.6

Exposure to Fetus from X-ray Studies

Head

Routine: < 50 mrad
Computerized axial tomography: < 100 mrad

Chest

Routine: < 50 mrad
Computerized axial tomography: < 1 rad
Mammography: < 50 mrad

Spine

Cervical: < 50 mrad
Thoracic: < 100 mrad
Lumbar/lumbosacral: 27-3,970 mrad

Abdominal

Upper GI series: 5-1,230 mrad
Cholecystography/cholangiography: 14-1,600 mrad
Barium enema: 28-12,600 mrad
Intravenous pyelography: 70-5,480 mrad
Pelvimetry: 220-5,480 mrad
Hysterosalpingography: 270-9,180 mrad

Extremities

Shoulder: 0.5-3.0 mrad
Other (excluding upper femur): < 50 mrad
Hips and femurs (proximal): 73-1,370 mrad

mrad = one thousandth of a rad

SOURCE:

Drugan, A., & Evans, M. (1988). Exposure of the pregnant patient to ionizing radiation. *Contemporary Ob/Gyn, 32* (4), 16-21. Reprinted with permission.

SIZE/DATES DISCREPANCY

Maureen T. Shannon

A size/dates (S/D) discrepancy exists when the uterine size (by clinical parameters) is either smaller or larger than is expected based on a client's <u>known</u> last normal menstrual period. There are two categories for size/dates discrepancies: 1) the uterine size is smaller than dates by LMP; or 2) the uterine size is larger than dates by LMP (Nichols, 1985; Varney, 1987).

Data Base

Subjective

- If the LMP is unknown or uncertain, the subjective signs and symptoms of pregnancy may not correlate with the estimated gestational age.

- May state that she feels more or less pregnant than her estimated gestational age.

- May note a rapid abdominal growth rate (in acute hydramnios or in ovarian cysts).

- May report an increased or decreased nutritional intake.

- May report a history of uterine fibroids or Rh disease.

- Client may have a family history of diabetes, multiple gestations, hypertension, or pre-eclampsia.

- In multiple gestation pregnancies, the client often reports a great deal of fetal movement.

- See subjective data contained in specific protocols for intrauterine growth retardation (IUGR), gestational trophoblastic neoplasia (GTN), gestational diabetes mellitus (GDM), and polyhydramnios.

Objective

- In true S/D discrepancy, serum or urine pregnancy tests are positive at the appropriate times.

- In true S/D discrepancy, the bimanual exam of the uterus done during the first trimester will usually correlate with the woman's known LMP.

- McDonald's measurements are 2 cm less than or 2 cm greater than what is expected for dates.

- Estimates of fetal weight are less than or greater than expected for gestational age.

- Two or more distinct fetal heart tones (FHTs) are noted by simultaneous auscultation done for 1 minute by 2 examiners (in multiple gestations).

- Absence of FHTs after the 12th week by dates (in molar pregnancy or missed spontaneous abortions)

- Ultrasound may reveal IUGR, fetal macrosomia, fetal anomalies, excessive amniotic fluid, etc.

- Maternal weight gain may be significantly increased or decreased for that point in the pregnancy.

- Fetus may be palpated in a transverse or oblique lie.

- Distended bladder of woman may be palpated.

- See objective data contained in specific protocols for IUGR, GTN, polyhydramnios, Rh isoimmunization, etc.

Assessment

- IUP with size less than dates or size greater than dates

- R/O Inaccurate dating

- R/O Transverse lie

- R/O IUGR

- R/O Polyhydramnios

- R/O Multiple gestations

- R/O GTN

- R/O Gestational Diabetes Mellitus

- R/O Fetal macrosomia

- R/O Fetal anomalies

- R/O Maternal fibroids, ovarian cysts, or tumors

Plan

Diagnostic Tests

- Ultrasound exam to help calculate gestational age; fetal size and growth patterns; presence of some fetal anomalies; presence of multiple fetuses; amount of amniotic fluid; presence of molar pregnancy; evidence of missed spontaneous abortion (SAB)

- Radioimmunoassay HCG level in suspected GTN or missed SAB

- Glucose screen on all patients, and a 3-hour GTT in patients with abnormal screens--see Gestational Diabetes Mellitus protocol.

- Maternal antibody titers in all patients at appropriate times--see Rh Isoimmunization protocol.

- Non-stress tests, contraction stress tests and/or biophysical profile of the fetus in patients with high-risk pregnancies (e.g., IUGR, postterm pregnancies, multiple gestations, polyhydramnios, etc.)

Treatment/Management

- Review the patient's pregnancy landmarks (e.g., date of LMP and possible conception, when subjective symptoms began, date of quickening, etc.) and the clinical parameters in the chart to confirm gestational age.

- Establish an accurate gestational age as soon as possible--ideally before the 20th week of pregnancy.

- Order an ultrasound exam on all pregnant patients with unknown or uncertain LMPs, patients taking oral contraceptives just before or during the possible time of conception, or if a S/D discrepancy exists.

- See specific protocols for the treatment/management of IUGR, multiple gestation, polyhydramnios, Rh isoimmunization, etc.

Consultation

- Required if S/D discrepancy is due to an abnormality (e.g., IUGR, multiple gestations, fetal anomalies, etc.).

- Referral to MD care if S/D discrepancy is based on an abnormality. In some situations (e.g., IUGR) client can be co-managed with MD.

Patient Education

- Education and counseling of a patient should be based upon the underlying cause of the S/D discrepancy.

    - If an abnormality is found, then the counseling of the patient is based upon the underlying problem (e.g., IUGR).

    - If no abnormality is found and fetal growth is within normal limits, then reassurance of the patient is all that is indicated.

- Educate the patient about the various tests that are being ordered, and interpret the test results for her.

- Nutrition counseling if the maternal weight gain is either less than or greater than it should be for that point in her pregnancy

Follow-up

- If S/D discrepancy evaluation reveals no problems and normal fetal growth, then continue routine prenatal care.

- If S/D discrepancy evaluation reveals an abnormality, then follow-up is per protocol for the specific problem (e.g., IUGR).

- Document in progress notes and problem list.

SUBINVOLUTION

Lucy Newmark Sammons

Subinvolution is the delayed or incomplete return of the uterus to normal dimensions following childbirth. Evaluation of the extent of involution is accomplished by palpation and bimanual examination. Normally, uterine fundal height moves from midway between the umbilicus and symphysis after third stage labor, to the level of the bony pelvis at two weeks, to nonpregnant uterine size at four to six weeks. Endometrial regeneration is complete by the third week, except at the placental site, where regeneration is complete about six weeks after delivery (Novy, 1987).

Common causative or contributing factors of subinvolution are endometritis, retained placental fragments, uterine overdistention from multiple gestation or polyhydramnios, fibroids, absence of lactation, or inadequate uterine drainage (Thomas, 1989; Willson, 1987). Recent use of immunohistochemical techniques suggest that subinvolution of the uteroplacental arteries may represent an abnormal interaction between maternal uterine cells and the fetal trophoblast manifesting itself as delayed involution (Andrew, Bulmer, Wells, Morrison, & Buckley, 1989).

Data Base

Subjective

- Client describes greater quantity and longer duration of bloody vaginal discharge than normal.

- Symptoms occur one week to several months postpartum, with maximal occurrence in second week (Andrews et al., 1989).

- Contributing/risk factors:

  - Increased maternal age

  - Multiparity

  - Current endometritis

  - History of polyhydramnios, fibroids, or multiple gestation current pregnancy

  - History of subinvolution previous pregnancy

  - Absence of lactation

- Hemorrhage may be abrupt in onset.

- Client may have symptoms of anemia--see Anemia protocol.

Objective

- Uterus enlarged, soft, boggy, possibly retrodisplaced

- Uterus generally freely movable

- Cervical os is patulous.

- Continuation of lochia rubra beyond the second to third week

- May have signs of concomitant infection--see Endometritis protocol.

- May have signs of anemia--see Anemia protocol.

Assessment

- Subinvolution
- R/O Retained placental fragments
- R/O Endometritis
- R/O Gestational trophoblastic neoplasia (GTN)
- R/O Anemia

Plan

Diagnostic Tests

- No definitive diagnostic tests
- Hemaglobin/hematocrit to assess anemia due to blood loss
- Other tests as indicated for suspicion of concomitant pathology, e.g., CBC, sedimentation rate, beta-HCG

Treatment/Management

- Methylergonovine maleate (Methergine) .2 mg tab <u>Sig</u>: tab i po tid x 2 days
- Referral for medical treatment of causative factors if indicated, e.g., removal of retained placental fragments, treatment of brisk hemorrhage, GTN. See protocols on Endometritis, GTN.
- May refer to MD if severely anemic--see Anemia protocol.

Consultation

- Medical consultation for prescription as necessary
- Medical consultation for collaborative management of underlying pathology

Patient Education

- Explain causes and therapeutic approaches for subinvolution.
- Preventive measures include enhancing normal uterine drainage by ambulation and upright positioning.
- Provide anticipatory guidance that ergot preparation may produce sensation of cramping; lochia is expected to decrease with treatment.
- Alert patient to signs of further complications: bleeding unresponsive or increases, fever or chills, etc.--see also Endometritis protocol.
- Advise patient to practice pelvic rest.

Follow-up

- Patient to contact provider in case of signs of further complications or failure to respond to therapy
- In absence of other morbidity, re-evaluate involution in one to two weeks.
- Document in progress notes and problem list.

SUBSTANCE ABUSE

Lucy Newmark Sammons

Substances with the potential for untoward effects on the pregnant woman and her baby, and hence of concern to the perinatal care provider, include 1) alcohol, 2) illegal drugs or chemicals, particularly cocaine and its derivatives; heroin; PCP; amphetamines; and marijuana; 3) legally available prescribed drugs, such as barbituates or narcotic analgesics, and 4) legally available non-prescription substances such as nicotine, caffeine, and over-the-counter drugs. This discussion will focus on substance abuse in the first three categories.

The principal addictive drug of concern today in obstetrics is cocaine (either alone, or in combination with alcohol or tranquilizers), replacing the previous focus on opiates and heroin (Keith, Donald, Rosner, Mitchell, & Bianchi, 1986). "Crack" is a particularly addictive form of cocaine, made by mixing a solution of cocaine hydrochloride with sodium bicarbonate, which is then smoked to produce high serum drug concentrations. Intravenous injection of cocaine with heroin, "speedball," is another common route of administration (Dombrowski & Sokol, 1990). While incidence figures for maternal perinatal substance abuse will vary based on the rigor and universality of assessment protocols and the breadth of the confirmatory toxicologic assays, estimates for both cocaine and excessive alcohol use are in the area of 10% of obstetric clients (Jessup & Roth, 1988).

Prenatal drug and alcohol abuse have multiple deleterious effects on the mother, and on her baby before and after birth (see Table 4.7, *Maternal/Fetal/Neonatal Effects of Substances Commonly Abused by Pregnant Women*, p. 224). Major potential maternal sequelae are cardiac, liver, and gastrointestinal damage; hypertension; preterm labor and birth (PTL and PTB); spontaneous abortion; placental abruption; cerebrovascular accident; and cardiac arrest. Major potential fetal/neonatal adverse outcomes include Fetal Alcohol Effects Syndrome (FAE); Fetal Alcohol Syndrome (FAS); addiction and acute withdrawal; stillbirth; intrauterine growth retardation (IUGR); low birthweight (LBW) and other consequences of prematurity; congenital anomalies; seizure disorders; meconium; multiple behavioral and feeding problems; developmental and learning disabilities; and increased rate for Sudden Infant Death Syndrome (SIDS). In addition, polydrug use and the addictive lifestyle subject the woman to increased risk of acquiring sexually transmitted diseases (STDs), gynecologic disorders, hepatitis, and HIV infection.

Data Base

Subjective

- Client may admit to current and/or past substance abuse; alternatively, a substance abuser may deny chemical dependency or addictive behaviors.

- Medical history may include:

  - Unexplained obstetrical/neonatal complications possibly associated with substance abuse (e.g., abruptio placenta, fetal death, FAS, IUGR, low birth weight infant, PTL, SIDS)

  - Use of mood-altering prescriptive drugs

  - Undocumented "seizure disorder," blackouts

  - Victim of physical or sexual abuse

- Menstrual irregularities

- Recent multiple sexually transmitted diseases

- Current obstetric care may present as:

  - Late unexplained registration for prenatal care

  - Noncompliance with keeping prenatal appointments or obtaining ordered laboratory tests, especially if coupled with frequent labor and delivery or emergency room drop-in visits

- Personal/family/partner psychosocial history may indicate:

  - Family or partner substance abuse

  - Dysfunctional family of origin

  - Psychiatric care history: inpatient or outpatient treatment, suicide attempt

  - Incarceration or arrest; drunk driving violations

  - Social instability or chaotic lifestyle: multiple, changing addresses and contact telephone numbers; homelessness; conflictual interpersonal relationships

  - Previous child(ren) cared for by foster parent or someone else other than woman herself

  - Vagueness or evasiveness in revealing history

Objective

- Toxicology screen, if obtained, is positive

- Client may demonstrate signs of current intoxication or drug use:

  - Alcohol on breath

  - Eye signs, as evaluated by general observation, pupil size measurement, pupil light reactivity, testing for nystagmus, and testing for convergence will vary from normal characteristics for major drugs of abuse (Tennant, 1988)

  - Speech slurred

  - Behavior inappropriate, suggestive of hallucinogenic use, bizarre, or agitated

  - Behavior combative, disruptive, abusive

  - Demonstrated mood swings, emotional lability

  - Unkempt appearance

- Medical indicators suggestive of history of or current substance abuse--physical examination or laboratory studies indicating (Jessup & Roth, 1988; Chasnoff, 1987):

  - General appearance of physical exhaustion, poor orientation

  - Cirrhosis, hepatitis

  - Pancreatitis

  - Hypertension

  - Gastrointestinal tract inflammation

  - Hematological disorders

  - Indicators of inadequate nutritional stores or current deficiency

220

- Cardiac arrhythmias, endocarditis, or other cardiac disease

- Cellulitis

- Phlebitis

- Sexually transmitted diseases, HIV infection

- Septicemia

- Pneumonia

- Withdrawal symptoms

- Observable track marks, abscesses, or edema, particularly in extremities

- Inflamed or indurated nasal mucosa

- Current pregnancy may include:

  - Signs of preterm labor

  - Inactive or hyperactive fetus

  - Inadequate weight gain

  - Vaginal bleeding or spotting

Assessment

- Substance abuse: specific drug/chemical or polydrug combination; prior to or during current pregnancy

- R/O Concomitant IUGR, anemia, STDs, HIV infection, vaginitis, and other general medical and obstetric complications associated with substance abuse (see listings under Objective Data Base) as indicated by data base

- R/O Drug withdrawal--symptoms of fatigue, headache, nausea, pelvic cramps are similar to early pregnancy (Ronkin, FitzSimmons, Wapner, & Finnegan, 1988)

Plan

Diagnostic Tests

- Toxicology screen for identification/quantification of drugs of abuse. Laboratories will vary as to which screening tests are available. Follow local specifications regarding sampling from urine, blood, or gastric sampling, and the volume of specimen required.

- Urinary retention times vary by drug, patient's physical condition and hydration, and route and frequency of drug use (Ronkin et al., 1988; Dombrowski & Sokol, 1990), with general times as follows:

Amphetamines	48 hours
Barbiturates	
Short-acting (secobartibal)	24 hours
Long-acting (phenobarbital)	2-3 weeks
Cannabinoids	
Moderate smoker	5 days
Heavy smoker (daily)	10 days
Chronic smoker	20 days
Cocaine	1-4 days
Opiates	2 days

- Future test modalities may include radioimmunoassays (RIA) of maternal hair and neonatal meconium for cocaine and illicit drug use.

Treatment/Management

- Assess all pregnant women for alcohol and substance abuse.

- Where risk factors are present, obtain screening test for drugs of abuse at intake or as soon as risk apparent. Obtain woman's consent; document if woman refuses to consent. Repeat toxicology screens each trimester or as indicated by previous results and interval history.

- Where heavy alcohol intake is known or suspected, obtain complete blood count with indices and liver function tests; institute daily recordings of urine dipstick ketone bodies; medically supervised detoxification will be required if consumption levels exceed 8 ounces of alcohol (1 pint of liquor) daily (Jessup & Green, 1987).

- Encourage Human Immunodeficiency Virus (HIV) antibody screening at intake.

- Screen for sexually transmitted diseases (gonorrhea, chlamydia, syphilis, condyloma) at intake and at 36 weeks.

- Additional screening for infection may include chest radiograph (Chasnoff, 1987).

- Obtain baseline sonogram at 20 weeks gestation, or at intake if woman registers later, to confirm dating and assess IUGR; additional sonograms at 30-32 weeks and 36-38 weeks; follow IUGR as needed--see IUGR protocol.

- Re-evaluate fetal surveillance plans at 28 and 34 weeks, e.g., fetal movement counts, NSTs, serial sonograms--see Antepartum Fetal Surveillance protocol.

- Refer to appropriate treatment program--see Follow-up section.

- Opiate-addicted women may be treated with methadone maintenance regimens of 20 mg or less daily (Chasnoff, 1986b).

- Provide supplemental iron.

- Attempt to establish trust relationship with woman through continuity of care by consistent provider; assure confidentiality as allowed by law.

- Provide contraceptive services consistent with woman's preferences and lifestyle.

- See also Patient Education.

Consultation

- Medical consultation and management by a multidisciplinary team required for confirmed cases of perinatal substance abuse

- Social Services consultation required

- Nutritional consult if indicated by serious nutritional deficits, eating disorder

Patient Education

- Educate all women about the effects of alcohol and substance abuse on themselves and their babies, during and after pregnancy.

- Educate women with identified abuse about the specific maternal and infant complications for which they are at risk; early warning signs should be periodically reviewed .

- Inform woman of possible screen for drugs during delivery period, and potential involvement of Children's Protective Services if drug or alcohol abuse is detected at birth (if notification procedures are employed at site; legal interpretations vary by institution).

- Provide and reinforce preterm labor detection and preterm birth prevention information.

- Educate patient regarding beneficial effects for herself and her baby of stopping substance abuse immediately.

- Inform woman of potential effects of drug and alcohol transmission through breastmilk if nursing is being considered; breastfeeding is contraindicated if mother continues to use cocaine, heroin and/or methadone (Chasnoff, 1987; Novy, 1987).

Follow-up

- Refer to available outpatient and inpatient treatment programs, with particular reference to antenatal/postpartum services; self-help groups such as alcoholics/cocaine/narcotics anonymous.

- Refer for nutritional consultation.

- Refer to pediatric care provider prenatally, with identification of high risk status.

- Refer to public health nursing services prenatally and postpartally as needed.

- Refer women who were active substance abusers during pregnancy to infant CPR courses in view of increased SIDS risk.

- Follow woman at 2 week intervals, or more often if needed, to 36 weeks, then weekly.

- Placement of infant with mother or with Child Protective Services will be dependent upon nature and extent of substance abuse, compliance with treatment program, local legal and hospital policies, and availability of alternate supportive services.

- Document problem, dates and nature of known substance exposures in problem list; document problem, education, counseling, and referrals made in progress notes .

Table 4.7

Maternal/Fetal/Neonatal Effects of Substances Commonly Abused by Pregnant Women

Drug Name (various forms)	Street Names	Maternal Effects	Fetal Effects	Neonatal/Infant Effects	Long-Term Effects
Alcohol/Ethanol Hard liquor, beer, wine, etc.	Alcohol, booze, etc.	Tolerance, intoxication, CNS depression, withdrawal, risk for seizures, end organ damage to liver, heart, CNS, stomach, etc. Alcohol withdrawal may cause: hypertension, tachycardia, and premature labor	Possible abnormalities in growth and development May result in Fetal Alcohol Syndrome or Fetal Alcohol Effects	Fetal Alcohol Effects (FAE) and Fetal Alcohol Syndrome (FAS) Three major characteristics: - Growth retardation - Central nervous system abnormalities including developmental and mental retardation - Structural abnormalities including characteristic facial, skeletal and organ defects Possible CNS depression and withdrawal with irritability, restlessness, agitation, and increased risk of neonatal mortality	Mental retardation, developmental delay, low IQ
Marijuana/THC	Grass, pot, weed, herb, joint, etc.	CNS depression, but can act as a stimulant; toxic to respiratory system and immune system Increased heart rate, hypotension May cause more complicated labor and delivery including prolonged or arrested deliveries, abnormal bleeding, meconimum staining, etc. THC use may impair sperm production in male	Reduced fetal weight gain, shorter gestation, some congenital anomalies	Possible neurological abnormalities resulting from CNS immaturity: - abnormal responses to light and visual stimuli - tremulousness - high pitched cry	Long-term effects not known
Prescription sedative-hypnotics (e.g., Valium, Xanax, Halcion, etc.)	Vals	Tolerance, CNS depression, respiratory depression Acute withdrawal with risk of premature labor	Drug accumulates in fetus at levels greater than in mother Fetal depression, abnormal heart rhythm, or even death Increased risk for cleft lip/palate	Drug and metabolites may remain in newborn for days or weeks longer than in mother; may result in lethargy, poor muscle tone, sucking difficulties, or even CNS depression; withdrawal may occur	Long-term effects not known
Amphetamines/ Stimulants	Crank, speed, meth, crystal, ice	CNS stimulation and increased cardio-respiratory activity: - increase heart rate - increased blood pressure - rapid respiration Anorexia, weight loss, insomnia Decreased blood flow to placenta Risk of AIDS with IV use	Possible growth retardation and fetal hypoxia	Possible withdrawal or intoxication Low birthweight Adequate studies are lacking.	Long-term effects not known
Cocaine/Crack	Coke, snow, freebase, base, rock, pasta, báse	CNS and cardiovascular stimulation: - increased heart rate - increased blood pressure - vascular constrictions Decreased blood flow to placenta Possible placental abruption and bleeding Premature labor	Growth retardation Fetal hypertension and distress Risk for intrauterine stroke Possible genito-urinary abnormalities Necrotizing enterocolitis	Intoxication and/or withdrawal - irritability/agitation - increased tone - tremors - jitters - inconsolability - increased respiration - risk for seizures Slower drug excretion in newborn Abnormal sleep and ventilatory patterns	Possible developmental delays Possible long-term deficits in attention and learning
Heroin/Opiates	Smack, "H," horse tar, China white	Tolerance, CNS depression Risk for AIDS and other infections with IV drug use Acute withdrawal and risk for spontaneous abortion or premature labor	Intrauterine growth retardation Risk of AIDS infection from mother	Addiction and "Neonatal Narcotic Withdrawal Syndrome" - hyperactivity - irritability/agitation - high pitched cry - increased tone - tremors - seizure risk Poor feeding; abnormal sleep and ventilatory patterns AIDS risk	Possible long-term neuro-behavioral deficits
PCP Phencyclidine	KJ, angel dust, Krystal, etc.	Hallucinatory, analgesic, depressant, and stimulating effects Agitation May complicate labor and delivery	Likely damage to CNS development	Intoxication and/or withdrawal Serious neurological and behavioral defects: - inconsolability - intense irritability - abnormal state control - abnormal muscle tone - tremors - inability to coordinate simple motor tasks - sensory input problems Microcephaly	Developmental delays Abnormalities in attention span and organizational abilities Possible learning problems Studies are preliminary.
Cigarettes (nicotine and other compounds in smoke)		CNS stimulation and respiratory damage	Reduced fetal oxygen supply Impaired fetal growth Increased risk for fetal distress and fetal demise Increased risk for spontaneous abortion and premature labor	Growth retardation Smaller head circumference Risk for congenital palate and heart defects Abnormal nursing	Long-term effects not clear.

© 1990 **Anthony J. Puentes M.D.** Reprinted with permission.

THYROID DISORDERS

Maureen T. Shannon

EUTHYROID OF PREGNANCY

Euthyroid of pregnancy is a term used to describe the "normal" enlargement of the thyroid gland often observed during pregnancy. This enlargement is diffuse, non-tender, and not more than twice the expected size for a normal thyroid gland. Furthermore, the patient does not report any signs or symptoms that may be associated with thyroid disease. This thyroid enlargement is attributed to the effects of pregnancy hormones on thyroid regulation and secretion. Although euthyroid of pregnancy is a very common physical finding, the possibility of hypothyroidism or hyperthyroidism should not be overlooked when evaluating any enlargement of the thyroid gland (Cunningham, MacDonald, & Gant, 1989).

Data Base

Subjective

- No personal or family history of thyroid disease

- No complaints of symptoms associated with thyroid disease

Objective

- Blood pressure--within normal limits (WNL)

- Pulse--WNL

- Thyroid gland--palpation may reveal diffuse, soft, non-tender enlargement not more than twice normal size without nodules

- Other components of physical examination--WNL

Assessment

- Euthyroid of pregnancy
- R/O Hypothyroidism
- R/O Hyperthyroidism
- R/O Thyroid mass

Plan

Diagnostic Tests

- TSH--will be WNL (should be less than 8 units/ml).

- T_3 resin uptake--decreased

- T_4 (Total)--increased

- T_4 (Free)--WNL (unchanged from nonpregnant levels)

Treatment/Management

- No treatment is indicated in euthyroid of pregnancy.

Consultation

- MD consultation is indicated in patients who are being evaluated for thyroid disease.

Patient Education

- Educate the patient regarding the tests that are being ordered.

- Discuss laboratory test results when they are obtained.

- Reassure the patient that this physical finding is very common during pregnancy and that it does not have any associated adverse effects on the mother or her infant.

Follow-up

- Routine prenatal follow-up visits are indicated unless thyroid disease is diagnosed.

- Document in problem list and progress notes.

HYPERTHYROIDISM

Hyperthyroidism is a disorder that occurs when there has been a chronic elevation of free thyroid hormone levels resulting in overstimulation of the basal metabolism (Mestman, 1985). This clinical syndrome is usually evident before a woman becomes pregnant, but initial episodes can occur during pregnancy. The most common cause of hyperthyroidism during pregnancy is Grave's disease, an autoimmune disorder (Abrams, 1989; Mestman, 1985). Other less common etiologies include toxic adenoma, multinodular goiter, viral thyroiditis, gestational trophoblastic neoplasia (GTN), iodine-induced hyperthyroidism, and hyperthyroxemia due to hyperemesis gravidarum (Abrams, 1989; Mestman, 1985).

Hyperthyroidism during pregnancy has been associated with an increased incidence of intrauterine growth retardation (IUGR) and low birth weight infants (Abrams, 1989; Mestman, 1985; Palmer, 1986). Neonatal hypothyroidism and goiter can result if large doses of antithyroid medications plus iodine therapy are used to treat maternal hyperthyroidism (Abrams, 1989; Mestman, 1985). Careful monitoring of maternal thyroid function tests (TFTs) and minimal doses of antithyroid medications have decreased the incidence of neonatal hypothyroidism. Monitoring of maternal TFTs should continue during the postpartum period, because there is an increased risk of thyroid storm occurring after delivery (Abrams, 1989; Mestman, 1985).

Data Base

Subjective

- May report a personal or family history of thyroid disease

- May report unintentional weight loss, palpitations, anxiety, fatigue, excessive perspiration, heat intolerance, diarrhea, muscle weakness, difficulty concentrating

Objective

- Weight--may be significantly less than expected for height and reported dietary intake

- Pulse--greater than 100 beats per minute at rest and will not decrease with a valsalva maneuver

- Thyroid gland--palpation may reveal a diffusely enlarged (2-5 times normal size), firm, non-tender thyroid.

- Auscultation over thyroid gland--may reveal a bruit.

- Hyperreflexia

- Pre-tibial edema

- Hair may feel fine and appear to be thinning.

- Plummer's nails (onycholysis)--loosening/detachment of the nails from the nailbeds may be observed.

- Skin may be warm and dry.

- Speech may be rapid and/or excited.

- Fundal height measurement--may be less than expected for gestation weeks.

- Tremors may be observed.

Assessment

- Enlarged thyroid--probably hyperthyroidism
- R/O Thyroid cancer
- R/O GTN
- R/O IUGR

Plan

Diagnostic Tests

- TSH--may be within normal limits (WNL) or decreased.
- Total T$_3$--increased
- Total T$_4$--increased
- Thyroid binding globulins--WNL
- Free T$_3$ index (FT$_3$I)--increased
- Free T$_4$ index (FT$_4$I)--increased
- Alkaline phosphatase--may be increased above the usual elevation expected during pregnancy.
- Microsomal antibodies--may be present in low titers.
- Ultrasonography--may reveal IUGR.
- Thyroid stimulating immunoglobulin (TSI) may be present in patients with Grave's disease and has been associated with transient neonatal thyrotoxicosis.

Treatment/Management

- MD consultation is indicated in patients who are being evaluated for thyroid disease. Refer to MD care patients who are diagnosed with hyperthyroidism.
- Treatment options for the patient with hyperthyroidism will be determined by the MD managing her care.

Consultation

- Consultation with an MD is mandatory in all suspected cases of hyperthyroidism.

Patient Education

- Education of the patient should include information regarding the possible cause(s) of the enlarged thyroid, the diagnostic tests that have been ordered and their results, the reason for fetal surveillance tests (if ordered), and the reason for consultation/referral to MD care.
- Treatment options, risks, side effects, and possible fetal/neonatal effects should be discussed with patient--ideally this should be done by the MD managing her care.
- Indications for neonatal thyroid function testing should be presented by the MD managing the patient's care and/or the pediatrician who will be caring for the infant after birth.
- Information regarding the signs and symptoms of thyroid storm and the possibility of its occurrence postpartum should be presented to the patient--ideally the MD managing her care should do this.

- The patient should be instructed about the possibility of breastfeeding while on antithyroid medications: if propylthiouracil is used, breastfeeding is possible, but if methimnazole is used, breastfeeding is contraindicated.

Follow-up

- Follow-up evaluations determined by the MD managing the patient's case
- Document in problem list and progress notes.

HYPOTHYROIDISM

Hypothyroidism is a deficiency in thyroid secretion resulting in a decreased basal metabolic rate. Hypothyroidism can be caused by an iodine deficiency, antithyroid medications, destruction of the gland (due to surgery or radioactive iodine), or Hashimoto's thyroiditis (Abrams, 1989). Although menstrual irregularities and anovulation are common problems in hypothyroid women, this does not preclude the possibility of conception. Many cases of documented hypothyroidism in pregnant women have been reported; however, these women usually reported very few symptoms of the disorder (Mestman, 1985). Since fetal and maternal thyroid functioning are independent of one another, there is no increased incidence of intellectual or physical abnormalities noted in infants who are born to hypothyroid mothers (Mestman, 1985).

Data Base

Subjective

- May report a personal or family history of thyroid disease

- May be asymptomatic

- May report fatigue, obesity, thinning of eyebrows/hair, facial or periorbital edema, thickened or coarse skin, numbness/ tingling of fingers, cold intolerance, constipation

Objective

- Excessive weight gain

- Pulse--decreased

- Dry skin (xerosis)

- Loss of hair from outer third of the eyebrows

- Exopthalmosis

- Goiter--may or may not be present.

- Deep tendon reflexes--delayed relaxation phase

- Dry, coarse-feeling hair

Assessment

- Possible hypothyroidism

- R/O Euthyroid of pregnancy

- R/O Thyroid mass

- Xerosis

Plan

Diagnostic Tests

- TSH--increased

- Free T_4 index--decreased

- AST or SGOT--may be slightly increased.

- ALT or SGPT--may be slightly increased.

- Serum cholesterol--may be elevated.

- CPK--may be elevated.

- Antimicrosomal and antithyroglobulin antibodies--elevated titers in patient's with autoimmune thyroiditis

Treatment/Management

- MD consultation is indicated in patients who are being evaluated for thyroid disease. MD management of a patient's thyroid disease is warranted.

- Thyroid replacement therapy should be determined by the MD consultant.

- Co-management by NP/NM/MD of patients responding to thyroid replacement therapy is possible.

Consultation

- Consultation with an MD is mandatory in all suspected cases of hypothyroidism.

Patient Education

- Education of the patient should include information regarding the possible diagnosis, the diagnostic tests ordered and their results (when available), and the reason for consultation with an MD. The need for repeat TFTs once thyroid replacement therapy has started should be explained to the patient.

- Reassure the patient regarding the lack of association between maternal hypothyroidism and any adverse fetal/neonatal effects.

- Discussion of any possible side effects of thyroid replacement therapy should be initiated by the MD managing the patient's hypothyroidism.

Follow-up

- Routine prenatal visits with NP/NM can continue as long as the patient is responding to thyroid replacement therapy.

- Follow-up evaluations and repeat TFTs to monitor thyroid replacement therapy should be determined by the MD managing the patient's hypothyroidism.

- Document in problem list and progress notes.

TRANSIENT POSTPARTUM THYROID DYSFUNCTION
(POSTPARTUM THYROIDITIS)

Transient postpartum thyroid dysfunction (postpartum thyroiditis) is a recently recognized autoimmune disorder occurring in 5-10% of pregnancies (Affonso, Andreyko, & Mills, 1987; Mestman, 1985). It is characterized by the development of hyperthyroidism approximately 3-4 weeks after birth and lasts for up to 4 months postpartum. This phase is followed by hypothyroidism and may last from 1-3 months. This disorder spontaneously regresses in 90% of patients, but may recur with a more protracted course in subsequent pregnancies. Pharmacologic therapy may be indicated in patients with clinical symptoms and laboratory evidence of hypothyroidism. It is important to recognize this disorder because its symptoms are often overlooked or dismissed as being the "expected" manifestations of a woman's psychological and physiologic adjustments during the initial postpartum months.

Data Base

Subjective

- Hyperthyroid Phase: see subjective section of Hyperthyroid protocol.

- Hypothyroid Phase: see subjective section of Hypothyroid protocol.

Objective

- Hyperthyroid Phase: see objective section of Hyperthyroid protocol.

- Hypothyroid Phase: see objective section of Hypothyroid protocol.

Assessment

- Transient postpartum thyroid dysfunction (postpartum thyroiditis)

- R/O Grave's disease

- R/O Postpartum depression

- R/O Sheehan's syndrome

Plan

Diagnostic Tests

- Hyperthyroid Phase: see diagnostic tests listed in hyperthyroid protocol.

  - Thyroid antimicrosomal antibody--titer is greater than 1:100 in approximately 50% of patients (Affonso et al., 1987).

- Hypothyroid Phase: see diagnostic tests listed in Hypothyroid protocol.

Treatment/Management

- Consultation with an MD is indicated when a patient is suspected of having transient postpartum thyroid dysfunction.

- Pharmacologic therapy of a patient is determined by the MD consultant.

- Repeat thyroid function tests (TFTs) should be done for two years postpartum. Appropriate intervals for these tests should be determined by the MD consultant.

Consultation

- Consultation with an MD is warranted for all patients who are suspected of having transient postpartum thyroid dysfunction.

Patient Education

- Eduction of the patient should include information regarding the possible cause(s) of her symptoms, the diagnostic tests ordered, and their results (when available).

- When the diagnosis of transient postpartum thyroiditis has been made, the patient should be educated regarding the course of the disorder, its possible treatments (if indicated), the likelihood that it will subside spontaneously and that it may recur following future births.

- Reassure the patient regarding the validity of her symptoms and inform her that no untoward long-term effects of this disorder are known (at this time).

Follow-up

- Follow-up evaluations of patients diagnosed with this disorder should be determined by the MD consultant.

- Document in problem list and progress notes.

TRIAL OF LABOR/VAGINAL BIRTH AFTER CESAREAN SECTION

Lisa L. Lommel

In the recent past, women who had a previous cesarean section were advised to have a repeat cesarean. This practice was encouraged out of fear of uterine rupture during subsequent labor. This belief prevented health care providers from offering a trial of labor and vaginal birth after cesarean (VBAC). It is currently believed that the risk of VBAC had been overestimated, and the trend toward trial of labor is now increasing.

The incidence of cesarean section in the United States is close to twenty-five percent of all deliveries. Approximately one-third of all cesarean operations are conducted as a repeat cesarean delivery (Martin, Morrison, & Wiser, 1988). The risk of uterine scar separation or rupture during labor is relatively low after a previous low-transverse incision (0.24 to 0.6 percent). The perinatal mortality rate in monitored patients undergoing a trial of labor is approximately 0.5 per 1,000 women (Martin et al., 1988). There has been no maternal deaths associated with rupture of low-transverse uterine scar for almost 60 years (Martin et al., 1988).

In contrast to the lower-uterine segment incision, a previous classic incision puts the women at significant risk for uterine rupture (4% incidence) (Haq, 1988). Because of this, one of the few consistent absolute contraindications to vaginal birth after cesarean is a prior classic incision (ACOG, 1988).

In 1982, 1985, and most recently in 1988, the American College of Obstetricians and Gynecologists Committee on Obstetrics: Maternal and Fetal Medicine formulated *Guidelines for Vaginal Delivery After a Previous Cesarean Birth*. The report recommends that women with one previous cesarean delivery and a low-transverse scar should be counseled to attempt VBAC. In addition, women with two or more previous caesareans (with low-transverse scar) may also attempt VBAC. Outlined are absolute contraindications including a known or strongly suspected classic uterine incision and patient refusal following full discussion and disclosure.

In properly selected patients, careful management of vaginal birth after cesarean entails less maternal and fetal risk than the risks associated with an elective repeat cesarean delivery.

Data Base

Subjective

- History of previous cesarean section(s) with low-transverse uterine incision
- Pregnant woman desires VBAC

Objective

- Data review to rule out inaccurate dating
- Fetal size, position, and presentation
- Pelvic size and adequacy
- Documentation of previous low-transverse scar from medical records

234

- No contraindications for vaginal delivery

Assessment

- Woman with previous low-transverse cesarean section desires VBAC
- Uterine size equal to dates
- No contraindications for vaginal delivery

Plan

Diagnostic Tests

- Obtain ultrasound as early as possible in the pregnancy to confirm dates.
- Electronic fetal monitoring during labor

Treatment/Management

- Discuss option for trial of labor in patients who meet criteria for VBAC.
- Initiate fetal movement counts at 28 weeks. See Fetal Movement Count protocol.
- Continue routine prenatal care.
- Electronic fetal monitoring in labor
- Availability of emergency cesarean delivery within 30 minutes from the time the decision is made until the surgical procedure is begun (ACOG, 1988)

Consultation

- MD consultation may be required to confirm eligibility for trial of labor.

Patient Education

- Explain the risks and benefit of VBAC to the patient and her partner.
- Encourage the patient and her partner to attend VBAC classes and become informed about VBAC.
- Explain what they may expect during labor including electronic fetal monitoring.
- Discuss situations that may necessitate a repeat cesarean delivery.

Follow-up

- Routine 6 week postpartum visit.
- Document that the patient is to undergo a trial of labor in progress notes and problem list.

Chapter 5

Hematologic Disorders

of Pregnancy

ABO INCOMPATIBILITY/IRREGULAR ANTIBODIES

Lisa L. Lommel

There are four major blood groups that belong to the ABO blood group system. These are blood group types A, B, AB, and O. Red blood cells have either antigen A, B, AB, or no antigen on the surface of their cells. Type A blood has A antigen, B has B antigen, AB has A and B antigens, and O contains no antigen. The antigens are all capable of inducing antibody production in an individual who does not have that antigen.

The mechanism by which ABO blood incompatibility occurs is the same as Rh erythroblastosis fetalis (see Rh Isoimmunization protocol). Unlike Rh isoimmunization, 40% to 50% of ABO incompatibilities occur in first-born infants. ABO incompatibility provides partial protection to Rh isoimmunization in the Rh-negative woman. Although not well understood, the mechanism is thought to involve the removal of fetal red blood cells from the maternal circulation at a faster rate and lowering the effective dose of antigen (Cook, 1982).

ABO incompatibility occurs in approximately 20% of all pregnancies. The majority of these cases are in blood group O mothers carrying a group A or B fetus. The group O mother has naturally occurring anti-A and anti-B antibodies in her blood that may cause fetal hemolysis. Because anti-A and anti-B antibodies do not readily pass from the mother to fetus, less than 10% of ABO incompatible pregnancies actually develop hemolytic disease which is never severe enough to cause fetal death. There is no definitive diagnostic test available for prenatal diagnosis of ABO incompatibility. The direct Coombs test (antibody screen) may be positive or negative and maternal antibodies are variable.

ABO hemolytic disease usually presents within 24 hours after birth with jaundice and variable elevation of the indirect bilirubin. Management of ABO hemolytic disease in the newborn (HDN) includes bilirubin surveillance and phototherapy. Exchange transfusion is necessary in only 1% of cases and serious fetal sequelae is extremely rare (Durfee, 1987).

Irregular antibodies occur in 1% to 2% of all pregnancies and are responsible for approximately 5% of hemolytic disease of the newborn (Barss, Frigoletto, & Konugres, 1988). The pathogenesis, management, and sequelae of HDN caused by irregular antibodies is similar to Rh erythroblastosis fetalis (see Rh Isoimmunization protocol). Sources of sensitization are also similar to those of the Rh antigen (i.e., fetal blood and/or transfused blood). The major difference from Rh disease is the involvement of both IgG and IgM class antibodies. The IgG antibodies readily cross the placenta allowing fetal antigen to enter the maternal blood circulation resulting in varying degrees of erythroblastosis fetalis which can lead to fetal death. The IgM antibodies do not cross the placenta, posing no threat to the fetus and requiring no follow-up. Table 5.1, *Hemolytic Disease Due to Irregular Antibodies* (pp. 242-243) outlines the known irregular antigens associated with HDN and the grade of severity of the disease caused by each antigen.

Data Base

Subjective

- Asymptomatic with ABO incompatibility
- Asymptomatic with irregular antibodies

Objective

- ABO incompatibility
  - Most often a blood type O mother
- Irregular antibodies
  - Positive antibody screen for irregular antibodies
  - If maternal screen is positive for antibody capable of causing HDN, document presence or absence of antigen in father of the baby.

Assessment

- ABO incompatibility
  - Rh-positive or Rh-negative mother with ABO incompatibility
- Irregular antibodies
  - Rh-positive or Rh-negative mother with irregular antibody
  - Irregular antibody not proven to cause HDN
  - Irregular antibody capable of causing HDN
    - father of baby negative or positive to the antigen

Plan

Diagnostic Tests

- Blood type, Rh type, and antibody screen at first prenatal visit on all patients.
- No specific tests available to detect ABO incompatibility prenatally.
- If the initial antibody screen is negative in Rh positive patients, a repeat antibody screen in later pregnancy is not usually recommended.
- Repeat antibody screen at 26-27 weeks gestation in Rh-negative women.
- If antibody screen is positive, the antibody should be identified by the laboratory.
- Obtain blood type and screen for the antigen in the father if the woman is positive for an antibody capable of causing HDN.

Treatment/Management

- Women with antibodies not proven to cause HDN require no further management except for type and crossmatch in labor (compatible blood may be difficult to find).
- Women with antibodies capable of causing HDN, with a father who is antigen negative for that specific antibody, require no further management.
- Women with antibodies capable of causing HDN, with a father who is positive for that specific antigen should be managed by amniotic fluid analysis and not by indirect Coombs titers. Coombs titers do not always correlate with fetal status and neonatal outcome (ACOG, 1986).

Consultation

- Refer to MD if patient has irregular antibody capable of causing HDN and the father is positive for that specific antigen. These patients may be candidates for Percutaneous Umbilical Blood Sampling (PUBS).

Patient Education

- If the mother is blood type O:

  - Explain the etiology and risk of ABO incompatibility.

  - Explain the process of HDN and management/treatment plans for the newborn after delivery.

- If the patient is antibody screen positive:

  - Give her a card identifying her Rh type, blood type, and irregular antibody.

  - Advise the patient to alert health care providers of her antibody status in the event of future pregnancies or blood transfusion.

  - Explain the risks for the fetus and management plans for the pregnancy.

  - Explain the importance of screening the father of the baby.

  - Discuss the meaning of a positive maternal and paternal antibody screen on subsequent pregnancies.

Follow-up

- Assure that the infant has adequate medical follow-up after delivery.

- Document in progress notes and problem list.

Table 5.1

Hemolytic Disease Due to Irregular Antibodies

Blood Group System	Antigens Related to Hemolytic Disease	Severity of Hemolytic Disease	Proposed Management
Lewis	Not a proved cause of hemolytic disease of the newborn		
I	Not a proved cause of hemolytic disease of the newborn		
Kell	K	Mild to severe with hydrops fetalis	Amniotic fluid bilirubin studies
	k	Mild	Expectant
	Ko	Mild	Expectant
	Kp^a	Mild	Expectant
	Kp^b	Mild	Expectant
	Js^a	Mild	Expectant
	Js^b	Mild	Expectant
Duffy	Fy^a	Mild to severe with hydrops fetalis	Amniotic fluid bilirubin studies
	Fy^b Not a cause of hemolytic disease of the newborn		
	Fy^3	Mild	Expectant
Kidd	Jk^a	Mild to severe	Amniotic fluid bilirubin studies
	Jk^b	Mild to severe	Amniotic fluid bilirubin studies
	Jk^3	Mild	Expectant
MNSs	M	Mild to severe	Amniotic fluid bilirubin studies
	N	Mild	Expectant
	S	Mild to severe	Amniotic fluid bilirubin studies
	s	Mild to severe	Amniotic fluid bilirubin studies
	U	Mild to severe	Amniotic fluid bilirubin studies
	Mi^a	Moderate	Amniotic fluid bilirubin studies
	Mt^a	Moderate	Amniotic fluid bilirubin studies
	Vw	Mild	Expectant
	Mur	Mild	Expectant
	Hil	Mild	Expectant
	Hut	Mild	Expectant
Lutheran	Lu^a	Mild	Expectant
	Lu^b	Mild	Expectant
Diego	Di^a	Mild to severe	Amniotic fluid bilirubin studies
	Di^b	Mild to severe	Amniotic fluid bilirubin studies
Xg	Xg^a	Mild	Expectant
P	$PP_1P^k(Tj^a)$	Mild to severe	Amniotic fluid bilirubin studies

Table 5.1 (continued)

Blood Group System	Antigens Related to Hemolytic Disease	Severity of Hemolytic Disease	Proposed Management
Public antigens	Yt^a	Moderate to severe	Amniotic fluid bilirubin studies
	Yt^b	Mild	Expectant
	Lan	Mild	Expectant
	En^a	Moderate	Amniotic fluid bilirubin studies
	Ge	Mild	Expectant
	Jr^a	Mild	Expectant
	Co^a	Severe	Amniotic fluid bilirubin studies
	Co^{a-b-}	Mild	Expectant
Private antigens	Batty	Mild	Expectant
	Becker	Mild	Expectant
	Berrens	Mild	Expectant
	Biles	Moderate	Amniotic fluid bilirubin studies
	Evans	Mild	Expectant
	Golzales	Mild	Expectant
	Good	Severe	Amniotic fluid bilirubin studies
	Heibel	Moderate	Amniotic fluid bilirubin studies
	Hunt	Mild	Expectant
	Jobbins	Mild	Expectant
	Radin	Moderate	Amniotic fluid bilirubin studies
	Rm	Mild	Expectant
	Ven	Mild	Expectant
	Wright^a	Severe	Amniotic fluid bilirubin studies
	Wright^b	Mild	Expectant
	Zd	Moderate	Amniotic fluid bilirubin studies

SOURCE:

Weinstein, L. (1982). Irregular antibodies causing hemolytic disease of the newborn: A continuing problem. *Clinical Obstetrics and Gynecology, 25* (2), 321-329. Reprinted with permission.

ALPHA THALASSEMIA

Winifred L. Star

The major normal adult hemoglobin, Hb A, is made up of 2 alpha and 2 beta globin chains. Minor adult hemoglobin, Hb A$_2$, is composed of 2 alpha and 2 delta globin chains. A small percentage of adult hemoglobin is Hb F or fetal hemoglobin which is composed of 2 alpha and 2 gamma globin chains. Normally each individual has 4 functioning alpha globin genes, 2 from each parent.

Alpha thalassemia syndromes are genetic disorders affecting the production of the alpha globin chains of normal hemoglobin. There are four possible states: silent carrier (one gene deletion), alpha thalassemia minor or trait (2 gene deletion), Hb H disease (3 gene deletion) or alpha thalassemia major (4 gene deletion). Silent carrier state is undetectable without specialized DNA studies. No clinical or hematologic abnormality will exist in this state. Individuals with alpha thalassemia trait have benign lifelong mild microcytic, hypochromic anemia with no clinical disease. Alpha thalassemia trait may coexist with a beta globin chain abnormality without adversely affecting (and occasionally improving) the clinical picture (e.g., sickle/alpha thalassemia). Hb H disease results in a chronic moderately severe hemolytic anemia. An enlarged liver or spleen and gallstones may develop. The anemia may become more severe in pregnancy and with infections. Alpha thalassemia major is incompatible with life. Hydrops fetalis with fetal or neonatal death will occur. To date, no cases of hydrops fetalis have been identified in the black population (Wintrobe, 1981). The location on the chromosome of the alpha gene deletion in blacks precludes the development of alpha thalassemia major.

Countries in which alpha thalassemia is prevalent include: China, the Philippines, Malaysia, Thailand, Cambodia, Laos, Vietnam, Burma, India and Sri Lanka. African and American blacks also may have certain forms of this hemoglobinopathy.

Data Base

Subjective

- Asymptomatic

- Patient may have awareness of abnormal lab results in past.

- With Hb H disease may have complaints related to hepatosplenomegaly and/or gallstones

- Ancestry indicative of prevalence of alpha thalassemia

Objective   (See Table 5.2, *Laboratory Values in Selected Anemias or Hemoglobinopathies*, p. 248)

Alpha thalassemia trait

- Hemoglobin normal or decreased

- RBC count normal or increased

- MCV below 80 fl (microcytosis)

- MCH below 26 pg (hypochromia)

- Mentzer index (MCV/RBC) usually less than l3

- Hemoglobin electrophoresis normal (normal A, A_2, and F) unless concomitant beta globin chain abnormality or Hb H disease

- Red cell morphology shows microcytosis, hypochromia, and aniso/poikilocytosis.

- Iron studies normal unless coexistent iron deficiency

- With concomitant sickle cell trait hemoglobin electrophoresis shows A and S bands of hemoglobin but % of S is less than with sickle cell trait alone; MCV is below 80.

Hemoglobin H Disease

- Hemoglobin in 7-10 gm/dl range

- MCV <80 fl

- MCH <26 pg

- Reticulocytes 5-10%

- Peripheral blood smear shows small misshapen red cells, microcytosis, hypochromia, and targeting.

- Hemoglobin electrophoresis of fresh blood shows 5-30% Hb H; or when blood incubated with Brilliant Cresyl Blue Stain, multiple small inclusions form in the red cell.

- Hb A_2 decreased

- Hb Bart's may be present in small amounts.

- Hepatosplenomegaly and/or gallstones or occasionally a more serious clinical picture (e.g., transfusion-dependent hemoglobinopathy)

- Disorder is mild in blacks.

Assessment

- R/O Alpha thalassemia trait (diagnosis of exclusion with normal A2, F, and iron studies)

- R/O Hb H disease

- R/O Coexistent iron deficiency anemia

- R/O Concomitant hemoglobinopathy

- R/O Hemoglobinopathy in father of baby

Plan

Diagnostic Tests (See Figure 5.1, *Evaluation of Microcytosis*, p. 249)

- CBC: MCV <80 fl, MCH <26 pg

- Hemoglobin electrophoresis with quantitative A_2 and F will be WNL (except in Hb H disease A_2 may be decreased).

- Serum iron and total iron binding capacity (TIBC) or ferritin to R/O iron deficiency. Serum iron/TIBC should be above 16% saturation or ferritin should be within normal limits if patient is not iron deficient.

- If hemoglobin, hematocrit, MCV, and MCH are extremely low, order a Brilliant Cresyl Blue dye study on freshly drawn blood to R/O Hb H disease.

NOTE: Hb H is a very unstable hemoglobin and precipitates rapidly; therefore electrophoresis and dye study must be done quickly on fresh blood samples. Lab should be notified prior to ordering of these tests to allow for appropriate set-up.

- If couple is non-black and mother has alpha thalassemia trait or Hb H disease, screen father of baby with CBC and hemoglobin electrophoresis with quantitative A_2 and F.

Treatment/Management

- No treatment for silent carrier state or alpha thalassemia trait.

- With Hb H disease anemia usually becomes worse in pregnancy (Hb may decrease to 4-5 gm/dl) therefore transfusion may be necessary.

- If coexistent iron deficiency anemia, treat according to protocol.

Consultation

- None required in alpha thalassemia trait with mild anemia

- Required for severe anemia (Hb below 10.0 gm/dl; Hct below 30%); consider MD referral or co-management.

- Required for Hb H disease; consider MD referral or co-management especially if anemia worsens in pregnancy.

Patient Education

- Stress importance of screening father of baby in non-black couples.

- If diagnosis of alpha thalassemia trait is made, discuss disorder and prenatal implications:

    - In Asian populations when both parents have alpha thalassemia trait, there is a 25% (1:4) chance that the fetus will be affected with alpha thalassemia major. This condition is amenable to prenatal diagnosis.

    - In the black population because of the location on the chromosomes of the absent genes in alpha thalassemia trait, there is no threat of alpha thalassemia major in the offspring when both parents have the trait.

- Discuss the possibility of blood transfusion for patients with severe anemia.

- "Designated donor" issues should be addressed. It has been shown that blood from a family member or friend is in general **not** as safe as blood from blood bank donors. Directed donors have more laboratory evidence of disease than blood bank volunteers and may not confess their ineligibility as blood donors when asked to donate by a friend or family member. Blood from the father of the baby may cause severe reactions when transfused to the mother because the mother may have been immunized to the father's gene products through pregnancy. First degree relative transfusions may (rarely) cause a fatal graft vs host reaction. In the instance of first degree relative donor-transfusion the blood is first irradiated to prevent this complication (Irwin Memorial Blood Bank, 1990). Check with local blood bank for particulars on designated donor procedures.

- Other information regarding transfusion includes: AIDS transmission via blood transfusion has been reduced to one in 50,000, hepatitis to one in 200 (chronic liver disease follows in 50% of cases, 20 of these will go on to cirrhosis); other rare causes of transfusion-related infection include malaria, syphilis and others; chills, fever, and/or hives occur in 2-3% of transfusions; more serious reactions which may result in shock or death are rare (Irwin Memorial Blood Bank, 1990).

Follow-up

- Refer to genetic counselor if father of baby also has hemoglobinopathy and couple is non-black.

- Genetics referral is advised when patient/couple desire(s) comprehensive education about the disorder.

- In coexistent iron deficiency, iron supplements should be continued for at least three months postpartum.

- Document in progress notes and problem list.

Table 5.2

Laboratory Values in Selected Anemias or Hemoglobinopathies

Type of Anemia

Factor	Iron Deficiency	Folic Acid Deficiency	Alpha Thalassemia	Beta Thalassemia	Sickle Cell Trait	G6PD Deficiency
Hb	↓	↓	↓	↓	Nl	↓
Hct	↓	↓	↓	↓	Nl	↓
RBC	↓	↓	Nl or ↑	Nl or ↑	Nl	↓
MCV	*Nl or ↓	↑	↓	↓	Nl	Nl
MCH	Nl or ↓	Nl or ↓	↓	↓	Nl	Nl
MCHC	Nl or ↓	Nl or ↓	↓	↓	Nl	Nl
Retic	Nl or ↑	Nl	Nl	Nl	Nl	Nl
Serum Fe	↓	Nl	Nl	Nl	Nl	Nl
TIBC	↑	Nl	Nl	Nl	Nl	Nl
Other findings	Iron saturation 16% or less; ferritin ↓	Folate ↓	Iron saturation greater than 16%; Nl Hb A & F; positive family history	Iron saturation greater than 16%; ↑Hb A₂; positive family history	Electrophoresis positive for S band, sickledex positive; positive family history	Bilirubin ↑

*Nl = normal

SOURCE:

Adapted from: Paterson, K. A. (1986). In J. D. Neeson & K. A. May (Eds.), *Comprehensive maternity nursing* (p. 502). Philadelphia: J. B. Lippincott Co. Reprinted with permission.

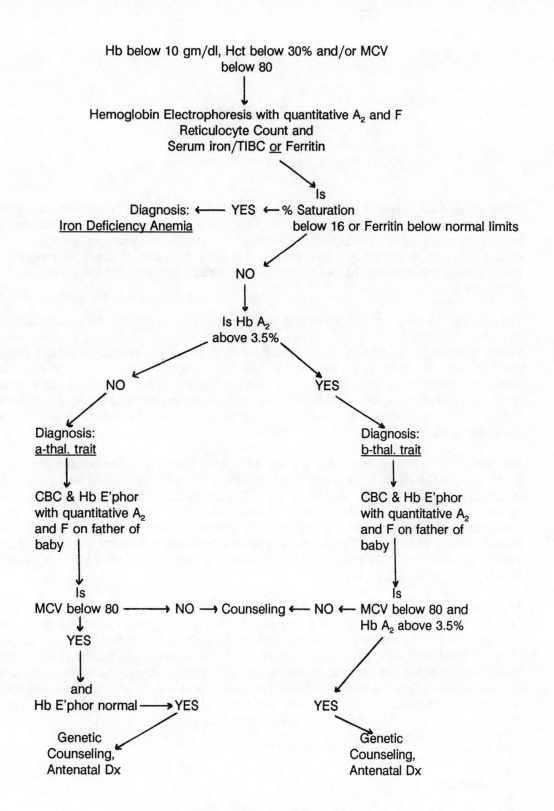

Figure 5.1. Evaluation of Microcytosis

SOURCE: Adapted from: Laros, R. K., & Golbus, M. S. (1977). Prenatal diagnosis of thalassemia trait. *University of Michigan Medical Center Journal, 43*(23). Reprinted with permission.

ANEMIA

Winifred L. Star

Anemia exists when there is a decrease in the amount of hemoglobin necessary to maintain the normal requirements of tissues for oxygen (Harvey, 1980). The World Health Organization defines anemia in pregnancy as a hemoglobin of less than 11.0 gm/dl. A hematocrit less than 31% is also indicative of anemia. Diagnostic classification of anemia is dependent upon the pathophysiologic mechanism responsible for the cell defect (Lubkin, 1982). This protocol will cover iron or folate deficiency anemia.

The status of pre-pregnant iron stores and the inadequacy of the average American diet contribute to an iron deficient state in many women. In pregnancy, the majority of true anemias are caused by iron deficiency. The total iron requirement during pregnancy is approximately 800 mg with the greatest need occurring during the second half due to increased red blood cell mass and the demands of the growing fetus. Despite increased gastrointestinal absorption in the latter trimesters, an unsupplemented diet will not provide more than one to two thirds of the normal requirements for iron. The recommended supplemental intake is 30-60 mg elemental iron/day (National Academy of Sciences, National Research Council, 1989).

Hemodilutional effects of pregnancy account for normal lowering of hemoglobin and hematocrit (H/H) values. Expansion of intravascular volume starts at 6 weeks gestation, peaks at about 28-34 weeks, and plateaus to term. Red blood cell (RBC) production increases at about 12 weeks and continues throughout pregnancy. Plasma volume (PV) expansion is faster and greater than RBC production with a resultant lowering of H/H. This is often termed "physiological anemia". Because of the individual variation in PV expansion true **anemia** is difficult to evaluate. A number of pregnant women with iron deficiency anemia will have lower PV expansions and their H/H will remain in the normal range (Dimperio, 1988).

The incidence of folate deficiency in the U.S. is 0.5-15% depending on the population (Biswas & Perloff, 1987). Three to four percent of women with anemia in pregnancy have a megaloblastic type secondary to folate deficiency. Cooking habits of the average American lead to the extreme loss of this nutrient from food; poor absorption of the vitamin is rare. Any condition which creates a folate demand above that required for normal pregnancy (e.g., sickle cell anemia) adds to the risk of folate deficiency anemia. Folate deficiency anemia is most likely to be revealed in late pregnancy or postpartum (Anderson, 1989). The recommended daily allowance is 800 mcg/day in pregnancy (National Academy of Sciences, National Research Council, 1989).

Data Base

Subjective

Risk factors

- Low socioeconomic status
- Underweight status
- Adolescence
- Multiparity (>5)

- Closely spaced pregnancies (<2 years birth - conception)
- Multiple gestation
- Cesarean section in prior pregnancy
- Major surgery in last year
- Chronic infectious process
- Malabsorptive state
- Blood loss
- Parasitic infection (except pinworms)
- Poor weight gain
- Inadequate nutritional intake of iron or folate-rich foods or supplements
- Vegetarian diet
- Pica
- Alcohol abuse

Symptomatology Patient may be asymptomatic or may complain of:

- Fatigue
- Weakness
- Irritability
- Nausea/vomiting
- Anorexia
- Dysphagia
- Low grade fever
- Exertional dyspnea or chest pain
- Increased heart rate
- Vertigo
- Syncope
- Visual disturbances
- Headaches
- Confusion
- Loss of concentration
- Increased need for sleep
- Loss of libido
- Paresthesias
- Cold-intolerance
- Tinnitus
- Food cravings (pica)
- Brittle nails

- Changes in bowel habits
- Sore tongue
- Weight loss

Obstetrical Complications Associated with Anemia

- Intrauterine growth retardation
- Abruptio placenta
- Pre-eclampsia/eclampsia
- Neural tube defects
- Preterm delivery
- Stillbirth
- Neonatal death
- Delayed wound healing

Objective   (See Table 5.2, *Laboratory Values in Selected Anemias or Hemoglobinopathies*, p. 248)

- Physical exam may reveal the following:
  - Skin: pallor
  - Hair: thin, brittle
  - Nails: brittle, ridging, koilonychia (spoon-shape)
  - Mouth/lips: cheilosis, glossitis
  - Heart: tachycardia, systolic heart murmur
  - Abdomen: splenomegaly (rare)
- Normal laboratory values - University of California laboratory.
  - Hemoglobin 12.0 - 16.0 gm/dl
  - Hematocrit 36 - 46%
  - Red blood cell count 4.0 - 5.2 million/mml
  - Red cell indices:

    MCV 80 - 100 fl

    MCH 26 - 34 pg

    MCHC 31 - 36 gm/dl
  - Reticulocytes 0.5 - 1.5% (or 33-137 K/mcl)
  - Ferritin 5 - 99 ng/ml
  - Transferrin 216 - 399 mg/dl
  - Serum iron (SI) 40 - 150 mcg/dl
  - Folate, RBC 165 - 170 ng/ml
  - Total iron binding capacity (TIBC) 300 - 450 mg/dl
  - SI/TIBC = greater than 16% saturation

- Hemoglobin electrophoresis:
  HbA = 95%
  HbA_2 = 3%
  HbF = 2%

- Laboratory changes consistent with anemia include the following:

  - Decreased H/H

  - MCV between 70-79 fl in iron deficiency; usually >110 fl in folate deficiency (macrocytosis may however be masked by iron deficiency/thalassemia)

  - Platelets may be normal, decreased or increased

  - Reticulocytes may be slightly increased or normal in iron deficiency

  - SI is reduced (<50 mcg/dl) and TIBC is increased (>400 mcg/dl) in iron deficiency

  - SI/TIBC <16%; usually <10% in iron deficiency

  - Ferritin <10 ng/ml in iron deficiency

  - Serum folate <165 ng/ml in folate deficiency

  - Peripheral red blood smear: in iron deficient states may see microcytosis, hypochromia, polychromatophilia, basophilia, poikilocytosis, anisocytosis, and target cells
    NOTE: Lab values may vary slightly from one lab to another.

Assessment

- R/O Iron deficiency/folate deficiency anemia

- R/O Hemodilutional effect of pregnancy

- R/O Concomitant hemoglobinopathy

- R/O Other causes of anemia as indicated (e.g., bone marrow failure, spherocytosis, G6PD, blood loss, chronic infection, malabsorptive syndromes)

Plan

Diagnostic Tests   (See Table 5.2, *Laboratory Values in Selected Anemias or Hemoglobino-pathies*, p. 248 and Figure 5.1, *Evaluation of Microcytosis*, p. 249)

- For patients with hemoglobin less than 10 gm/dl, hematocrit less than 30%, and/or MCV less than 80 fl order reticulocyte count, hemoglobin electrophoresis with quantitative A_2 and F, SI and TIBC or ferritin.
  NOTE: Patient must be off iron for at least 24 hours prior to SI/TIBC. Ferritin levels may be drawn without reference to the time of the last iron ingestion.

- Calculate % saturation of SI/TIBC.

- If MCV above 80 fl order serum folate; may also consider ordering serum B_{12} if patient a strict vegetarian to R/O vitamin B_{12} deficiency (a rare condition).

Treatment/Management

- Prevention of anemic states includes routine early administration of prenatal vitamins and iron once a day.

NOTE: Iron is best absorbed on an empty stomach and without other minerals ingested at the same time. The presence of minerals in the prenatal vitamin may significantly impair iron absorption; therefore, supplemental iron should be given alone and at a different time from ingestion of the vitamin (Dimperio, 1988).

- The goal of therapy in iron deficiency anemia is to correct the nutrient deficit and replenish the stores. When iron deficiency is diagnosed, increase iron supplementation to three times a day.

- If not tolerated without food iron is best taken with meat, fish, poultry, or vitamin C-rich foods. Three forms of iron are available and vary according to the amount of elemental iron they provide:

  - Ferrous gluconate 320-325 mg (36 mg elemental iron)

  - Ferrous sulfate 300-325 mg (60 mg elemental iron)

  - Ferrous fumarate 200 mg (67 mg elemental iron)

- Parenteral iron therapy is rarely necessary. Its use should be strictly reserved for absolute contraindications to oral intake or proven failure of the oral route to correct the deficit (Anderson, 1989).

- If the H/H is in the low normal pregnancy range but all other indices are within normal limits, diet counseling and routine supplementation (one vitamin, one iron/day) is probably sufficient therapy. Patient probably has greater than average hemodilution (Dimperio, 1988).

- If H/H normal but other indices consistent with iron (or folate) deficiency the patient probably has hemoconcentration superimposed upon anemia and may benefit from appropriate supplementation (Dimperio, 1988).

- A low H/H in association with an elevated MCV is indicative of folic acid deficiency. The addition of folacin to a dose of 500 mcg - 1 mg is to be prescribed in folate deficient patients (Dimperio, 1988).

- Perform a 24-48 hour diet recall. Ideally, patient to be referred to a nutritionist.

- Nutritional counseling to include discussion of iron/folate rich foods: animal protein (liver, red meat), deep green leafy vegetables, fruits, iron-fortified cereals, dried peas and beans, seeds and nuts. Assess intake of substances which interfere with iron absorption such as milk, tea, spinach, and fiber-foods. See Nutrition protocol for additional information.

Consultation

- Required if patient fails to respond to iron/folate/vitamin supplementation and nutritional counseling.

- If hemoglobin remains below 10 gm/dl or hematocrit below 30%, patient may be referred to MD for further care or co-managed.

Patient Education

- Discuss implications of anemia and the rationale and importance of proper supplementation.

- Offer nutrition counseling as described above.

- Encourage good health maintenance.

- Discuss side effects of iron supplementation: nausea, constipation, diarrhea, black or tarry stool, skin rash, stained teeth from liquid iron.

- Warn patients to keep iron out of reach of children!

- For patients who are having difficulty tolerating iron supplements due to GI distress offer these suggestions: take after meals; crush tablet and add to food or a tasty drink; try liquid iron or time-released capsule; spread iron ingestion out over the course of the day. Provider should consider changing the form of iron (e.g., ferrous gluconate rather than ferrous sulfate) as indicated (Dimperio, 1988). A stool softener may be necessary for patients with severe constipation.

- Discuss possibility of blood transfusion for patients with severe anemia who may require replacement during delivery or in puerperium. See Alpha Thalassemia protocol for discussion of blood transfusion issues.

Follow-up

- As a general rule, repeat CBC and reticulocyte count in about 2-4 weeks after initiating therapy. (Hemoglobin will increase 7-10 days following therapy; the reticulocyte count will begin to increase after 5-7 days and will peak between 10-14 days.

- It is important to carefully assess how the patient is taking her supplements and if she is tolerating them.

- Patients not responding to therapy should be evaluated for other causes of anemia (e.g., hemoglobinopathies, chronic disease states, inflammatory process, blood loss, etc.).

- Additional routine labs should be ordered as indicated by return visit protocol.

- Patient should remain on therapeutic iron/folate supplements for 3-4 months postpartum to replenish iron/folate stores.

- Document in progress notes and problem list.

BETA THALASSEMIA

Winifred L. Star

Beta thalassemia is a hereditary condition characterized by decreased production or absence of the beta chains of hemoglobin, usually due to a mutation of the beta globin genes. Normally each individual has 2 functioning beta globin genes (one pair). One gene is inherited from each parent.

In beta thalassemia minor or trait (heterozygotic state), a person has one gene for the production of the usual amount of beta chains and one gene for a decreased amount. There are at least four different manifestations of beta thalassemia distinguishable by hemoglobin electrophoresis. Persons with the trait have a lifelong microcytic, hypochromic anemia which may be more pronounced in infancy and during pregnancy. Severe anemia is unusual, however, and if present iron or folate deficiency should be suspected. Mild to moderate splenomegaly occurs in one-third of cases of beta thalassemia trait (Bunn, Forget, & Ranney, 1977).

In beta thalassemia major or Cooley's anemia (homozygotic state) a person has two genes for decreased or absent production of beta chains. The clinical picture is more severe in the homozygotic state. Severe hemolytic anemia begins within a few months after birth and a regular transfusion program is necessary. Progressive hepatosplenomegaly and bony structure abnormalities develop. Infection is common. Physical growth and development is below normal, menarche and secondary sex characteristics absent. Intellectual development is unaffected, however. Iron overload (hemosiderosis) is common due to the transfusion regimen and damage to major organs occurs as a result. With proper care patients may live to their twenties. A variation of homozygous beta thalassemia major is entitled beta thalassemia intermedia. Individuals (especially blacks) with this form of the disorder have a milder clinical course requiring few or no transfusions (Bunn et al., 1977).

An individual may acquire a thalassemia gene for a given globin chain on one chromosome and a gene for a structural variant of the same type of globin chain on the other chromosome, resulting in an interacting thalassemia. An example of this is sickle/beta thalassemia, a form of sickle cell anemia with a milder course. (Other hemoglobins which interact unfavorably with beta thalassemia trait are C, and E.) On the other hand, when a beta chain abnormality is inherited with a structural variant for another globin chain (such as in alpha thalassemia trait), the clinical severity of the condition is similar to the heterozygous state for the structural variant. This is referred to as a noninteracting thalassemia (Bunn et al., 1977).

Beta thalassemia trait is commonly found in people of Mediterranean origin (especially Greeks and Italians -- 1 in ten), Asians (1 in 25), Africans, American blacks (1 in 50), West Indians and to a lesser extent in people from India, Thailand and the Middle East.

This protocol will cover assessment and management of women with beta thalassemia trait.

Data Base

Subjective

- Asymptomatic
- May have awareness of abnormal lab results in past

256

- May have complaints related to enlarged spleen

- Ancestry indicative of prevalence of beta thalassemia

Objective   (See Table 5.2, *Laboratory Values in Selected Anemias or Hemoglobinopathies*, p. 248)

- Mild anemia: hemoglobin (Hb) 1-2 gm/dl lower than normal for age and sex (usually 10-11 gm/dl in most patients)

- RBC count may be increased above the normal range.

- MCV <80 fl (microcytosis)

- MCH <26 pg (hypochromia)

- Peripheral blood smear may show target cells, ovalocytes, aniso/poikilocytes and basophilic stippling.

- Hb A_2 increased

- May have elevated Hb F (50% of cases).

- Bone marrow may show mild erythroid hyperplasia.

- Iron studies normal unless coexistent iron deficiency

- Variants of heterozygous beta thalassemia:

  - Delta beta thalassemia or F thalassemia: Hb A_2 normal or slightly decreased, Hb F increased to 5-20%

  - Delta-beta thalassemia with normal Hb A_2 & F: difficult to distinguish clinically from heterozygous beta thalassemia suspected by clinically significant beta thalassemia syndrome in offspring; globin synthesis studies may be necessary to make diagnosis

  - Hb Lepore trait: normal Hb A_2, slight elevation of Hb F, and 5-15% Hb Lepore

- In sickle/beta thalassemia the hemoglobin electrophoresis reveals 60-90% Hb S, 0-30% Hb A, 1-20% Hb F, and increased Hb A_2 (Bunn et al., 1977).

Assessment

- Beta thalassemia trait

- R/O Coexistent iron deficiency anemia

- R/O Concomitant hemoglobinopathy

- R/O Hemoglobinopathy in father of baby

Plan

Diagnostic Tests (See Figure 5.1, *Evaluation of Microcytosis*, p 249)

- CBC: MCV <80 FL, MCV <26 pg

- Hemoglobin electrophoresis with quantitative A_2 and F: A_2 will be >3%, F may be >2%

- Serum iron and total iron binding capacity (TIBC) <u>or</u> ferritin. Serum iron/TIBC should be above 16% saturation or ferritin should be within normal limits if patient not iron deficient. NOTE: Iron deficiency anemia can cause a decrease in Hb A_2 in a patient with beta thalassemia trait. The A_2 levels in beta thalassemia with coexistent iron deficiency may thus fall in the normal range and confuse the laboratory picture of the thalassemia.

- Screen father of baby with CBC and hemoglobin electrophoresis with quantitative A_2 and F if mother has beta thalassemia trait.

Treatment/Management

- No treatment for beta thalassemia trait

- If coexistent iron deficiency anemia treat according to protocol.
  NOTE: In cases of iron deficiency anemia where microcytosis and hypochromia persist after iron replacement, suspect beta thalassemia. Hb A_2 will return to elevated levels in beta thalassemia patients after correction of a coexistent iron deficiency.

Consultation

- None required in beta thalassemia trait with mild anemia

- Required for severe anemia (Hb less than 10 gm/dl or Hct less than 30%); consider MD referral or co-management

- MD care of patients with sickle/beta thalassemia

Patient Education

- Stress importance of screening father of baby.

- If diagnosis of beta thalassemia trait is made discuss disorder and prenatal implications.

  - If both mother and father of baby have beta thalassemia trait there is a 25% (1:4) chance that the fetus will have beta thalassemia major. This condition is amenable to prenatal diagnosis for most families.

  - If one parent has beta thalassemia trait and the other parent has another beta chain hemoglobin trait (e.g., sickle cell trait), there is a 25% (1:4) chance that the fetus will have sickle/beta thalassemia.

Follow-up

- Ensure prompt referral to genetic counselor if father of baby also has hemoglobinopathy. Extended family studies are often needed before prenatal diagnosis can be made.

- Genetics referral is advised when patient/couple desire(s) comprehensive education about the disorder.

- Document in progress notes and problem list.

GLUCOSE-6-PHOSPHATE DEHYDROGENASE DEFICIENCY

Maureen T. Shannon

Glucose-6-Phosphate Dehydrogenase (G6PD) deficiency is an x-linked hereditary erythrocyte enzyme deficiency which is passed on to the male offspring of female carriers (Cunningham, MacDonald, & Gant, 1989; Fischbach, 1988). Although the female carriers are usually asymptomatic, this enzyme deficiency can result in an acute, usually mild, hemolytic anemia when the affected person ingests specific drugs (sulfonamides, nitrofurantoin, primaquine) or foods (fava beans); or is exposed to viral or bacterial infections. Although there are more than 50 variants of this disorder, the major types include: Type A (found in Blacks) and the Mediterranean type (found in Greeks, Sardinians and Sephardic Jews) (Cunningham et al., 1989; Fischbach, 1988).

Data Base

Subjective

- Usually the patient is asymptomatic.

- May complain of fatigue (especially if she also has iron deficiency anemia).

Objective

- Decreased erythrocytes, hematocrit, & hemoglobin with normal MCV and iron studies (if iron deficiency anemia is not present)

- G6PD results less than normal amount (normal values vary and depend on the laboratory used)

Assessment

- G6PD deficiency

- R/O Iron deficiency anemia

- R/O Hemoglobinopathy

Plan

Diagnostic Tests

- CBC

- G6PD--if low hematocrit, hemoglobin, & erythrocytes with normal MCV and iron studies, order G6PD. Results will be less than normal values established by a specific laboratory.

- Hb electrophoresis with quantitative A_2 and F (if not already done)

Treatment/Management

- Continue routine prenatal care.

- If co-existent iron deficiency anemia or hemoglobinopathy, then treat per appropriate protocol.

- If infections or fevers develop during a patient's care, do not prescribe sulfonamides or nitrofurantoin.

Consultation

- Not required unless severe anemia exists

Patient Education

- Explain and interpret tests to the patient and discuss importance of partner screening.
- Educate the patient about G6PD deficiency and factors which may trigger an acute hemolytic anemia.

Follow-up

- Prenatal screening for partner
- Recommend mother and father talk with pediatrician before the birth of their infant to establish rapport and discuss possible implications (during neonatal and infancy periods) if the infant has G6PD deficiency.
- Routine 6-week post-partum follow-up for mother
- Document in progress notes and problem list.

Rh ISOIMMUNIZATION

Lisa L. Lommel

The Rh factor is an inherited antigen confined to the surface of red blood cells. Rh antigens are grouped into three pairs: Dd, Cc, and Ee. The presence of the D antigen determines that an individual is Rh-positive. The absence of D determines that an individual is Rh-negative. The presence or absence of this factor is important when an Rh-negative mother is carrying a Rh-positive fetus.

Rh isoimmunization is characterized by the Rh-negative woman who produces IgG antibodies in response to Rh-positive fetal red blood cells entering the maternal circulation. These antibodies readily cross the placenta and destroy the erythrocytes of the fetus (erythroblastosis fetalis) causing hemolytic disease of the newborn. Erythroblastosis fetalis is usually manifested in one of three ways: neonatal anemia, kernicterus, or generalized edema (hydrops fetalis). The perinatal mortality rate for hydrops fetalis is high. Early intervention, before the onset of hydrops fetalis, greatly improves neonatal outcome.

Hemolytic disease of the newborn can vary from mild to severe. It is characterized by the presence of edema, anemia, hepatomegaly, splenomegaly, and placental enlargement. The severity of HDN will depend on several factors: the maternal immune response to the fetal blood antigen, the amount of antigen infused into maternal circulation, the ABO group of the fetus (see ABO Incompatibility/Irregular Antibody protocol), and the gestational age at which maternal antibody response and hemolysis become significant (Lloyd, 1987). The severity of HDN in subsequent pregnancies of Rh-positive fetuses is usually equal to or greater than that of the previous pregnancy (ACOG, 1986).

Rh isoimmunization occurs whenever an Rh-negative woman is exposed to Rh-positive erythrocytes in her circulation and produces IgG antibodies against these Rh-positive cells. Administering Rh immune globulin (RhIG) within 72 hours of exposure can prevent this formation of antibodies and has been effective in reducing the incidence of Rh isoimmunization. However, Rh isoimmunization can still occur if an inadequate dose of RhIG is given or if RhIG is not given when it is indicated (Lloyd, 1987). Rh immune globulin is not useful if the mother has already developed D antigen antibodies. It is important to screen all pregnant women for Rh status and offer antenatal and postpartum RhIG to non-sensitized Rh-negative mothers to prevent isoimmunization in subsequent pregnancies.

Pregnancies complicated by Rh isoimmunization should be managed by a physician. Management includes serial amniocentesis to evaluate the level of bilirubin in the amniotic fluid. High levels of bilirubin measured in conjunction with fetal gestational age (Liley graph) can estimate the severity of hemolytic disease of the newborn. Fetuses that are considered severely affected may undergo intrauterine fetal transfusions to reduce the risk of death until sufficient pulmonary maturity exists for delivery.

Data Base

Subjective

- History of Rh-negative status

- Rh-negative woman with history of fetal-maternal hemorrhage caused by:

  - vaginal or cesarean delivery (as little as 0.1 ml of fetal blood in the maternal circulation can produce an immune response)

  - amniocentesis

  - chorionic villi sampling

  - ectopic pregnancy

  - antepartum hemorrhage

  - manual removal of the placenta

  - placenta previa

  - abruptio placentae

  - external version

  - pregnancy induced hypertension/pre-eclampsia

  - fetal demise

  - multiple pregnancy

  - abdominal trauma

  - traumatic delivery

- History of previous pregnancy with rising titers, and /or affected fetus or infant

- History of blood transfusion

- Father of baby's Rh type unknown or Rh-positive

- Usually asymptomatic

Objective

- Non-sensitized Rh-negative mother

- Sensitized Rh-negative mother

- Presence or absence of rising antibody titer

- Documentation of father of baby's Rh type

Assessment

- Rh-negative mother, sensitized or non-sensitized

- Rh-positive father or status unknown

- Rising antibody titer

- Document procedures performed in the pregnancy (i.e., S/P amniocentesis, CVS)

Plan

Diagnostic Tests

- Blood type, Rh type, and antibody screen (indirect Coombs test) at first visit on all patients

<u>Non-sensitized Rh-negative patient</u>

- Screen father of baby for blood type and Rh type if certain of paternity (otherwise assume he is Rh-positive).

- Antibody screen of Rh-negative mothers at 26-27 weeks of gestation

<u>Sensitized Rh-negative patients</u>

- Refer to MD.

Treatment/Management

<u>Non-sensitized Rh-negative patient</u>

- If the father of the baby is Rh-negative, no further testing is necessary. The fetus will be Rh-negative.

- If the father of the baby is Rh-positive, administer 300μg of Rh-immune globulin at 28-29 weeks gestation to patients whose antibody screen is negative at 26-27 weeks. Administration of 300μg of RhIG protects against approximately 30 ml of fetal whole blood or 15 ml of fetal red blood cells in the maternal circulation.

- Administer 300μg of RhIG to patients who undergo a second trimester amniocentesis. These patients should also receive the standard dose of 300μg of RhIG at 28-29 weeks gestation.

- Administer 300μg of RhIG to patients who undergo a third trimester amniocentesis when delivery is not expected within 48 hours of the procedure. If delivery occurs within 48 hours, only a standard postpartum dose of 300μg is recommended.

- Administer 300μg of RhIG to patients who have a spontaneous or therapeutic abortion of greater than 12 weeks gestation. A dose of 50μg of RhIG is adequate in pregnancies terminated before 13 weeks gestation, ectopic pregnancies, or after chorionic villi sampling.

- If 300μg of RhIG is given at 28-29 weeks gestation, a repeat antibody titer at 36 weeks is not recommended. Approximately 20% of antibody titers performed at 36 weeks will be positive due to passively acquired antibodies from RhIG (ACOG, 1984).

- Administer 300μg of RhIG within 72 hours after delivery to patients whose newborns are found to be Rh-positive after cord blood sampling.

- If a patient experiences a high-risk pregnancy or delivery which is known to be associated with greater amounts of fetal to maternal bleeding (i.e., abruptio placentae, placenta previa, cesarean delivery, intrauterine manipulation, or manual removal of placenta), screening should be done to test for the amount of fetal cells in the maternal circulation. After calculating the volume of the fetal-maternal bleed (Kleihauer-Betke test), additional RhIG should be given at the rate of 300μg for every 30ml of fetal blood detected (Fleischer, 1989; Sutton et al., 1988; ACOG, 1984).

Consultation

- MD management is required of isoimmunized patients.

Patient Education

- Discuss Rh factor and implications for the fetus.

- Explain to women the risks and benefits of RhIG immunization.

- Provide her with a card that identifies her as Rh-negative and any RhIG immunizations she received.

- Advise her to alert her health care providers that she is Rh-negative in the event of future pregnancies or blood transfusions.

- Advise patient that reaction to RhIG is rare and is usually localized to the site of injection. A slight temperature elevation may be experienced.

- Discuss the risks to the fetus, need for amniocentesis, possibility of intrauterine transfusions, and management by MD in Rh-isoimmunized patients.

Follow-up

- Document in progress notes and problem list to alert intrapartum health care provider to administer RhIG postpartum to non-sensitized patients whose infants are Rh-positive.

SICKLE CELL TRAIT

Winifred L. Star

Sickle cell trait occurs when a person has one gene for normal hemoglobin A (2 alpha, 2 beta chains) and one gene for hemoglobin S (2 alpha, 2 beta S chains). An individual with sickle cell trait has 34% to 54% hemoglobin S, the rest hemoglobin A. Persons with sickle cell trait are rarely anemic and for the most part are asymptomatic and in good health. Several conditions may be associated with sickle cell trait: bacteriuria, hematuria, hyposthenia, and splenic infarction at altitudes greater than 7,000 feet. Sickle cell trait occurs in about 8% of American Blacks; it is also found in Africans, Italians, Middle Easterners and Indians.

Data Base

Subjective

- May have awareness of diagnosis

- Generally asymptomatic

- May report history of: urinary tract infections, hematuria, pyelonephritis in pregnancy

- Ancestry indicative of prevalence of sickle cell trait

Objective   (See Table 5.2, *Laboratory Values in Selected Anemias or Hemoglobinopathies*, p. 248)

- CBC normal. If coexistent iron deficiency anemia or other hemoglobinopathy, indices may reveal low MCV and low MCH.

- Hemoglobin electrophoresis shows 34-54% Hb S. In patients with concomitant alpha thalassemia or iron/folate deficiency the % of Hb S may be less.

- Sickle prep or sickledex positive for presence of S hemoglobin

- Iron studies are normal unless coexistent iron deficiency.

- Urinalysis may show microscopic evidence of hematuria and/or bacteriuria. Urine culture may be positive for significant pathogen.

Assessment

- Sickle cell trait
- R/O Coexistent iron deficiency anemia
- R/O Concomitant hemoglobinopathy
- R/O Asymptomatic bacteriuria
- R/O Hemoglobinopathy in father of baby

Plan

Diagnostic Tests

- CBC and hemoglobin electrophoresis with quantitative A_2 and F to be ordered on all blacks at first prenatal visit.

- If electrophoresis shows presence of Hb S in mother, screen father of baby with CBC and hemoglobin electrophoresis with quantitative A_2 and F.

Treatment/Management

- No treatment for sickle cell trait

- Order complete urinalysis and culture with sensitivities each trimester and as indicated by urine dipstick, to R/O asymptomatic bacteriuria.

- Treat asymptomatic bacteriuria according to protocol.

- If coexistent iron deficiency anemia treat according to protocol.

Consultation

- None required for sickle cell trait

- Required if patient has severe anemia secondary to other causes (Hb below 10.0 gm/dl or Hct less than 30%); consider MD referral or co-management

- Refer patients with sickle cell disease to MD.

Patient Education

- Stress importance of screening father of baby.

- Discuss disorder and prenatal implications: if both mother and father of baby have sickle cell trait there is a 25% (1:4) chance that the fetus will have sickle cell anemia. This condition is amenable to prenatal diagnosis.

- Educate patient regarding symptoms of urinary tract infection and advise prompt disclosure to health care provider.

Follow-up

- Refer to genetic counselor if father of baby also has hemoglobinopathy.

- Genetics referral is advised when patient/couple desire(s) comprehensive education about the disorder.

- In coexistent iron deficiency, iron supplements should be continued for at least three months postpartum.

- Document in progress notes and problem list.

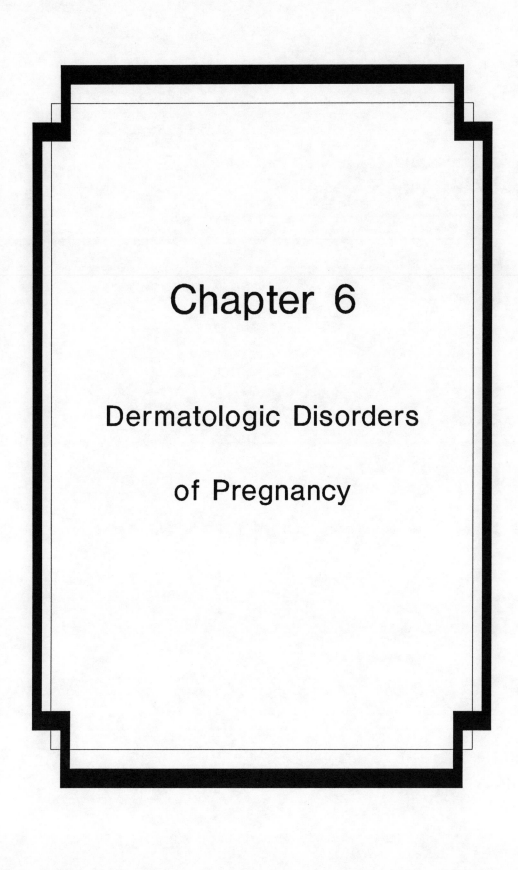

Chapter 6

Dermatologic Disorders

of Pregnancy

HERPES GESTATIONIS

Maureen T. Shannon

Herpes gestationis is a rare dermatological condition of pregnancy the etiology of which is unknown. Despite its name, there is no causal relationship between this condition and the herpes virus. The clinical manifestations of this disorder are immunologically induced and mediated by an IgG anti-basement membrane antibody (a C3 complement component) (Braverman, 1988).

Herpes gestationis is characterized by the eruption of extremely pruritic blister-like lesions beginning in the second or third trimester. These lesions usually begin as erythematous, urticarial papules or plaques that develop vesicles or bullae peripherally/circumferentially (Abrams, 1989; Braverman, 1988; Sodhi & Sausker, 1988). They may be single lesions or in groups that may eventually coalesce to form circular patterns. The vesicles and bullae will eventually crust and heal without scarring (Abrams, 1989).

Initially, the pruritis and lesions are distributed over the patient's abdomen and trunk, but can progress to involve the entire cutaneous surface of her body. The lesions will persist until delivery with regression occurring within a few weeks postpartum. Opinions vary regarding the possible increased perinatal mortality associated with this disease; however, it has been observed that in most instances it will resolve without adverse effects to the mother or infant (Braverman, 1988). Herpes gestationis lesions can develop in the newborns of patients affected with this condition, but it usually regresses spontaneously and without complications. It has also been noted to recur in subsequent pregnancies, during oral contraceptive use, and during menstrual cycles (Braverman, 1988).

Data Base

Subjective

- May report a history of herpes gestationis in a previous pregnancy
- Complains of severe itching of trunk and abdomen in the second or third trimester (can occur during the first trimester if a recurrent episode)
- May report development of erythematous papules, plaques, or blisters

Objective

- Observation of erythematous urticaria-like papules, vesicles, or bullae on abdomen and/or trunk initially; and on other cutaneous surfaces after the initial eruption
- May have signs of secondary infection of lesions (rare)

Assessment

- Herpes gestationis
- R/O Erythema multiform
- R/O Papular dermatitis of pregnancy
- R/O Pemphigus vulgaris

- R/O Impetigo herpetiformis
- R/O Herpes zoster
- R/O Disseminated herpes simplex

Plan

Diagnostic Tests

- Histologic examination of specimen taken from lesions will reveal the classic dermatologic effects of herpes gestationis.
- May have an increased IgG.

Treatment/Management

- Consultation with an MD is warranted in all suspected cases of herpes gestationis with transfer of care indicated in patients diagnosed with severe forms of this condition.
- Co-management of patient with MD is possible in less severe forms of this condition.
- Pharmacologic management by MD may include corticosteroid therapy and/or pyridoxine.

Consultation

- Required in all patients suspected of having herpes gestationis

Patient Education

- Education of the patient who is experiencing this condition should include information about this dermatologic condition; how it will probably progress during the pregnancy; the likelihood of complete regression without complications or scarring a few weeks after delivery; and that this condition may recur in subsequent pregnancies, during menstrual cycles, or if oral contraceptives are used.
- Educate the patient about the very remote possibility that her infant may have similar lesions after birth, but that these lesions will usually regress without scarring or complications.
- Discuss proper skin hygiene, and the signs and symptoms of possible secondary infection of lesions.
- Pharmacologic therapy options should be discussed with the MD prescribing the medication(s).

Follow-up

- Follow-up evaluations of patients with herpes gestationis is per MD recommendation and depends upon the severity of the condition and the pharmacologic agent(s) prescribed.
- Document in problem list and progress notes.

IMPETIGO HERPETIFORMIS

Maureen T. Shannon

Impetigo herpetiformis is a very rare dermatologic condition similar to, if not a form of, generalized pustular psoriasis (Abrams, 1989). The actual etiology of this condition is unknown. It can occur at any time during pregnancy and is characterized by the abrupt eruption of painful erythematous plaques and patches that are rapidly covered with sterile pustules (Abrams, 1989; Braverman, 1988). The distribution of the eruptions can involve any part of the body; however, they usually develop in the periumbilical area, lower abdomen, inner thighs, inguinal areas, axilla, and between the breasts (Braverman, 1988). Painful lesions of the oral mucosa can also develop. Systemic manifestations that usually accompany each eruption include fever, arthralgias, lethargy, leukocytosis, hypocalcemia, and splenomegaly (Abrams, 1989; Braverman, 1988). This condition usually spontaneously regresses after delivery, but can recur in subsequent pregnancies. Initial reports of this condition have associated it with an increased maternal mortality rate.

Data Base

Subjective

- History of condition occurring in previous pregnancy
- Complains of eruption of painful red rash with pustules (may be anywhere on the body)
- Complains of lethargy
- Complains of tender joints when eruption developed
- May complain of painful oral lesions

Objective

- Observation of erythematous papules or plaques with superficial pustules on lower abdomen, groin, inner thighs, or in mouth (however, may be observed anywhere on the body)
- Temperature--will be elevated if lesions are erupting.
- Joints may be tender to palpation.
- Palpation of abdomen may reveal splenomegaly.

Assessment

- Impetigo Herpetiformis
- R/O Herpes gestationis
- R/O Pemphigus vularis

Plan

Diagnostic Tests

- White blood cell count--elevated with an increased neutrophil count

271

- Serum calcium--decreased

- Cultures of pustules--no growth of bacteria or viruses unless there is secondary infection of the lesions

- Biopsy with histologic examination will reveal the presence of "spongiform pustules of the epidermis" (Braverman, 1988, p. 533).

Treatment/Management

- Consultation with and transfer of care to an MD is mandatory because patients diagnosed with this condition require hospitalization for fluid and electrolyte replacement, administration of systemic cortisteroids, and close maternal/fetal surveillance.

Consultation

- Consultation with an MD is mandatory in all patients who are suspected of having impetigo herpetiformis.

Patient Education

- Education of the patient with this condition should include the probable course of impetigo herpetiformis, its treatment, and its possible recurrence in future pregnancies. This information should be presented by the MD managing the patient's care.

Follow-up

- Follow-up evaluations of patients diagnosed with this condition are per MD recommendation.

- Document in problem list and progress notes.

PAPULAR DERMATITIS OF PREGNANCY

Maureen T. Shannon

Papular dermatitis of pregnancy is a rare pruritic condition of unknown etiology that can occur anytime during pregnancy. The characteristic eruption of this condition consists of discrete, single erythematous papules approximately 3-5 mm in diameter. The papules are scattered throughout the body, will appear excoriated (secondary to the pruritis), and will heal within 10 days after eruption leaving areas of hyperpigmentation (Braverman, 1988). This condition is also characterized by elevated urinary chorionic gonadotropin levels, decreased plasma cortisol levels, and decreased urinary estriol levels during the last trimester (Braverman, 1988). Papular dermatitis of pregnancy will abate with delivery or during the early post-partum period; however, it may recur in subsequent pregnancies. Initial reports regarding an increased fetal loss associated with this dermatologic condition are controversial.

Data Base

Subjective

- History of papular dermatitis of pregnancy occurring in a previous pregnancy
- Complains of severe itching
- Reports eruption of papules on body
- Reports hyperpigmentation at sites where papules have healed

Objective

- Observation of discrete, individual erythematous papules with excoriation throughout body
- May observe hyperpigmented areas where papules have healed

Assessment

- Papular dermatitis of pregnancy
- R/O Allergic reaction
- R/O PUPPP syndrome
- R/O Scabies
- R/O Xerosis

Plan

Diagnostic Tests: The following laboratory test results will confirm the diagnosis (Braverman, 1988):

- Urinary chorionic gonadotropin level--increased during the third trimester
- Plasma cortisol level--decreased during the third trimester
- Urinary estriol level--decreased during the third trimester

Treatment/Management

- Consultation with an MD is indicated. Due to the initial reports of possible increased fetal loss associated with this condition, referral to MD care is indicated.

- Pharmacologic therapy should be determined by the MD, and usually includes high doses of systemic corticosteroids.

- Nonpharmacologic therapy can include the use of oatmeal baths to decrease the discomfort, and wearing of loose fitting clothing to reduce skin irritation.

Consultation

- Required in all patients suspected of having papular dermatitis of pregnancy

Patient Education

- Education of the patient should include information about the course, treatment options, and the possible recurrence of the condition in subsequent pregnancies.

- Discussion regarding the questionable association of this condition with an increased incidence of fetal loss should involve the MD managing the patient's care.

Follow-up

- Follow-up evaluations of patients with papular dermatitis of pregnancy is per MD recommendation.

- Document in problem list and progress notes.

PRURIGO GESTATIONIS

Maureen T. Shannon

Prurigo gestationis is a dermatologic condition of unknown etiology occurring in 2% of pregnancies. It is characterized by the eruption of small excoriated, pruritic papules on the extensor surface of the patient's extremities, and occasionally on her abdomen, trunk, and shoulders (Abrams, 1989; Braverman, 1988; Lamberg, 1986). The eruptions usually begin during the latter half of the second trimester through the beginning of the third trimester. This condition will spontaneously regress after delivery, although this process may take up to 3 months; and it may recur in subsequent pregnancies (Abrams, 1989; Lamberg, 1986). There are no known associated maternal or fetal complications.

Data Base

Subjective

- History of condition in a previous pregnancy

- Complains of itching

- Complains of a papule-like rash on the extensor surfaces of the extremities, and possibly the abdomen, trunk, and shoulders

- Reports the symptoms began after the twentieth week of pregnancy

Objective

- Observation of erythematous, excoriated papular lesions on the extensor surfaces of the extremities; may also observe the eruption on the abdomen, trunk, and shoulders

Assessment

- Prurigo gestationis

- R/O Papular dermatitis of pregnancy

- R/O Allergic reaction

- R/O Scabies

- R/O PUPPP syndrome

Plan

Diagnostic Tests: No specific diagnostic tests will confirm the diagnosis; however, tests may be ordered to R/O other dermatologic conditions as indicated.

Treatment/Management

- Consultation with an MD is warranted in order to R/O other dermatologic conditions (e.g., papular dermatitis of pregnancy).

- Symptomatic treatment can include calamine lotion to affected areas, oatmeal baths to reduce discomfort, and wearing loose fitting clothing to decrease skin irritation.

- Pharmacologic therapy may include antihistamines and/or topical corticosteroids. The agent and dose to be used should be determined by the MD consultant.

Consultation

- Consultation with an MD is recommended to R/O other dermatologic conditions.

Patient Eduction

- Education of the patient with this dermatologic condition should include information regarding the expected course and regression after delivery; the possibility of recurrence in subsequent pregnancies; and the fact that it is not associated with any adverse maternal or fetal complications.

- Education regarding the pharmacologic options available should be discussed (including risks versus benefits of specific medications) if pharmacologic treatment is being considered.

- Review proper skin hygiene to decrease the likelihood of secondary infection of lesions.

Follow-up

- Routine prenatal follow-up visits
- Document in problem list and progress notes

PRURITIC URTICARIAL PAPULES AND PLAQUES OF PREGNANCY

Maureen T. Shannon

Pruritic urticarial papules and plaques of pregnancy (PUPPP) syndrome is a pruritic dermatologic condition of unknown etiology that begins in the third trimester and slowly regresses during the first few weeks postpartum (Lamberg, 1986). It is characterized by the development of discrete erythematous papules, plaques, and hive-like patches over the abdomen, thighs, and occasionally the buttocks, legs, and arms (Abrams, 1989; Lamberg, 1986). These pruritic eruptions are rarely seen above the mid-thorax, and are never present on the face (Abrams, 1989). PUPPP syndrome is observed primarily in primigravidas and recurrence in subsequent pregnancies is rare. There are no adverse maternal, fetal, or neonatal effects associated with this condition (Abrams, 1989; Lamberg, 1986).

Data Base

Subjective

- Complains of itching of abdomen, thighs, and possibly buttocks, legs, and/or arms
- Reports the development of hive-like or vesicular lesions over the abdomen, thighs and/or buttocks, arms, legs

Objective

- Observation of discrete erythematous papules, plaques, and hive-like patches on the abdomen, thighs, and/or buttocks, arms, legs
- May observe a thin pale halo surrounding the papules (Braverman, 1988)
- Examination of upper trunk, neck, and face will reveal the absence of a similar eruption

Assessment

- PUPPP syndrome
- R/O Allergic reaction
- R/O Papular dermatitis of pregnancy
- R/O Herpes gestationis

Plan

Diagnostic Tests: No specific laboratory changes occur that would further confirm the diagnosis; however, tests can be ordered to R/O other possible diagnoses (e.g., herpes gestationis).

Treatment/Management

- Consult with MD to confirm diagnosis and R/O other possible dermatologic conditions (e.g., herpes gestationis).

- Application of a topical antipruritic (e.g., calamine lotion) may relieve itching in mild-moderate pruritis.

- Severe cases of PUPPP syndrome may require the use of topical or systemic corticosteroids or antihistamines to relieve the pruritis. Consult with an MD regarding the type of medication and dose indicated.

- Oatmeal baths may help to relieve the discomfort.

- Avoidance of tight fitting clothing will help decrease irritation.

Consultation

- Indicated to confirm diagnosis, R/O other dermatologic conditions, and determine if topical and/or systemic corticosteroids or antihistamines are to be prescribed.

Patient Education

- Education of the patient should include information about the course of PUPPP syndrome, treatment options, and the fact that it probably will not recur in subsequent pregnancies. Reassure the patient that the condition will not adversely affect her or her fetus.

- Review proper skin hygiene to decrease the possibility of secondary infection of the lesions.

Follow-up

- Routine prenatal follow-up visits

- Document in problem list and progress notes.

PRURITIS GRAVIDARUM

Maureen T. Shannon

Pruritis gravidarum is a very common cause of pruritis occurring during pregnancy, and is due to intrahepatic cholestasis with the accumulation of bile salts. This condition is characterized by abdominal pruritis without evidence of any lesions except for scratch marks (Lamberg, 1986). Approximately 2-3 weeks after the pruritis begins, jaundice may develop (Lamberg, 1986). The initial episode of pruritis gravidarum usually begins during the third trimester, but may occur any time after the twentieth week of gestation (especially in patients who report this condition having occurred in previous pregnancies). An increased incidence of preterm labor and low birthweight infants has been reported in some patients who have pruritis gravidarum with cholestatic jaundice (Abrams, 1989); however, overall maternal and fetal mortality rates have not been affected by this condition. Regression of pruritis gravidarum occurs shortly after delivery.

Data Base

Subjective

- May report a history of pruritis gravidarum in previous pregnancies
- Complains of mild-severe abdominal itching
- May report jaundice

Objective

- Direct observation of the skin will reveal an absence of lesions where pruritis is reported
- May observe scratch marks in areas where pruritis is reported
- May observe jaundice of skin, sclera

Assessment

- Pruritis gravidarum
- R/O Hepatitis
- R/O Biliary obstruction
- R/O Scabies
- R/O Allergic reaction

Plan

Diagnostic Tests

- Alkaline phosphatase--will usually be 2-4 times the normal nonpregnant values (Lamberg, 1986; Braverman, 1988).
- Total bilirubin--may be increased (Lamberg, 1986; Braverman, 1988)
- Hepatitis screen--within normal limits

- Serum transaminases--within normal limits (Braverman, 1988)

Treatment/Management

- Oatmeal baths should be recommended to help soothe the itching.

- Pharmacologic modalities should be determined by the MD consultant and may include antihistamines and/or cholestyramine (an agent used to bind bile salts that theoretically may decrease the pruritis, but has not been found to be very effective in actual use). Cholestyramine binds fat-soluble vitamins and may necessitate additional fat-soluble vitamin supplementation in patients using this agent for long periods of time (Lamberg, 1986; Braverman, 1988).

Consultation

- Consultation with an MD is indicated in all suspected cases of pruritis gravidarum.

- Co-management with MD is possible if there is no evidence of biliary obstruction.

Patient Education

- Education of the patient should include the etiology of pruritis gravidarum; diagnostic tests that have been ordered and their results; the probable course of this condition; the anticipated remission after delivery; and possible recurrence in subsequent pregnancies or if the patient uses oral contraceptives.

- The signs and symptoms of preterm labor should be discussed with all patients, especially patients suspected of having cholestatic jaundice.

- Nonpharmacologic therapy to reduce the itching should be discussed with the patient and should include oatmeal baths and the avoidance of tight fitting clothing.

- Medication options (risks versus benefits) should be discussed with the patient.

- Reassure the patient that this condition should not adversely affect the fetus, especially if preterm labor and low birthweight are prevented.

Follow-up

- Follow-up evaluations of patients is per MD recommendation and will be determined by whether or not cholestatic jaundice is evident.

- Document in problem list and progress notes.

Chapter 7

Infectious Diseases

in Pregnancy

CHLAMYDIA

Winifred L. Star

Chlamydiae are a group of highly specialized gram-negative bacteria, differentiated from other microorganisms by a unique developmental cycle. The genus *chlamydia* is divided into two species. *C. psittaci* causes a variety of infections in birds and mammals. *C. trahomatis* includes the agents which cause trachoma (serotypes A-C), sexually transmitted diseases and inclusion conjunctivitis (serotypes D-K), and those causing lymphogranuloma venereum [LGV] (serotypes L-1, L-2, L-3). Clinical manifestations associated with chlamydial infection are similar to gonococcal infection. The major mode of transmission is sexual. Like other sexually transmitted diseases (STDs), chlamydial infections are epidemic in the U.S.

In the female, chlamydial infection is associated with mucopurulent cervicitis, urethritis, Bartholinitis, perihepatitis and postpartum endometritis. Acute salpingitis or pelvic inflammatory disease (PID) is the most significant sequelae of chlamydial infection. PID increases the risk of subsequent ectopic pregnancy and tubal factor infertility. About 20-40% of sexually active women have chlamydial antibody titers. The prevalence of chlamydia in the endocervix of asymptomatic women ranges from 3-26%. This high prevalence is due to several factors: minimal or no symptoms, a long incubation period (10 days), and the presence of a persistent carrier state (ACOG, 1985).

Infection rates during pregnancy vary from 2-47% depending upon the population studied (Rettig, 1988). The U.S. national average is thought to be 5% (Gibbs & Sweet, 1989). In utero transmission of chlamydia trachomatis has not been shown. There is a 60-70% chance that infants born through the birth canal of an infected mother will contract chlamydia. Twenty-five to fifty percent of exposed infants will develop conjunctivitis in the first two weeks of life and 10-20% will develop pneumonia (Gibbs & Sweet, 1989).

There is controversy regarding adverse pregnancy outcome in the mother with chlamydial infection. Some studies have documented an association between cervical chlamydial infection and preterm premature rupture of membranes, preterm labor and delivery, low birth weight, increased perinatal mortality, and postpartum endometritis. Other studies do not support these claims (Gibbs & Sweet, 1989). Clearly, more research in this area is indicated.

Data Base

Subjective

<u>Risk factors</u>

- Ages 15-24 (teenagers less than 18 years of age more likely than older adolescents to be infected)
- Blacks, Navajo women, Alaskan Eskimos have higher prevalence
- Lower socioeconomic status
- Single status
- Less education
- Early age at first intercourse

- Cervical eversion (may be associated with oral contraceptive use)
- Coinfection or previous infection with gonorrhea
- Other concomitant STD
- Use of non-barrier contraceptives
- Increased number of lifetime sexual partners
- Multiple sexual partners
- New sexual partner within the preceding 3 months
- Partner with recently diagnosed urethritis
- Pregnancy

Symptoms

- Asymptomatic state **common**
- Patient may complain of:
    - conjunctival irritation, redness
    - pharyngeal soreness
    - vulvar irritation
    - abnormal vaginal discharge
    - abnormal bleeding or spotting
    - dysuria
    - urinary urgency, frequency
    - dyspareunia
    - dysmenorrhea
    - abdominal/pelvic pain
    - rectal pain
    - inguinal adenopathy
- In a patient with PID fever, chills, malaise, nausea, and vomiting may be present.
- Partner(s) may have symptoms of urethral discharge, dysuria, epididymal pain/swelling, rectal pain/discharge, inguinal adenopathy

Objective

- Vital signs as indicated
- Eye, throat exam as indicated
- Abdominal exam: may have tenderness and/or redound tenderness; may have palpable masses, inguinal adenopathy
- Pelvic exam:
    - BUS: abnormal discharge, swelling may be present
    - External genitalia: erythema, edema, excoriation may be present

- Vagina: abnormal discharge may be present

- Cervix: erythema, edema, friability, eversion, mucopurulent discharge, cervical motion tenderness may be present

- Uterus: note size, shape, consistency, mobility, tenderness

- Adnexa: assess ovaries, presence of masses/tenderness

- Recto/vaginal: assess presence of masses/tenderness

Assessment

- Chlamydia trachomatis
- R/O Gonorrhea
- R/O Other concomitant STD
- R/O Vaginitis
- R/O Urinary tract infection
- R/O Urethral syndrome
- R/O Conjunctivitis
- R/O PID (unlikely in pregnancy)
- R/O Fitz-Hugh-Curtis syndrome [perihepatitis] (unlikely in pregnancy)
- R/O Cervical intraepithelial neoplasia (CIN)

Plan

Diagnostic Tests

- Pap smear as indicated (preferable not to do in presence of cervicitis unless patient unlikely to follow-up for care)

- Wet mounts to be performed. NaCl slide may show >10 WBCs/HPF.

- "Gold standard" for diagnosis is culture. Endocervical (columnar) cells are required. Special media and proper handling is important. Check with individual lab for details.

- Additional diagnostic tests may include:

- fluorescein-conjugated monoclonal antibody assay (MicroTrak): less sensitive than culture but relatively specific; good for use in high risk populations where culture not available

- enzyme immunoassay (Chlamydiazyme): similar to above in sensitivity/specificity; best for use in high prevalence settings where culture not available

- microimmunofluorescence assay (Micro-IF): detects IgG, IgM antibodies; not useful as a tool to diagnose acute infection because of the high background rate of antichlamydial antibodies; helpful epidemiologic tool in large populations to identify previous infection

- NOTE: Use of the various diagnostic tests is site-specific and may depend upon chlamydial prevalence in a given population. The sensitivity of all currently available tests is substantially less than 100%; false-negative tests occur. False-positive results may occur with nonculture tests (CDC, 1989).

- Gonococcal cultures to be done

- VDRL or RPR for syphilis to be done

- HIV-antibody test to be offered

- Additional labs as indicated (e.g., CBC, sedimentation rate, urinalysis, urine culture & sensitivities)

Treatment/Management

- Ideally all pregnant women should have cervical cultures for chlamydia and gonorrhea and serologic testing for syphilis at the first prenatal visit. Cultures should be repeated late in the third trimester (36 weeks) if previous positive or at high risk for STD.

- The treatments listed below are taken from: Centers for Disease Control (1989). Sexually transmitted disease guidelines. *Morbidity and Mortality Weekly Report, 38*(S-8), 27-29.

<u>Treatment of C. trachomatis in Pregnancy</u>

- Erythromycin base 500 mg po qid x 7 days. If not tolerated:

- Erythromycin base 250 mg po qid x 14 days **or**

- Erythromycin ethylsuccinate 800 mg po qid x 7 days **or**

- Erythromycin ethylsuccinate 400 mg po qid x 14 days. If erythromycin not tolerated:

- Amoxicillin 500 mg po tid x 7 days (limited data regarding efficacy)

- All sexual contacts within 30 days of symptom-onset should be examined and tested, and treated prophylactically. Refer to CDC guidelines for treatment of non-pregnant individuals.

Consultation

- For prescription as necessary

- For diagnosis of conjunctivitis, PID, Fitz-Hugh-Curtis syndrome

Patient Education

- Discuss cause, mode of transmission of infection, incubation period, symptoms, potential complications and neonatal implications.

- Stress compliance with treatment regimen.

- Discuss importance of evaluation and treatment of partner(s).

- Advise abstaining from intercourse until treatment of both patient and partner completed.

- Address STD prevention, provide guidelines for safer sex practices, encourage careful screening of sex partners and committed use of condoms (especially with new/multiple/non-monogamous partners).

- Allow patient to ventilate her surprise, anger, fear etc. as indicated.

Follow-up

- "Because antimicrobial resistance of C. trachomatis to recommended regimens has not been observed, test-of-cure evaluation is not necessary when treatment has been completed" (CDC, 1989, p. 28).

- If utilized, test-of-cure cultures should not be obtained until 3-6 weeks after treatment. Positive re-cultures require re-treatment of patient and all interim sex partners.

- *C. trachomatis* and *N. gonorrhoeae* cultures and serologic tests for syphilis should be repeated in the third trimester (~ 36 weeks) especially if at high risk for STD or if previous positive cervical culture(s) during pregnancy.

- Public health reporting: confidential morbidity and mortality report to be filed with the Department of Public Health for all patients diagnosed with chlamydia.

- Alert delivery room personnel of positive culture if patient in labor at time of diagnosis.

- Refer patients with CIN for colposcopy.

- Refer patients with conjunctivitis to ophthalmologist.

- Document in progress notes and problem list.

CONDYLOMATA ACUMINATA

Lisa L. Lommel

Condylomata acuminata, also known as genital or venereal warts, is primarily a sexually transmitted disease (STD) caused by the human papillomavirus (HPV). This double-stranded DNA virus belongs to the papovavirus family and has the ability to remain latent. There are over 60 known serotypes of HPV to date that cause a variety of clinical wart syndromes. Human papillomavirus serotypes 6 and 11 are responsible for the majority of benign anogenital disease and usually present as papillary condylomas and, less frequently, as flat condylomas. Serotypes 16, 18, 31, 33, 35, and 39 usually result in flat condylomas and have been associated with premalignant and malignant anogenital disease. More than 90% of cervical neoplasia has been strongly associated with these latter serotypes (Schneider, 1988). Co-factors such as herpes simplex virus, smoking, and pregnancy are thought to contribute to HPV related neoplasias (Gissman, 1989). Human papillomavirus related neoplasia can also occur on the vulva and penis and in the vagina and anus (Buscema et al., 1988) (Krebs, 1989).

Genital HPV infections are one of the most common sexually transmitted diseases in the United States. Occurrence rates are highest in the sexually active young adult population age 15-29 years. The incubation period to clinical appearance of warts or subclinical lesions may range from one month to several years (Richart et al., 1988). Transmission rates are difficult to establish because of the latent nature of the disease. It is thought that up to 85% of women whose partners have condylomata will develop the lesion (Richart et al., 1988).

Treatment of HPV infection includes a variety of localized destructive and immunotherapies. Reoccurrence of clinical lesions are common after destructive therapy because HPV associated lesions are surrounded by a diffuse area of subclinical infection. Repeated treatments are often needed to achieve stable remission. However, it has been reported that destructive therapy will lead to remission in up to 85% of patients (Krebs, 1989). Spontaneous regression of genital lesions may be accomplished by a host immune response. Lasting clinical remission has been achieved by localized destruction of obvious lesions and the body's cellular immune response (Reid & Campion, 1989).

The incidence, prevalence, and replication of HPV in pregnant women is higher than non-pregnant women. The relative state of immunosuppression during pregnancy greatly contributes to these factors (Ferenczy, 1989). Condylomata in pregnancy may become large enough to impede delivery. Premature rupture of membranes, or chorioamnionitis due to secondary infection of condylomas by vaginal and rectal bacteria may occur. Rarely will the fetus become infected during delivery (Schwartz, Greenberg, Daoud, & Reid, 1988; Ferenczy, 1989).

Juvenile laryngeal papillomata (JLP) can occur in children exposed during delivery. The exact incidence of JLP is unknown but it is believed to be rare. There is an estimated 150 to 300 cases per year in the United States (Ferenczy, 1989). Juvenile laryngeal papillomata can produce mortality or significant long-term morbidity in affected children (Schwartz et al., 1988). External anogenital and conjunctival lesions can develop in offspring after contact during delivery. Congenital genital lesions have also been reported (Ferenczy, 1989).

Routine viral screening and typing for detection of HPV is not yet standard practice. Evaluation for signs and symptoms of HPV infection can be accomplished for women by history, Pap smear, and physical examination. Further evaluation will be limited by practice site availability of laboratory techniques, colposcopy, and experienced clinicians. The only definitive diagnostic test for presence of HPV is by histological evaluation of a biopsy.

Data Base

Subjective

- Majority of patients are asymptomatic

- Presence of vulvar lesion on self or lesion on sex partner

- Vulvar pruritus, burning, and/or bleeding

- Dyspareunia

- Profuse vaginal discharge and/or pruritus

- Accompanying signs and symptoms of vaginitis

- History of abnormal or suspicious Pap smear

Risk factors may include (Stone, 1989; Horn, 1989):

- Young age (peak age 20-24)

- History of genital warts

- Concomitant and/or history of STD

- Oral contraceptive use

- Positive exposure by sexual contact

- Multiple sexual partners

- Pregnancy

- Cigarette smoking

- Immunosuppressed state

Objective

- Latent disease is defined by absence of morphologic abnormalities.

- Subclinical infection usually appears as flat condylomata most often affecting the cervix followed by the vulva, vagina, and anal epithelium. Flat condylomatas appear as 1 to 4 mm in diameter flat-topped, papules usually not seen without the application of acetic acid to produce acetowhitening and the use of magnification.

- Clinically apparent lesions appear as flat condylomatas or acuminata. Acuminata present as small 2 to 3 mm in diameter soft, papillary growths occurring singly or in clusters. Older and larger lesions may have a cauliflower-like appearance.

- Vagina and introitus usually present with multiple, fine, finger-like projections.

- Squared-off keratotic papules may be seen on non-mucosal dry areas of the groin.

- Lesions of varying presentation may be seen in the mouth, larynx, or conjunctivae.

- Bleeding and/or excoriation of the lesions may be present due to irritation from clothing or scratching.

- Signs of concomitant vaginitis or STD

Assessment

- Condylomata acuminata
- R/O Condylomata lata of secondary syphilis
- R/O Molluscum contagiosum
- R/O Folliculitis
- R/O Vaginitis
- R/O Concomitant STD
- R/O Cervical intraepithelial neoplasias (CIN)

<u>Acetowhitening may be due to</u>:

- HPV infection
- Variation of normal epithelium
- Tissue inflammation secondary to vaginitis
- Allergic or contact dermatitis
- Microtrauma
- Post-treatment areas (up to 6 months)
- Lichen sclerosis et atrophicus
- Pantyhose or tight pants
- Hyperkeratosis

Plan

Diagnostic Tests

- Examination of genital tissue is facilitated by applying liberal amounts of 5% acetic acid (ordinary white vinegar) with large cotton swabs. Acetic acid causes the larger nuclei of proliferating epithelium to appear opaque (acetowhitening) because it causes the cytoplasm of the cells to shrink. Flat lesions not ordinarily seen and papillary lesions will be enhanced after 1 to 5 minutes of exposure to acetic acid. Magnification (with magnifying glass or colposcope) will further aid in evaluation (Buck et al, 1989). Acetowhitening is <u>not</u> diagnostic of HPV infection (see Assessment for differentials)--it serves to increase the index of suspicion in an otherwise unsuspicious area. Further evaluation is necessary for all suspicious lesions.

- A Pap smear of the cervical transformation zone is used as a screening technique. Because of false negatives, a negative Pap does not indicate absence of disease. The Pap smear should not be the only technique for cervical evaluation where there is evidence of disease elsewhere or if the cervix is not normal-appearing.

- A colposcopy and directed biopsy can confirm HPV infection in acetowhite or suspicious lesions. Biopsy for diagnosis is required in all cases except the most obvious classical condylomata acuminata (Krebs, 1989). The colposcopy and/or biopsy is performed by a trained health care provider.

- A viral screening kit which determines the presence of serotypes 6, 11, 16, 18, 31, 33, and 35 is available for clinical use. The screening kit cannot distinguish one serotype from another. A viral typing kit is available for clinical use and tests for specific serotypes.

- Prepare wet mounts for presence of vaginitis

- VDRL, gonorrhea, and chlamydia cultures

- Additional cultures as indicated (e.g., herpes simplex virus)

Treatment

- Treatment of the cervix should be conducted by those with specific training in colposcopy and treatment methods. The procedure usually involves laser and/or cryotherapy.

- Trichloracetic acid in concentrations of at least 50% to 85% in ethanol solution (70%) may safely treat non-cervical individual lesions in pregnancy. Under controlled magnification, the solution is applied with a small cotton tipped or pointed wooden applicator to the surface of the wart lesions and a small amount of surrounding skin. The acid does not need to be washed off after application. A moderate to intense burning sensation may be felt by the patient for 5 to 10 minutes after application. Applications may be repeated every seven to fourteen days depending upon individual healing time.

- Liquid nitrogen (-196°C) applied by freezing the cotton tip of a swab and then touched on a lesion can be used in pregnancy. This technique requires repeated applications, causes significant localized discomfort, tissue necrosis, and occasional bleeding (Ferenczy, 1989; (Buck et al, 1989).

- Podophyllin and 5% 5-fluorouracil in cream (Efudex) should <u>not</u> be used in pregnancy because they may be absorbed into the vascular system and cause serious complications in the mother and fetus (Ferenczy, 1989).

- Interferon therapy should <u>not</u> be used in pregnancy because it may interfere with normal liver, bone marrow, and immune functions (Ferenczy,1989).

- Electrocautery, cryocautery and laser therapy are the therapies of choice for resistant or extensive lesions in pregnancy. These techniques are performed by the physician when appropriate.

- Treat concomitant vaginal infection or STD as appropriate.

Consultation

- Consult with physician as necessary.

- Referral to trained health care provider for colposcopy and directed biopsy

- Referral required for treatment of the cervix and electrocautery, cryocautery or laser therapy.

Patient Education

- Explain about the virus, its transmission, and consequences.

- Discuss the link with cervical cancer and need for follow-up.

- Explain that warts can be cured especially when treatment of the patient and partner occur simultaneously.

- Explain that although the warts are curable, recurrences are common as the virus can live in normal appearing cells.

- Inform patient prior to treatment regarding post-treatment pain associated with specific therapies.

- Advise patient to call her health care provider if signs of infection appear such as redness, increased pain or presence of pus.

- Advise patient that sexual partner(s) should be evaluated and treated for HPV infection.

- Advise abstinence or use of latex condoms <u>and</u> vaginal spermicide for intercourse. Spermicidal condoms should be used for at least 6 months after both partners are lesion free. Nonoxynol-9 has been shown to be viricidal to the HPV virus (Buck et al, 1989).

- Advise the patient to keep the vulva clean and dry; a damp environment enhances growth of the warts.

- Advise the patient to wear cotton underwear and loose fitting clothes.

- Advise maintenance of a healthy lifestyle to aid the immune system including diet, rest, stress reduction, and exercise.

- Explain importance of proper thorough treatment of concomitant vaginitis or STD.

- Discuss feelings that the patient may have regarding her experiences with this infection.

Follow-up

- Self examination and semi-annual or annual health exams are recommended to assess disease reoccurrence.

- Follow-up Pap smear schedules will vary between sites. It is suggested that if the cervix is treated, a Pap smear should be done 4 to 6 months after the first. After 2 negative Pap smears at 6 month intervals an annual schedule can be followed (Buck et al, 1989).

- At least annual Pap smears should be done on women who have been treated for HPV/CIN infection.

- Document in problem list and progress notes.

CYTOMEGALOVIRUS

Winifred L. Star

Cytomegalovirus (CMV) is the most common viral infection in pregnancy. Two to thirty percent of pregnant women excrete the virus from the cervix and 0.5-2.5% of all newborns have CMV at birth. Approximately 50% of reproductive age females are susceptible to CMV; seroconversion occurs mostly between the ages of 15-35. When present, CMV is persistently excreted and thus can be communicable for extended periods. Similar to herpes simplex virus, CMV may become latent after primary infection and be reactivated at a later time. The means of primary CMV acquisition is not known. The virus is sexually transmitted (Gibbs & Sweet, 1989).

Perinatal infection with CMV has multiple sources: transplacental, *in utero* (due to ascending infection from an infected cervix), and vaginal. Breast milk is also a potential source of CMV although no correlation between breastfeeding and viral excretion in infants has been shown (Gibbs & Sweet, 1989).

In utero infections are of major concern. Congenital infections can occur after either primary or recurrent maternal infection. Most women who excrete virus in pregnancy do so as a result of recurrent infection, thus intrauterine CMV infection more often follows recurrent maternal infection. On the other hand, primary infection is more often associated with severe congenital CMV (Gibbs & Sweet, 1989). The timing of infection during pregnancy is important in determining fetal effects. First or second trimester CMV infection will result in more severely affected infants. Effects on the offspring include CNS and perceptual disabilities, mental retardation, seizures, spastic diplegia, optic atrophy, blindness, and sensorineural deafness (Gibbs & Sweet, 1989).

Data Base

Subjective

- Incidence of CMV infection highest in lower-income, young, primiparous, less educated, unmarried women

- Majority of infections asymptomatic

- Symptoms of infection may include a mononucleosis-like syndrome with:

    - abrupt onset of spiking temperature

    - malaise

    - myalgias

    - chills

    - mild pharyngitis

    - minimal lymphadenopathy

Objective

- Maternal signs may include: leukocytosis, lymphocytosis, abnormal liver function tests, negative heterophile.

- Congenitally infected infants may present with: hepatosplenomegaly, jaundice, thrombocytopenia, purpura, optic atrophy, cerebral calcifications, chorioretinitis, microcephaly.

- About 80% of congenitally infected neonates have IgM antibody in the first few months of life.

Assessment

- Cytomegalovirus infection
- R/O Mononucleosis
- R/O Other perinatal viral infection

Plan

Diagnostic Tests

- Indirect hemagglutination tests (IHA), enzyme-linked immunosorbent assay (ELISA), fluorescent antibody (FA), and neutralization tests are available.

- A single positive test does not indicate recent or current infection as 50% of adults have antibody to CMV.

- A primary infection may be diagnosed with acute and convalescent titers on paired sera. A significant rise in titer between first and second specimens indicates acute infection.

- IgM antibody can be detected if the infection has occurred within the previous 60 days.

- Isolation of CMV from the urine or cervix is the best means of establishing the presence of the virus.

Treatment/Management

- To date there is no known treatment for CMV infection.

- Treatment of the mono-like syndrome in the mother is purely symptomatic.

- No satisfactory therapy exists for the congenitally-infected neonate. Antiviral agents have been tried in infants with severe infection.

Consultation

- MD consultation required
- Depending upon site-specific protocol, patient may be managed by the MD.

Patient Education

- Because the majority of maternal infections are not diagnosable, counseling is difficult.

- Pregnancy termination should be presented as an option in cases where primary infection is documented in the first 20 weeks of gestation.

- Counseling a woman who has given birth to an infant with CMV is also difficult. The incidence of recurrence is not known. In general subsequent cases are less severe.

- Information on congenital effects should be presented to the patient so she has time to prepare for the outcome.

Follow-up

- Psychosocial support and referrals to appropriate services should be important considerations.
- Document in problem list and progress notes.

GENITAL HERPES SIMPLEX VIRAL INFECTIONS

Maureen T. Shannon

Genital herpes simplex viral infections can be caused by two different types of herpes virus. Type II herpes simplex virus (HSV-2) is responsible for the majority of the genital infections observed; however, between 7-50% of genital infections can be caused by herpes simplex virus type I (HSV-1); (Straus et al., 1985).

In pregnancy, maternal infection with HSV-2 can have adverse effects on both the mother and the fetus. Pregnant patients rarely will have dissemination of primary HSV-2 infection from either the genital or oral site to the viscera causing hepatitis with or without coagulopathy, thrombocytopenia, leukopenia, and/or encephalitis (Stagno & Whitley, 1985). The observed mortality rate among these pregnant patients affected by dissemination of primary HSV-2 infection has been noted to be as much as 50%, with a fetal wastage rate of 50% also (although the fetal deaths were not always associated with maternal deaths) (Stagno & Whitley, 1985). Furthermore, there has been a 25-30% spontaneous abortion rate observed in patients who experience a primary HSV-2 infection before the 20th week of pregnancy (Connell & Tatum, 1985; Stagno & Whitley, 1985).

Primary genital infection, symptomatic, recurrent local infections, or asymptomatic viral shedding of HSV-2 by pregnant patients near term are of major concern because of the possible transmission of the virus to the fetus or newborn. The most severe sequelae of HSV neonatal infections involve the CNS or visceral organs, with severe disability and/or death of these infants reported to be between 10-50% (even with antiviral therapy) (Stagno & Whitley, 1985). Between 40 and 70% of infected infants are born to asymptomatic patients (Connell & Tatum, 1985). However, multiple factors influence an infant's risk of developing HSV infection, with premature and low birth weight infants noted to be at greater risk than term infants. A risk of neonatal HSV infection in excess of 50% has been noted to occur in pregnant patients who deliver when early stages of a primary HSV infection are occurring (Brown, Berry, & Vontner, 1986). In pregnant patients with recurrent HSV infection who have shedding of the virus at the onset of labor, the risk of the development of neonatal herpes infection has been estimated to be less than 5% (Brown et al., 1986). One of the reasons for this low percentage is the fact that pregnant patients with recurrent HSV infection (and their fetuses) develop antiherpes antibodies which exert a protective effect on the fetus, especially if the antibody levels are elevated (greater than 1:35); (Brown et al., 1986).

Controversy still exists regarding the most effective means of preventing neonatal HSV infections. Until recently, weekly HSV cultures beginning at 34-36 weeks gestation in patients with a history of recurrent HSV were recommended as a means of screening for asymptomatic HSV shedding near term. However, it has been documented that this practice is not predictive of asymptomatic reactivation of HSV infection at the time of delivery (Arvin et al., 1986). Additionally, it was determined that many patients were undergoing cesarean sections, with their associated increased morbidity and mortality rates, for questionable benefits. Therefore, it is recommended that weekly antepartum cultures of patients with a history of recurrent HSV infection be discontinued, and that the method of delivery for these patients be determined by the presence or absence of suspicious genital lesions and the status of their membranes at the time of delivery. Cesarean sections should be performed on patients in labor who present with suspicious genital lesions and whose membranes are intact or have ruptured within four hours of surgery (Maslow & Bobitt, 1988). If these patients report that their membranes ruptured more than four hours before surgery can be performed, then a vaginal delivery can be permitted because the organisms may have already ascended into the uterus and exposed the infant to HSV infection. Consideration should be given to obtaining HSV cultures from mothers and their infants at the time of delivery because this may be an important means of identifying infants who have been exposed to HSV during the intrapartum period. Documentation of a positive culture result will definitively diagnose neonatal herpes infection and may expedite the initiation of antiviral therapy in infants affected by this disease.

Data Base

Subjective

<u>Primary infection</u>: Approximately 50% of patients with primary HSV-2 infections are asymptomatic (Connell & Tatum, 1985).

- Exposure to infected person

- Viremia (chills, headache, myalgia, malaise, generalized lymphadenopathy, elevated temperature)

- Itching and/or burning at the site of the infection

- Painful genital lesions (papules, vesicles, ulcerations, pustules with crusts)

- Inguinal lymphadenopathy

- Dyspareunia

- Leukorrhea

- Symptoms resolve within 2-4 weeks

<u>Recurrent infection</u>: Asymptomatic viral shedding by pregnant patients with recurrent genital HSV-2 infections is 3-12% (Stagno & Whitley, 1985).

- History of previous episodes

- Hyperesthesia of the area where the lesions will develop

- Itching and/or burning of the affected site

- Painful genital, anal or thigh lesions

- Leukorrhea

- Dysuria

- Dyspareunia

- Symptoms resolve within 7-10 days

Objective

- Elevated temperature (primary HSV-2)

- Inguinal and generalized lymphadenopathy (primary HSV-2)

- Splenomegaly (primary HSV-2)

- Atypical lymphocytosis (primary HSV-2)

- Altered fetal growth by fundal measurements and sonogram (intrauterine growth retardation can occur in pregnant patients with primary HSV-2 infections--see IUGR protocol)

- Painful lesions of the vulva, vagina, perianal area, and/or thighs (may be papules, vesicles, ulcerations, pustules or crusts)

- Cervical lesions and some vaginal lesions resemble mucous patches, or bleeding lesions with central necrosis and elevated borders; or a generalized cervicitis may be evident.

- Pap smear of vesicular fluid may reveal giant multinucleated cells with inclusion bodies (indicates a viral infection but is not <u>diagnostic</u> of HSV-2).

- Serologic studies reveal an elevation of neutralizing antibodies in convalescent serum (however, this is not specific for genital infections).

- HSV culture of the base of the lesion or cervix is positive (diagnostic of HSV infection or shedding).

- VDRL, gonorrhea (GC), and chlamydia cultures--may or may not be positive

Assessment

- Genital HSV infection (either primary or recurrent)

- R/O Herpes zoster

- R/O Allergic reaction

- R/O Other sexually transmitted diseases (e.g., chancroid, syphilis)

- R/O Other causes of cervicitis (e.g., chlamydia)

Plan

Diagnostic Tests

- HSV culture of genital lesions & cervix

- Pap smear

- Serology (e.g., RPR or VDRL)

- Cervical culture for gonococcus and chlamydia

- Sonogram if suspected IUGR (may occur with disseminated primary HSV infections)

Treatment/Management

- There is no cure for HSV infections.

- Acyclovir is not recommended for use in pregnant women unless disseminated infection occurs (Cunningham, Macdonald, & Gant, 1989).

- Keep lesions dry and clean. Can use Campho-phenique lotion, compresses of cold milk, colloidal oatmeal, or Domeboro's solution which should be applied every 2-4 hours.

- If no genital lesions are present at the time of labor then a vaginal delivery may be attempted.

- A cesarean section is indicated if HSV lesions are present at the time of labor and if the membranes are intact or have ruptured within four hours of surgery.

Consultation

- Required if a pregnant patient experiences primary HSV infection during pregnancy whether or not she exhibits signs and symptoms of disseminated disease.

Patient Education

- Regarding plan of care during prenatal period (e.g., explanation of tests, interpretation of results, etc.)

- Explain the importance of immediately notifying labor and delivery if the patient experiences rupture of membranes (ROM) at a time when HSV lesions are present.

- Teach symptomatic treatment for HSV lesions.

- Teach/review perineal hygiene.

- Educate patient about the importance of abstaining from oral/genital sexual intercourse during active infections; and advise the use of condoms during latent periods to prevent transmission of HSV.

- Reiterate the importance of annual Pap smears.

Follow-up

- Routine prenatal follow-up unless complications develop

- Pap smear at 6 week post-partum visit and then annually

- Document in progress notes and problem list.

GONORRHEA

Winifred L. Star

Gonorrhea, the most commonly reported communicable disease, is caused by *Neisseria gonorrhoeae*, a gram-negative diplococci. One million cases/year are reported but it is estimated that about 3 million occur. The infection presents more frequently in males versus females (1.5:1) with rates of infection varying among different populations (Fogel, 1988). The incidence of gonorrhea in pregnancy has been reported to be between 0.5-7% (Gibbs & Sweet, 1989). Coinfection with *chlamydia trachomatis* occurs in 25-50% of nonpregnant women. Infectious states are often asymptomatic.

Transmission of gonorrhea occurs sexually (in the majority of cases) via genital-genital, oral-genital, and anal-genital contact (Fogel, 1988). The risk of transmission from an infected male to an exposed female is estimated to be 80-90%, with an incubation period of 3-5 days (Gibbs & Sweet, 1989). Perinatal complications of gonococcal infection may include premature rupture of membranes, preterm delivery, chorioamnionitis, neonatal sepsis, intrauterine growth retardation, and maternal postpartum sepsis. A more recently recognized manifestation of gonococcal infection in pregnancy is the amniotic infection syndrome. This manifests as placental, fetal membrane, and umbilical cord inflammation occurring after premature rupture of membranes and is associated with infected oral/gastric aspirate, leukocytosis, neonatal infection, and maternal fever (Gibbs & Sweet, 1989). Infants born through a gonococci- infected birth canal are at high risk for ophthalmic infection and infection at other body sites. Neonatal gonococcal ophthalmia is extremely contagious and may lead to blindness if left untreated; however, routine neonatal prophylaxis has reduced the rate of this infection.

The most common clinical presentation of gonorrhea in pregnancy is disseminated gonococcal infection (DGI). DGI occurs in 0.5-3% of all patients and can be mild or lead to chronic disability or death (Wilson, 1988). Risk in pregnancy increases in the second and third trimester. DGI occurs in two stages. The first is characterized by a dermatitis, the second by a septic arthritis. Treatment depends upon the severity of the presentation, and in some cases is carried out in the hospital (Gibbs & Sweet, 1989).

In recent years treatment for gonorrhea has been complicated by antibiotic-resistant strains. Resistance can be of three types: 1) penicillinase-producing *Neisseria gonorrhoeae* (PPNG); 2) chromosomally mediated resistant *Neisseria gonorrhoeae* (CMRNG); and 3) tetracycline-resistant *Neisseria gonorrhoeae* (TRNG). "PPNG are gonococcal strains that have acquired an extrachromosomal element which encodes for beta-lactamase, an enzyme that destroys the beta-lactam ring of penicillin" (CDC, 1987, p. 1S). PPNG is a significant problem in San Francisco, California, and this area is now considered hyperendemic. Cases of PPNG have been reported in most states. It is now estimated that approximately 2% of all gonococcal infections are penicillinase-producing (Spence, 1988). In contrast to PPNG, CMRNG strains do not produce beta-lactamase. Resistance in these cases is not limited to penicillin and can include resistance to tetracycline, cephalosporins, spectinomycin, and other aminoglycosides. In most instances CMRNG strains have not been associated with treatment failure (CDC, 1987). In cases of TRNG, treatment with tetracycline alone will not be effective.

300

Data Base

Subjective

<u>Risk factors</u>
- Young age (peak incidence 18-24 years)
- Single
- Black race
- Lower socioeconomic status
- Inner city dweller
- Multiple sexual partners
- Partner with sexually transmitted disease (STD)
- History of STD
- Concomitant STD
- History of pelvic inflammatory disease (PID)
- No contraceptive use

<u>Symptoms</u>
- Patient may be asymptomatic or may complain of:
    - vulvar pruritus/irritation
    - swelling of labia majora
    - abnormal vaginal discharge
    - abnormal bleeding
    - dysuria
    - urinary urgency/frequency
    - dyspareunia
    - dysmenorrhea
    - menstrual irregularity
    - lower abdominal/pelvic pain or low backache
    - rectal pruritus/fullness/pressure/pain
    - anal discharge
    - tenesmus
    - pus/blood in stool
    - sore throat
    - nausea/vomiting/diarrhea
    - fever
    - malaise
    - inguinal/cervical adenopathy

- joint/tendon pain

- migratory polyarthritis

- Partner(s) may have symptoms of urethral/rectal discharge, dysuria, frequency, redness of urethral meatus, epididymal pain/swelling, lower abdominal pain, rectal pain, tenesmus, pus/blood in stool.

- Obtain complete menstrual history, sexual history (including sexual orientation/practices, date of last sexual contact, number of partners, partner STD/symptom history), and medical history.

Objective

- Vital signs as indicated

- Throat exam as indicated

- Exam of skin as indicated (in general, and especially volar aspect of arms/hands//fingers). Look for vesicles/pustules with hemorrhagic base.

- Extremity exam as indicated. Look at knees, ankles, and wrists for swelling/redness. Pus may be aspirated from affected joints.

- Abdominal exam: may have tenderness and/or rebound tenderness; may have palpable masses, inguinal adenopathy

- Pelvic exam:

    - BUS: abnormal discharge, swelling/abscess formation may be present

    - External genitalia: erythema, edema, excoriation may be present

    - Vagina: abnormal discharge, blood, pus may be present

    - Cervix: purulent discharge, edema, erythema, friability, cervical motion tenderness may be present

    - Uterus: note size, shape, consistency, mobility, tenderness

    - Adnexa: assess ovaries, presence of masses/tenderness

    - Recto/vaginal: assess discharge/bleeding, presence of masses/tenderness

Assessment

- Gonorrhea (may be oral, cervical, rectal)

- R/O Disseminated gonococcal infection (DGI)

- R/O Chlamydia trachomatis

- R/O Other concomitant STD

- R/O Vaginitis

- R/O Urinary tract infection (UTI)

- R/O Urethral syndrome

- R/O PID (unlikely in pregnancy)

- R/O Cervical intraepithelial neoplasia (CIN)

- R/O Group A beta-hemolytic streptococcal pharyngitis

- R/O Endocarditis/Meningitis (rare)

302

Plan

Diagnostic Tests

- Pap smear as indicated (preferable not to do in presence of cervicitis unless patient unlikely to follow-up for care)

- Wet mounts to be performed. NaCl slide may show >10 WBCs/HPF.

- Cervical cultures for gonococcus (GC) and chlamydia to be done. For optimum GC yield, two consecutive endocervical (or endocervical and rectal) specimens should be obtained. A single specimen will miss 10% of gonococcal infections (Gibbs & Sweet, 1989). Cultures are considered the "gold standard" for diagnosis of gonorrhea.
  NOTE: Use Thayer-Martin media for GC and place promptly in CO2 incubator, candle jar, or biological chamber system (self-sealing plastic bags) that use CO2-generating pills. All GC isolates should be screened for beta-lactamase production. (Endocervical cells are necessary for chlamydia culture).

- Pharyngeal and rectal cultures as indicated.

- Gram stain is not sensitive enough to detect gonorrhea in women and should be used only in trained hands.

- Rapid diagnostic tests (enzyme-linked immunosorbent assays and fluorescent antibody techniques) are now commercially available and may be useful in high-prevalence populations (Spence, 1988).

- Serologic tests have been used but sensitivity/specificity are poor.

- VDRL or RPR for syphilis to be done.

- Additional labs as indicated (e.g., CBC, sedimentation rate, urinalysis, urine culture & sensitivities, HIV-antibody).

Treatment/Management

- Ideally all pregnant women should have cervical cultures for GC and chlamydia and serologic testing for syphilis at the first prenatal visit. Cultures should be repeated late in the third trimester (36 weeks) if previous positive or at high risk for STD.

- The treatments listed below are taken from: Centers for Disease Control (1989). Sexually transmitted diseases treatment guidelines. *Morbidity and Mortality Weekly Report*, *38*(S-8) 21-27; and the Department of Public Health, City and County of San Francisco, *Medical Alert - PPNG in San Francisco*, November 6, 1989.

<u>Treatment of Gonococcal Infections in Pregnancy</u>

- Ceftriaxone 250 mg IM (effective for all sites of GC infection)

  - PLUS-

- Erythromycin base or stearate 500 mg po qid x 7 days **or**

- Erythromycin ethylsuccinate 800 mg po qid x 7 days (to cover coexisting chlamydia)

For patients allergic to cephalosporins give:

- Spectinomycin 2.0 grams IM **followed by** erythromycin as above

NOTE: Cross-reactivity of third-generation cephalosporins and penicillin in penicillin-allergic patients is rare. Ceftriaxone should be withheld in those patients with a history of anaphylactic or histamine response to penicillin (City and County of San Francisco, Department of Public Health, 1989).

- Ideally pregnant women should be treated for chlamydia on the basis of a positive culture; however, if chlamydia testing is not available treatment for coexisting chlamydia should be prescribed.

- Patients with both gonorrhea and syphilis as well as contacts of patients with syphilis should be treated for syphilis according to CDC guidelines. See Syphilis protocol.

- Observe patients for 30 minutes after administration of IM medication.

- Hospitalization is recommended for patients with disseminated gonococcal infection. Specific treatment for this condition is beyond the scope of this protocol.

- In nonendemic PPNG areas (<1% prevalence) gonococcal infections can be treated with regimens with proven efficacy for penicillin-sensitive organisms (Spence, 1988). This should be combined with medication to cover coexisting chlamydia. Examples are:

  - Aqueous procaine penicillin G (APPG) 4.8 million units IM (accompanied by probenecid 1.0 grams po)

  - Ampicillin 3.5 grams po **or** Amoxicillin 3.0 grams po (accompanied by probenecid 1.0 grams po)

    - PLUS -

  - Erythromycin as above

- All sexual contacts within the preceding 30 days should be examined and cultured, and treated prophylactically. Refer to CDC guidelines for treatment of non-pregnant individuals.

Consultation

- For prescription as necessary

- For disseminated gonococcal infections, PID, endocarditis, meningitis

Patient Education

- Discuss cause, mode of transmission of infection, incubation period, symptoms, potential complications and neonatal implications.

- Stress compliance with treatment regimen and importance of follow-up cultures to determine cure.

- Discuss importance of evaluation and treatment of partner(s).

- Advise abstaining from intercourse until negative follow-up culture.

- Address STD prevention, provide guidelines for safer sex practices, encourage careful screening of sex partners and committed use of condoms (especially with new/multiple/non-monogamous partners).

- Allow patient to ventilate her surprise, anger, fear etc. as indicated.

Follow-up

- Follow-up cervical <u>and</u> rectal cultures for gonorrhea should be obtained 4-7 days after treatment is completed.

- Patients treated with spectinomycin should have a serologic test for syphilis in 1 month as this medication has not been shown to be effective for treatment of this STD.

- Patients at high risk for STD should be recultured for GC and chlamydia at about 36 weeks. A VDRL or RPR should also be repeated in the third trimester for all high risk women.

- Public health reporting: confidential morbidity and mortality report to be filed with the Department of Public Health for all patients diagnosed with gonorrhea.

- Recurrence of gonorrhea after one of the above prescribed treatment regimens may be due to reinfection rather than treatment failure. Advise of need for improved compliance with prevention and partner treatment.

- Alert delivery room personnel of positive culture if patient in labor at time of diagnosis.

- Refer patients with CIN for colposcopy.

- Document in progress notes and problem list.

GROUP B STREPTOCOCCUS

Winifred L. Star

Group B streptococcus (GBS), also known as *streptococcus agalactiae*, is a facultative gram positive cocci. There are 5 serotypes (Ia, Ib, Ic, II & III). GBS infection is the most common cause of neonatal sepsis in the U.S. with mortality rates as high as 50%. Vertical transmission to the fetus generally occurs during labor and delivery with increased rates in women with dense vaginal colonization (Boyer & Gotoff, 1988).

Maternal morbidity from Group B streptococcus infection includes premature rupture of membranes (PROM), preterm labor and delivery, amnionitis, and endomyometritis. One to five percent of urinary tract infections in pregnancy may be caused by GBS (Gibbs & Sweet, 1989; Dinsmoor, 1990). Colonization rates of the genitourinary tract in pregnancy range from 5% to 30%. Sexual transmission of the organism is common. Carriage patterns in pregnancy may be either transient, intermittent, or persistent. Rectal and urethral carriage of GBS provide reservoirs for recurrent cervical and vaginal colonization. Cultures performed during gestation, however, may not predict colonization status at the time of labor and delivery (Dinsmoor, 1990). Fluctuations in the presence of the organism may make effective antibiotic therapy difficult to evaluate and resolution of the organism may occur without therapy (Eschenbach, 1985). Antenatal antibiotic prophylaxis or suppression does not consistently reduce maternal colonization.

Neonatal clinical syndromes of early- or late-onset disease may occur following GBS transmission. The incidence of early-onset infection ranges from 1.1-3.7/1000 live births and is increased in PROM (>18-24 hours), preterm delivery, prolonged labor, endometritis, maternal fever, and low levels of maternal type-specific antibody (Boyer & Gotoff, 1988; Dinsmoor, 1990). Manifestations of pneumonia, septicemia, and meningitis usually occur within 12 hours of birth but may develop anytime in the first week (Gibbs & Sweet, 1989; Dinsmoor, 1990). Mortality is high -- somewhere in the 50-70% range. Late-onset disease starts after the first week of life and onset is more gradual. Incidence is half that of early-onset disease. Factors playing a role in late-onset infection include vertical transmission, nosocomial (i.e., nursery) or community acquisition. This form of the disease may result in multiple sites of localized infection, meningitis, and bacteremia. Mortality is generally 15-30% (Gibbs & Sweet, 1989; Dinsmoor, 1990). Many infants with meningitis will have long-term neurological sequelae (Dinsmoor, 1990).

Data Base

Subjective

- Risk factors associated with increased maternal rates:

    - Less than 20 years of age

    - Caucasian race

    - Low socioeconomic status

    - Multiple sexual partners

    - Sexual partner(s) positive for carriage of group B strep

    - Prolonged premature rupture of membranes

- Preterm labor/delivery
- Low birth weight
- Amnionitis
- Endomyometritis (especially postcesarean section)

- Neonatal colonization from infected mother, nosocomially, or via community acquisition

- Neonatal complications of sepsis, pneumonia, meningitis

- Symptoms of maternal infection may include: fever, chills, uterine tenderness, dysuria, and urgency.

Objective

- Signs of maternal or neonatal infection as described above

- Cervical, urine, or rectal culture positive for GBS

- Other positive tests may include: fluorescent-antibody test, latex agglutination test, gram stain

Assessment

- Group B streptococcus (GBS)

- R/O PROM

- R/O Preterm labor

- R/O Amnionitis/Endomyometritis

- R/O Urinary tract infection

Plan

Diagnostic Tests

- Routine antenatal screening specifically for GBS is not recommended at the present time. Antenatal cultures may not correlate with the presence of GBS at the time of labor and vice versa.

- Cervical cultures and/or rapid latex agglutination tests may be performed in the following circumstances: prolonged PROM (>18-24 hours), premature labor, prolonged labor, maternal fever.
  NOTE: The combined use of cervical and rectal cultures may improve the predictive value of the cultures (Boyer & Gotoff, 1988). Rapid agglutination test results can be available in 60 minutes (Brady, Duff, Schilhab, & Herd, 1989).

- Routine urine culture to be performed at initial prenatal visit. May repeat in third trimester for high risk patients.

Treatment/Management

- Standards for management for maternal carriage of GBS vary from institution to institution.

- Antenatal antibiotic prophylaxis or suppression is not routinely recommended due to the lack of success with reducing maternal carrier rates (Gibbs & Sweet, 1989).

- Intrapartum antibiotic therapy with intravenous ampicillin (2 grams q 6 hours) for patients with GBS is indicated in cases of premature rupture of membranes, preterm labor or delivery, and/or maternal fever.

Consultation

- Required

Patient Education

- Discuss the etiology, transmission, and transient nature of the organism.

- Discuss implications of GBS for the pregnant woman and the neonate.

- Inform patient of the non-standardized approach to therapy and counsel according to the practices at individual facility.

- Encourage use of condoms during sexual intercourse to decrease the potential for sexual transmission.

- Advise that partners with symptoms of sexually transmitted disease seek evaluation and treatment.

- Discuss preterm birth prevention at about 20-22 weeks and thereafter. See Preterm Birth Prevention protocol.

Follow-up

- Alert delivery room and nursery personnel regarding maternal colonization if patient in labor (preterm or term).

- In all cases document in progress notes and especially problem list.

HEPATITIS B

Lisa L. Lommel

Viral hepatitis is a systemic infection that primarily affects the liver. There are currently four clinically similar diseases that are distinct etiologically and epidemiologically (Edwards, 1988).

Hepatitis A
Also known as "infectious hepatitis," hepatitis A has a brief incubation period of 15-50 days. It is usually transmitted by fecal or oral routes. The virus is detectable in blood and stool in the late incubation period, but disappears within one week of disease onset. Hepatitis A is self-limiting, does not cause a chronic state and is rarely fatal (Schreeder, 1988).

Hepatitis B
Also known as "serum hepatitis," the incubation period varies from 20-180 days. It is transmitted by way of infected blood, serum, or other body fluids. It can be transmitted through a break in the skin, by way of mucous membranes, parenteral, or perinatal exposure. It is rarely transmitted through fecal-oral routes. Hepatitis B is associated with certain high-risk populations. Approximately ten per cent of patients with acute hepatitis B will develop a chronic carrier state. A carrier is defined as an inidividual who is HBsAG-positive on at least 2 occasions 6 months apart. There are three catagories of chronic carrier hepatitis B infection including chronic asymptomatic carrier state, chronic persisitent hepatitis, and chronic active hepatitis. Chronic active hepatitis and chronic persistent hepatitis occurs in 1 to 2 per cent of all infections and may predispose an individual to cirrhosis or hepatocellular carcinoma (Schreeder, 1988).

Delta Hepatitis
Delta hepatitis is a defective virus that depends upon the presence of hepatitis B for replication. Delta hepatitis only occurs in individuals who are acutely or chronically infected with hepatitis B. Risk factors for Delta hepatitis are identical to those for hepatitis B. Coinfection or superinfection of Delta hepatitis with hepatitis B is an important factor in hepatitis morbidity.

Non-A Non-B Hepatitis
Non-A non-B hepatitis is diagnosed by exclusion of the hepatitis A and hepatitis B infections. It is caused by at least two different agents with varying modes of transmission and incubation periods. In the United States, non-A non-B hepatitis is the major cause of post-transfusion hepatitis due to screening for hepatitis B. This infection can produce a chronic persistent hepatitis, but leads to cirrhosis and chronic active hepatitis less frequently than hepatitis B.

The virus identified as most threatening to the fetus and neonate is hepatitis B. Hepatitis B is caused by a large DNA virus and is associated with three antigens and their associated antibodies (Table 7.1, *Hepatitis B Nomenclature*, p. 314). Detection of these antigens and antibodies at various times in the course of the disease is helpful in tracking hepatitis B infection (Table 7.2, *Practical Laboratory Guide for the Differential Diagnosis of Viral Hepatitis*, p. 315; Figures 7.1, *Serologic Diagnosis: Acute Hepatitis B* and 7.2, *Serologic Course of the Chronic HBsAg Carrier*, p. 316).

Perinatal transmission of Hepatitis B virus from mother to infant is one of the most efficient modes of infection. Transmission of the virus through the placental membrane is thought to be rare because of the relatively large size of the virus. Neonatal infection is also rare when maternal hepatitis infection is resolved during the first and second trimesters. Transmission most often occurs in mothers who have an acute hepatitis infection late in the third trimester or during the intrapartum and postpartum periods from exposure to HBsAg positive vaginal secretions, blood, amniotic fluid, saliva, and breast milk (Klein, 1988).

Infants born to mothers who are both HBsAG and HBeAG-positive (denotes highly infectious state) have a 70%-90% chance of acquiring perinatal hepatitis B infection. It is estimated that 85%-90% of infected infants will become chronic carriers. Twenty-five percent of chronic carriers will die from primary hepatocellular carcinoma or cirrhosis of the liver (CDC, 1988). In the United States, approximately 16,500 births occur to HbsAG-positive women each year and an estimated 3,500 of these infants will become chronic carriers.

Although hepatitis B is more endemic in certain populations and risk groups, screening only those individuals have omitted up to 35% of HBsAG-positive mothers. Current recommendations suggest screening for the presence of HBsAg on all women as early as possible in pregnancy. Testing mothers for other markers is not necessary, since infants of mothers who are only HBsAG-positive may become infected and develop severe hepatitis B infection (CDC, 1988).

Treatment strategies for hepatitis B infection include evaluation of the infected mother by a physician for the presence of liver disease. The exposed infant should be given hepatitis B immunoglobulin and a series of hepatitis B vaccines. This regime has been found to be 85%-95% effective in preventing neonatal infection when given correctly (CDC, 1988). Screening and vaccination of susceptible household members and sexual partners of hepatitis B carriers is also recommended.

Data Base

Subjective

- Women at risk for hepatitis B infection include those of Asian, Pacific, or Eskimo descent (whether or not U.S. born) and women born in Haiti or sub-Saharan Africa.

- Past history of acute or chronic liver disease

- Work or treatment in a dialysis unit

- Work or residence in institutions for the mentally retarded

- Previous rejection as blood donor

- History of multiple blood transfusions

- Occupational exposure to blood or blood products

- Household contact with hepatitis B carrier or hepatitis patient

- History of multiple sexually transmitted diseases (STDs)

- History of intravenous drug use

- Prodromal symptoms may include anorexia, fatigue, nausea, and vomiting

- Acute hepatitis B infection symptoms may include weight loss, headache, myalgia, photophobia, coryza, abdominal pain, jaundice, fever, rash, pruritus, and arthralgias.

Objective

Acute hepatitis B

- Fever of 38°C to 39°C

- Skin spiders, petechiae, palmar erythema, needle tracts, ecchymosis
- Dark urine and/or clay-colored stool
- Jaundice, icteric conjunctiva
- Bleeding gums/mucous membranes, palatial petechiae
- Enlarged, tender liver
- HBsAG positive
- Elevations of AST (SGOT), ALT (SGPT)
- Wet mounts and/or blood tests may be positive in presence of concomitant STD.

Chronic hepatitis B (carrier state)

- Usually asymptomatic
- HbsAg positive
- May be HBeAG positive
- May have elevated liver function studies

Assessment

- HBsAG positive, acute infection vs chronic carrier state
- R/O hepatitis A
- R/O hepatitis non-A non-B
- R/O concomitant STD

Plan

Diagnostic Tests

- Test all women during the early prenatal period with a HBsAG screen.
- If HBsAG is positive order HBeAG, anti-HBe, anti-HBc, SGOT, alkaline phosphatase, and liver panel per consult with physician
- If HBsAG is negative in early pregnancy and the mother could possibly be in the "window period" of infection after exposure to hepatitis or high-risk behavior occurring during the pregnancy (e.g., parenteral drug abuse), a repeat HBsAG should be ordered in the third trimester.
- Wet mounts, cervical cultures, and/or additional blood tests as appropriate for STDs

Treatment

- Pregnancies complicated by acute viral hepatitis are usually managed on an outpatient basis.
- There is no specific therapy but advise patient to:
  - increase bedrest
  - high protein, low-fat diet
  - adequate hydration
  - avoidance of medications metabolized in the liver

- Hospital management is indicated when there is:

  - intractable nausea and vomiting

  - severe anemia

  - prolonged prothrombin time

  - low serum albumin

  - serum bilirubin greater than 15mg/100ml

  - associated condition such as diabetes

- Women with definite exposure to hepatitis B should be given hepatitis B immunoglobulin (HBIG) 0.05-0.07 ml/kg as soon as possible within a 7 day period after exposure, with a second identical dose given 30 days after the first.

- Women who are chronic hepatitis B carriers should have evaluation of their liver function studies, be counseled regarding the implications of the laboratory results, and referred to an internist for evaluation if elevations in liver enzymes exist.

- Infants born to women who are HBsAG-positive during pregnancy should be treated with HBIG (0.5 mL) when stable (preferably within the first 12 hours of birth). Ten μg of plasma-derived or 5 μg of yeast-recombinant vaccine should be given at the same time as the HBIG (or within the first 7 days after birth). Repeat vaccine at one and 6 months of age.

- Household members and sexual partners of HBsAG-positive mothers should be screened for hepatitis and vaccinated if negative.

Consultation

- MD consultation required for acute hepatitis, or abnormal liver function tests

- Refer postpartum, HBsAG-positive women to physician for on-going evaluation.

Patient Education

- Explain meaning of hepatitis B infection including transmission, state of infectivity, and sequelae.

- Explain importance of immunoprophylaxis for infant, household members, and sexual contacts.

- Advise that breastfeeding is not contraindicated if the infant was immunized.

- Inform of hygienic practices that will reduce the transmission to others:

  - wash hands with soap and water after using the toilet

  - carefully dispose of tampons, peripads, bandages in plastic bags

  - do not share razor blades, tooth brushes, manicure tools, or needles

  - have male sex partner use a condom if unvaccinated and without hepatitis B

  - avoid sharing of saliva through kissing, or sharing of feeding bowls and utensils

  - inform all health care providers of carrier state

  - wipe up blood spills immediately with detergent and water

- Discuss with the patient her feelings regarding this infection.

Follow-up

- If HBsAG-positive, give hepatitis letter recommending infant immunization and follow-up for patient and family.

- Encourage the women to obtain follow-up care for herself and family.

- A public health nurse referral may assist the family with preventive care and teaching in the home.

- Note hepatitis status on the problem list and progress notes.

Table 7.1

Hepatitis B Nomenclature

Term	Abbreviation	Comment
HBV	Hepatitis B virus	Etiologic agent of "serum" hepatitis; also known as Dane particle.
HBsAG	Hepatitis B surface antigen	Earliest serologic marker of acute HBV infection, dectectable in large quantities in serum, several subtypes identified.
HBeAG	HBV antigen	Early indicator of acute, active infection. Presence denotes the most infectious period.
HBcAG	HBV core antigen	Not detectable in blood but is detectable in the nuclei of infected hepatocytes.
Anti-HBs	Antibody to HBsAG	Not detectable until weeks or months after the disappearance of HBsAG in the serum. Indicated past infection with an immunity to HBV, passive antibody from HBV immune globulin, or immune response from HBV vaccine.
Anti-HBe	Antibody to HBeAG	Indicated low infectivity of HBsAG-positive serum.
Anti-HBc	Antibody to HBcAG	Indicates past infection with HBV at some undefined time.

© 1990 L. L. Lommel

Table 7.2

Practical Laboratory Guide for the Differential Diagnosis of Viral Hepatitis

Clinical Interpretation	IgM Anti-HA	HBsAg	HBeAg	Anti-HBe	Anti-HBc	Anti-HBs
Acute HA	+	-	-	-	-	-
Incubation period or early acute HB	-	+	+	-	-	-
Acute HB	-	+	+	-	+	-
Fulminant HB	-	+	-	-	+	+/-
Convalescence from acute HB	-	-	-	+	+	+/-
Chronic HB	-	-	-	+	+	+/-
Persistent HB carrier state	-	+	-	+	+	-
Past infection with HB virus	-	-	-	-	+	+
Infection with HB virus without detectable (excess) HBsAg	-	-	-	-	+	-
Immunization without infection	-	-	-	-	-	+
Non-A/non-B hepatitis by exclusion of markers for HA and HB	-	-	-	-	-	-

SOURCE:

Sweet, R. L., & Gibbs, R. S. (1985). *Infectious diseases of the female genital tract* (p. 195). Baltimore: Williams & Wilkins. Reprinted with permission.

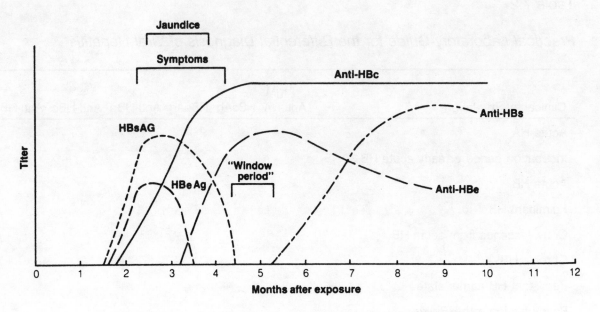

Figure 7.1. Serologic Diagnosis: Acute Hepatitis B.

SOURCE:

Clark, D., & Kao, H. (1983). Meaning markers for Hepatitis Dx and Px. *Contemporary Ob/Gyn, 21,* 31-50. Reprinted with permission.

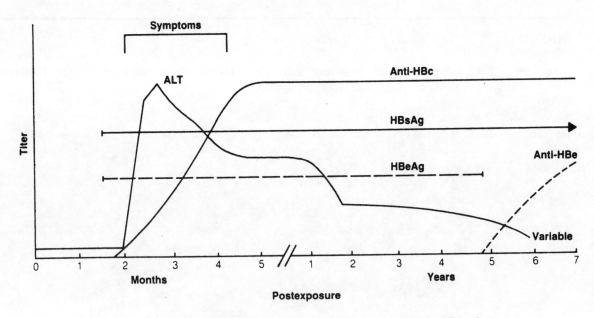

Figure 7.2. Serologic Course of the Chronic HBsAg Carrier

SOURCE:

Clark, D., & Kao, H. (1983). Meaning markers for Hepatitis Dx and Px. *Contemporary Ob/Gyn, 21,* 31-50. Reprinted with permission.

HUMAN IMMUNODEFICIENCY VIRUS INFECTION SCREENING

Maureen T. Shannon

Human immunodeficiency virus (HIV) infection constitutes a spectrum of symptoms and disease processes that begins when a person is inoculated with HIV. HIV is a retrovirus that can infect several cells in the body including the T_4 lymphocytes, macrophages, and neural cells of a person, resulting in the development of immune deficiency and neurologic problems. Transmission of HIV can occur by exposure to an infected person's blood, semen, or cervico-vaginal secretions (Vogt et al., 1986); through blood products (e.g., factor VIII); through use of contaminated needles; transplacentally (Lapointe et al., 1985); or through breastmilk (Ziegler, Cooper, Johnson, & Gold, 1985).

Persons who have been exposed to HIV infection can be divided into four categories: 1) Persons who have a negative HIV antibody test result in the incubation stage of the infection; 2) Persons who are HIV antibody positive but who are asymptomatic; 3) Persons who have AIDS-Related Complex (ARC) and have developed a cluster of certain chronic, severe physical symptoms (specifically, fever with night sweats; nonspecific diarrhea; extreme weight loss; persistent generalized lymphadenopathy; fatigue; and yeast infections--usually of the mouth); and 4) Persons who actually have acquired immunodeficiency syndrome (AIDS) (Buckingham & Rehm, 1987).

In order for the diagnosis of AIDS to be made, two criteria must be met: 1) There must be the presence of a reliably diagnosed disease which is at least moderately indicative of an underlying cellular immunodeficiency (e.g., *Pneumocystis carinii* pneumonia, chronic *Cryptosporidium* enteritis, Kaposi's sarcoma, etc.); and 2) There must be the absence of a known underlying cause for the person's reduced resistance to the disease (e.g., the absence of immunosuppressive drugs, Hodgkin's disease, etc.) (Castro, Hardy, & Curran, 1986).

The first reported case of AIDS in the United States was in 1978, and occurred in a previously healthy homosexual man. Since that time, the majority of AIDS cases (more than 70%) have been reported in homosexual men (Castro et al., 1986). However, in recent years an increased incidence of the disease has been noted in both male and female intravenous drug users (IVDU), hemophiliacs, recipients of blood transfusions, the sexual partners of persons with AIDS or persons who are at risk for developing AIDS, and the infants born to women who are HIV antibody positive. In March 1990, the Centers for Disease Control (CDC) reported that 12,744 women in the United States have been diagnosed as having AIDS (10% of total AIDS cases), 80% of whom are of reproductive age (CDC, 1990). More than 70% of these women are Black or Latina. The prevalence of asymptomatic HIV infection in women is estimated to be between 70,000-140,000. The long-term implications of this disease in women is of major concern since approximately 80% of AIDS cases reported in children are due to the transmission of HIV from infected mothers (American Academy of Pediatrics, 1988). Women who are in high-risk categories for exposure to HIV are:

- Intravenous drug users (IVDU) or persons who share needles for other reasons (e.g., skin popping)

- Sexual partners of AIDS patients or persons who are at risk for developing AIDS (e.g., IVDUs, hemophiliacs, etc.)

- Sexual partners of bisexual men

- Women with a history of multiple sexual partners since 1978, especially if they are from areas where there is a high incidence of AIDS (e.g., New York, California, Florida, New Jersey, Texas)

- Recipients of blood products (1/1/79 to 6/1/85)

- Donor inseminated women (unless the donor has been screened since 1/1/79)

- Mothers of perinatally infected infants

- Women who have resided in geographic areas where AIDS is endemic--Africa (e.g., Zaire, Malawi, Rwanda) and Haiti

- Health care workers with occupational exposure (e.g., needlestick)

Because many women who test positive for HIV are not aware that they are in high-risk categories, all pregnant women should be appropriately counseled and offered testing. In the U.S., the overall perinatal transmission rate for HIV is 35% (Scott, 1989).

Currently, there is no known cure for AIDS. The overall mortality rate has been reported to be 51%; but figures vary depending upon the type of opportunistic diseases encountered and the time from the diagnosis of AIDS (e.g., as time from the diagnosis of AIDS increases the mortality rate increases) (Castro et al., 1986).

Data Base

Subjective

- May give a history indicating a high risk category

- May be asymptomatic

- May complain of symptoms of ARC: fever with night sweats; chronic, severe diarrhea; excessive weight loss; fatigue; generalized lymphadenopathy; yeast infection--especially of the mouth

- May request HIV antibody testing without giving a history of high-risk exposure or symptoms of the disease

- May give a history of hospitalization for, or treatment of, an opportunistic infection associated with HIV infection (e.g., *Pneumocystic carinii* pneumonia)

Objective

- May not have any physical manifestations of AIDS or ARC

- May be febrile

- May be underweight

- May have enlarged lymph nodes (greater than 1 cm) palpable in 2 or more extrainguinal areas

- May have evidence of oral candidiasis--white patches and ulcers of the mouth

- May have evidence of pulmonary disease (e.g., pneumonia --increased bronchophony, egophony, and whispered pectoriloquy; presence of rales or crackles; etc.)

- May have red to purplish macular or papular skin lesions

- HIV antibody test may be positive.

- CBC with differential may reveal leukopenia, lymphopenia, and a decreased Hb/Hct.

- Platelet count may be decreased.
- Assay for IgA and IgG may be elevated.

Assessment

- HIV antibody positive
  NOTE: Some institutions do not utilize this assessment in charts in order to ensure confidentiality of the patient's results. Often "Hepatitis B Precautions", "H/A Precautions" [Hepatitis/AIDS Precautions], or "Body Fluid Precautions" are written without alluding to the HIV antibody status of the patient.)

- Anemia (if present)

- Persistent generalized lymphadenopathy (if evident)

- AIDS (if evident--see above note under HIV antibody positive)

- ARC (if evident--see above note under HIV antibody positive)

- IVDU (if appropriate)

- Partner of IVDU, AIDS or ARC patient, hemophiliac, bisexual man (if appropriate)

- History of blood transfusion (give date)

- History of multiple sexual partners (if appropriate)

- History of occupational exposure (give date)

Plan

Diagnostic Tests (Many of these tests will be ordered after consultation with an MD.)

- CBC with differential

- HIV antibody screen

- T-cell counts (T_4/CD_4 count, T_8/CD_8 count, T_4:T_8/CD_4:CD_8 ratio) if strong suspicion of HIV infection

- Hepatitis B screen

- PPD (with Candida skin test as control)

- Toxoplasmosis titer

- Chest x-ray (if pulmonary disease is suspected)

- Assay for IgA and IgG (as indicated)

- Stool specimens if chronic, severe diarrhea

- Bacterial, viral or fungal cultures as indicated by the presence of specific disease symptomatology

- Antepartum testing as indicated depending on the status of the pregnancy (e.g., if intrauterine growth retardation is present then appropriate antenatal testing should be utilized--see specific protocols for indicated testing)

Treatment/Management

- In patients with positive HIV antibody status, AIDS or ARC, referral to MD care is warranted. Co-management of asymptomatic HIV seropositive patients is possible in some institutions.

Consultation

- Required in all patients who are HIV antibody positive or who have symptoms of ARC or AIDS

Patient Education

- Regarding the limitations of the test (e.g., the possibility of a false positive or negative result). Written informed consent should be obtained before the HIV antibody test is done. If the patient desires anonymous testing, this can often be obtained at a public health department.

- Regarding the confidentiality of reporting the test results. The results of an HIV antibody test should be given in person to the patient (not over the phone or by mail) in order to maintain confidentiality of the results, and to offer the patient support and further information should the test be positive.

- Patients with positive HIV antibody tests should be counseled by knowledgeable health care workers about the implications for the mother and her fetus. Education regarding how to prevent transmission to her family members and/or sexual partner(s) is imperative. Information about confidential or anonymous testing of her partner should also be given.

- In patients with negative HIV antibody tests, extensive education regarding preventive measures to decrease the risk of exposure to HIV should be done, and should be appropriate to the situation (e.g., use of condoms and nonoxynol nine spermacides; stopping I.V. drug use; stopping use of contaminated needles if an IVDU; how to sterilize needles if an IVDU; etc.) Consider repeat testing in 3 months of patients in whom a false negative result is suspected or of those who continue high-risk behaviors.
  NOTE: Generally, a person infected with HIV will have a positive HIV antibody test result 2-12 weeks after infection with the virus. However, in some individuals seroconversion has not been evident until 6 months or more after their last known exposure. Therefore, consider re-testing a woman with a history of recent high-risk behaviors/factors, even if she has a documented negative antibody test.

Follow-up

- Patients with positive HIV antibody tests who are symptomatic of HIV infection require follow-up care with an MD.

- Referral of patients at risk, patients with positive HIV antibody status, or patients with AIDS or ARC to a social worker and/or to community resources that have been established (e.g., the San Francisco AIDS Foundation Hotline telephone numbers 415-863-AIDS or 1-800-FOR-AIDS).

- Results of an HIV antibody test are confidential. In many institutions HIV antibody test results are not charted as such, but "Hepatitis B Precautions," "H/A Precautions," or "Body Fluid Precautions" are written in the chart to alert the staff that certain preventive measures should be employed when handling blood or other bodily fluids from the patient. Each institution should devise their own system of documentation in such a manner as to protect both the patient's confidentiality and the staff.

- In California, disclosure of HIV test results among health care workers involved in direct care of an HIV positive patient is legally permitted, but should be done with discretion in order to maintain patient confidentiality and prevent discriminatory treatment of the patient and her infant.

320

LISTERIA

Winifred L. Star

Listeria monocytogenes is a small gram-positive rod frequently confused with a diptheroid. The organism, a facultative anaerobe, is not species-specific and can be recovered from multiple sources: water, milk, soil, dust, plants, animals, and birds. Listeriosis epidemics have been described in the literature but in most cases the source and route of infection can not be identified. The mode of transmission in generalized maternal infections is probably via ingestion of listeria-contaminated food. Sexual and fecal-oral transmission is possible. Two to five percent of pregnant women may harbor listeria in the vagina. Most infections are asymptomatic and may result in GI or genital tract carriage (Bobbit, 1984; Chapman, 1986; Valkenburg, Essed, & Potters, 1988).

Maternal listeriosis is a rare but significant cause of spontaneous abortion, intrauterine death, premature labor, and neonatal sepsis (Barresi, 1980). When infection occurs the clinical manifestations are nonspecific, with complaints similar to flu-like upper respiratory or gastrointestinal disorders.

Neonatal listeriosis has two distinct clinical entities: early and late-onset types. Early-onset disease which is acquired in-utero manifests within five days of birth as septicemia, with associated perinatal death in 20-50% of cases. Late-onset disease occurs one to four weeks after delivery through a colonized birth canal (Boucher & Yonekura, 1986). Premature delivery and infection can result from either transplacental (secondary to maternal bacteremia) or ascending spread of infection. Listeria, unlike other perinatal infections has not been associated with other complications such as developmental abnormalities, SGA infants, or persistent postnatal infection (Bobbit, 1984).

Data Base

Subjective

- Maternal symptoms are usually mild and may include:
    - nausea, vomiting, diarrhea
    - chills, fever (usually low-grade)
    - malaise, fatigue
    - rhinorrhea
    - coryza
    - pharyngitis
    - pruritis
    - urinary tract symptoms
    - abdominal pain
    - vaginal bleeding
    - uterine contractions
    - malodorous/discolored leakage of amnionic fluid

- Alternately, may present with symptoms of meningitis, or adult respiratory distress syndrome (ARDS).

Objective

- Any of the following may be present:

    - abnormal vital signs

    - purulent conjunctiva

    - injected pharynx

    - cutaneous purple lesions of the throat, urethra, or vagina

    - cervical adenopathy

    - signs of labor (preterm or term)

    - amnionitis with malodorous/stained amnionic fluid

    - fetal heart rate abnormalities during labor (e.g., late decelerations; absence of accelerations)

    - maternal cultures (genital, blood or other) positive for *L. monocytogenes*

    - culture-positive neonate

    - placental abscesses; placenta culture-positive for *L. monocytogenes*

Assessment

- Listeria monocytogenes
- R/O Other perinatal infectious disease
- R/O Viral syndrome
- R/O UTI
- R/O Endometritis
- R/O Septicemia

Plan

Diagnostic Tests

- No reliable serologic test currently available
- Listeria-positive cultures of throat, cervix, vagina, urine, stool, or blood confirms diagnosis.

Treatment/Management

- Consider blood and cervical cultures on any pregnant woman for acute, severe febrile illness.

- If *L. monocytogenes* is identified antibiotic treatment should be instituted. In general, the treatment of choice is a broad-spectrum antibiotic (e.g., ampicillin) given IV. Sensitivity testing should serve as a guide to appropriate antibiotic selection, however. Erythromycin may be used in penicillin-allergic individuals. Treatment should continue for 7-10 days.

- Preterm labor in a febrile mother is generally allowed to progress.

- Delivery by cesarean section is recommended for fetal distress.

- A pediatric team should be standing by in the delivery room to assess the infant.

- Multiple neonatal cultures should be obtained prior to antibiotic treatment of the newborn. The antibiotic of choice is ampicillin in combination with an aminoglycoside (gentamicin, kanamycin).

Consultation

- Required in all cases

- Generally, the patient with listeria will be managed by an MD.

Patient Education

- Educate to the nature of the infection, transmission, perinatal implications, and management.

- Ideally, the primary physician caring for the patient will discuss the perinatal issues with her.

Follow-up

- Repeat maternal cultures (blood and cervical) should be obtained following antibiotic therapy.

- Document in problem list and progress notes.

MEASLES

Winifred L. Star

Measles or rubeola is the most communicable childhood viral infection. It is spread by droplets to a susceptible individual. Incubation time is from 10-14 days. An attenuated measles vaccine has been in use in the U.S. since 1963 which has reduced the incidence of the disease significantly.

Maternal measles is less common than either chickenpox or mumps. An increased mortality among pregnant women with measles, usually secondary to pneumonia, has been reported. Research on measles indicates an increased rate of prematurity if disease onset is in late gestation. Increased risk of spontaneous abortion and teratogenicity have not been proven. Measles appearing in the newborn or in the first 10 days of life is considered to be acquired transplacentally; later onset measles is postnatally acquired. Congenital measles has a mortality rate of 32%. This rate may be even higher in preterm infants.

Complications of measles include otitis media, croup, bacterial pneumonia, encephalitis, thrombocytopenic purpura, myocarditis, and subacute sclerosing panencephalitis (Gibbs & Sweet, 1989).

Data Base

Subjective

- Symptoms of acute measles include the following:

    - Prodrome of fever and malaise 10-11 days postexposure

    - Coryza, sneezing, conjunctivitis, and cough follows within 24 hours

    - Koplik's spots appear after prodrome: tiny papular white lesions with erythematous halos in lateral buccal mucosa

    - Maculopapular rash on head, neck, behind ears spreading to trunk, upper then lower extremities 12-14 days after exposure

Objective

- Fever

- Observation of rash as described above

- Complications of measles may be present. See introductory section.

Assessment

- Measles (Rubeola)
- R/O Other viral exanthem
- R/O Complications of measles

Plan

Diagnostic Tests

- No specific tests.
- If pneumonia present - sputum Gram stain and culture

Treatment/Management

- Symptomatic relief.
- Antibiotic therapy for otitis media or pneumonia based on results of Gram stain and culture
- Passive immunization with immune serum globulin (ISG) 0.25 ml/kg IM given as soon as possible postexposure to susceptible pregnant women
- Infants should be given 0.25 ml/kg of ISG if born to women with measles in the last few weeks of pregnancy or in the first week postpartum.
- Live measles vaccine is **contraindicated** in pregnancy. Nonpregnant individuals should receive live vaccine 8 weeks after passive prophylaxis.
- Infants having received ISG should be immunized with live measles vaccine after 12 months of age.

Consultation

- Required. Patient may be managed by NP/NM.

Patient Education

- Educate regarding etiology of infection and signs and symptoms of complications.
- Educate regarding signs and symptoms of preterm labor. See Preterm Birth Prevention protocol.
- Reassure regarding fetal implications. Discuss course of congenitally acquired disease in the neonate (may range from mild to rapidly fatal). Postnatally acquired infection, however, is usually mild.
- Offer suggestions for symptomatic relief.

Follow-up

- Routine prenatal care
- Observation for complications
- Document in progress notes and problem list.

MUMPS

Winifred L. Star

Mumps is a viral disease of childhood affecting the parotid and salivary glands. It is transmitted by droplets and saliva to susceptible individuals. The incubation period is from 14-18 days. Only 10% of mumps cases occur in persons older than 15 years of age.

In pregnancy mumps is more common than chicken pox or measles. The infection is fairly benign if acquired during this time, however. Studies have reported a twofold increase in spontaneous abortion if mumps occurs during the first trimester. Complications of prematurity, intrauterine growth retardation, or perinatal mortality are not significant. Teratogenicity is unproven. The major concern has been the postulation between maternal mumps infection and the later development of congenital cardiac anomalies [e.g., endocardial fibroelastosis] (Gibbs & Sweet, 1989). More studies are required to support or refute this concern.

Complications of mumps are uncommon. Morbidity may include orchitis, aseptic meningitis, pancreatitis, mastitis, thyroiditis, myocarditis, nephritis, and arthritis (Gibbs & Sweet, 1989).

Data Base

Subjective

- Symptoms of mumps include:

    - Prodrome of fever, malaise, myalgia, anorexia

    - Bilateral (usually) parotitis within 24 hours of prodrome

Objective

- Fever

- Red, swollen Stensen's duct

- Parotid gland swelling

- Submaxillary glands may be swollen in some cases.

- Complications as described in introductory section may be present.

Assessment

- Mumps

- R/O Other viral illness

- R/O Complications of mumps

Plan

Diagnostic Tests

- None indicated

Treatment/Management

- Symptomatic relief.
- Cold or heat applied to the parotid glands may alleviate discomfort.
- Live mumps vaccination is contraindicated in pregnancy.
- Nonpregnant individuals may be immunized with the Jeryl Lynn live vaccine.

Consultation

- Required. Patient may be managed by NP/NM.

Patient Education

- Discuss etiology and benign nature of the infection.
- Offer suggestions for symptomatic relief.
- Advise of potential complications and need to inform health care provider if signs of more serious disease occur.
- Reassure regarding fetal implications. Educate regarding signs and symptoms of spontaneous abortion if mumps contracted in the first trimester.

Follow-up

- Routine prenatal care
- Observation for complications
- Document in progress notes and problem list.

PARVOVIRUS

Winifred L. Star

The human parvovirus (B19) was discovered in 1975 and was subsequently implicated as the primary etiologic agent of erythema infectiosum (fifth disease). B19 is a cause of transient aplastic crisis in patients with chronic hemolytic anemias and is associated with acute arthritis (Kinney & Kumar, 1988).

Fifth disease most commonly occurs in childhood and is characterized by features similar to the flu. A "slapped cheek" rash which spreads to the trunk and extremities in a lacelike pattern may appear. Thirty to sixty percent of adults are seropositive. The respiratory tract is the likely portal of entry and the incubation period is from 4-20 days (Mead, 1989).

Adverse pregnancy outcomes attributed to parvovirus include spontaneous abortion, hydrops fetalis, and stillbirth. B19 infection does not appear to be teratogenic, although at the present time only limited data regarding perinatal effects is available (Kinney & Kumar, 1988). According to one study the risk of fetal death after maternal infection is estimated to be <10% (Mead, 1989).

Data Base

Subjective

- Woman may report:

    - fever, malaise, myalgias

    - upper respiratory symptoms

    - "slapped cheek" facial rash; reticulated trunk and extremity rash

    - pruritis

    - adenopathy

    - exposure to household member or schoolage child with fifth disease or viral syndrome (outbreaks usually occur in late winter or early spring)

    - no symptoms (15-35%)

Objective

- Appearance of maternal fever or rash as described above

- Maternal serum positive for human parvovirus B19 immunoglobin M (IgM) antibody

- Elevated MSAFP levels

- Nonimmune hydrops fetalis characterized by:

    - ascites

    - pericardial/pleural effusion

    - myocarditis

    - myositis of skeletal muscle

328

- leukoerythroblastic response of liver, spleen, kidney

- bone marrow aplasia and hemolysis

- heart failure

- anemia

- low red and white cell counts in peripheral blood (Kinney & Kumar, 1988)

- Human parvovirus B19 DNA in fetal organs

- Eosinophilic nuclear inclusions with peripheral condensation of chromatin in erythroid precursors of infected woman (Mead, 1989)

- Hemosiderin deposition in intercellular space in liver on histologic exam of fetal tissue (Maeda et al., 1988)

Assessment

- Parvovirus (B19) infection

- R/O Other perinatal infection

Plan

Diagnostic Tests

- IgM antibody: detected by ELISA or radioimmunoassay in 90% of cases by third day following symptom-onset; titer falls 30-60 days after illness-onset, can persist for $\geq$ 4 months; most sensitive test to detect recent infection (Mead, 1989)

- IgG antibody: appears by day 7, persists indefinately; presence of only IgG indicates previous infection and immune status (although infection may have occurred as recently as 4 months prior) (Mead, 1989)

- Presence of both IgM and IgG suggests recent exposure, from 7 days to 6 months previously (Mead, 1989).

NOTE: Serologic tests for B19 IgM and IgG are available in research labs and at the CDC's Division of Viral Diseases which will accept specimens from State Health Departments (Kinney & Kumar, 1988; Mead, 1989). Since the lab will report both IgM and IgG antibody results only a single specimen obtained between 4 days and 4 weeks of symptom-onset or 2 weeks post exposure will suffice to establish the serologic diagnosis of acute infection (Mead, 1989).

Treatment/Management

- B19 infection should be accurately diagnosed utilizing data obtained from the maternal history, and physical and laboratory examinations.

- There are no available medications to treat parvovirus infection or a vaccine to prevent it. At this time routine prophylaxis with immune globulin is not recommended.

- Weekly MSAFP levels following onset of infection-- elevated levels precede hydrops fetalis and fetal death

- Serial ultrasonography to assess hydrops fetalis

- Consider percutaneous umbilical blood sample (PUBS) to assess fetal B19 IgM and fetal hematologic indices.

- If fetal hydrops is demonstrated, intrauterine transfusion may be considered to alleviate severe anemia (Berstein & Capeless, 1989).

Consultation

- Required in all cases of suspected or confirmed parvovirus infection
- Patient may be managed by MD in some settings.

Patient Education

- Explanation of the etiologic and perinatal effects of parvovirus infection should be done by the NP/NM or MD managing the case.
- Psychological support of the woman/couple during the diagnostic work-up and management phase is warranted.

Follow-up

- The CDC does not recommend excluding pregnant women from schools where an outbreak of fifth disease has occured. Pregnant women should receive serologic testing if exposed.
- Public health measures would include follow-up of outbreaks of rash illness in schools to establish an exact diagnosis. This would be carried out by the Public Health Department.
- Pathologic examination of hydropic fetuses is warranted to assess B19 infection.
- Psychosocial support of the woman/couple is important. Psychological and social services should be utilized as indicated.
- Document problem in progress notes and problem list.

RUBELLA

Winifred L. Star

Of all the viruses causing congenital infections, rubella is one of the best known and investigated. The association of maternal rubella infection and the occurrence of congenital birth defects was identified by N. McAllister Gregg, an Australian ophthalmologist in 1941. Fetal infection may occur at any stage of pregnancy, although the mechanism by which the virus causes fetal damage is not well-understood. Congenital rubella syndrome (CRS) includes many features: the classic triad of cataracts, deafness, and congenital heart disease; IUGR; CNS disease; mental retardation; pneumonitis; bony lesions; immunologic disorders; chromosomal anomalies; hepatitis; and thrombocytopenic purpura (Freij, South, & Sever, 1988). Miscarriage and stillbirth may also occur secondary to rubella virus insult. Other defects, largely endocrinopathies, are not noticeable at birth but develop later from continued viral replication (Zeichner & Plotkin, 1988). The outcome of fetal infection depends upon the time in pregnancy in which the mother becomes infected. The overall risk of CRS is about 20-25% if primary maternal infection occurs in the first trimester (ACOG, 1981; Gibbs & Sweet, 1989). During second to third trimester exposure the incidence of CRS drops to <1% (ACOG, 1981).

Acute rubella infection is droplet-spread from infected respiratory secretions. (Manifestations of the infection are described in the Subjective section below.). The infection is most common among children 5-9 years, and occurs mostly in the springtime. Widespread use of the rubella vaccine has resulted in dramatic declines in incidence rates in the U.S. Subsequently, the number of infants born with CRS has also declined. However, surveys indicate that 12-24% of postpubertal individuals are still susceptible to rubella infection (Freij et al., 1988).

Maternal viremia must occur for fetal/placental infection to take place. Although uncommon, rubella infection can occur in women with previously naturally acquired infection or in vaccine recipients (Freij et al., 1988). Fetal risk from maternal reinfection is small.

Rubella vaccine

The vaccine currently available in the U.S. is the RA 27/3 strain; a live attenuated rubella virus which simulates natural infection. Antibody levels are present in >95% of vaccinees for at least six years without significant decline (ACOG, 1981). Rubella vaccine is known to cross the placenta and may potentially infect the fetus during the early stages of development. However, data collected by the CDC since 1979 has shown no evidence that the vaccine administered to pregnant women causes CRS (CDC, 1989). Because of the **small** theoretical risk to the fetus, the Immunization Practices Advisory Committee (ACIP) of the Public Health Service continues to state: 1) pregnancy remains a contraindication to rubella vaccine because of the theoretical, albeit small, risk of CRS; 2) reasonable precautions should be taken to preclude vaccination of pregnant women, including asking women if they are pregnant, excluding those who say they are, and explaining the theoretical risk to others; and 3) if vaccination occurs within 3 months before or after conception, the risk of CRS is so small as to be negligible; thus inadvertent vaccination of a pregnant woman should not be a reason in itself to consider interruption of pregnancy (CDC, 1989).

Data Base

Subjective

- Susceptible client may report exposure to individual with rubella.
- Subclinical infection exists in large proportion of individuals.
- Occurrence 14-21 days following exposure of susceptible individual
- Features of symptomatic disease include:
    - mild prodrome: malaise, low-grade fever, headache, conjunctivitis
    - rash appearing 1-5 days after prodrome: macular, beginning on face, behind ears; spreading downward over 1-2 days; disappearing over 3 days
    - postauricular, suboccipital, and posterior cervical lymphadenopathy
    - transient arthralgias
    - arthritis (uncommon) (Freij et al., 1988)

Objective (see also Diagnostic Tests section)

- Documentation of signs and symptoms of acute viral illness in pregnant woman
- Viral shedding from nasopharynx occurs 1 week before and 1 week after rash onset and persists for 6-12 months.
- Low-level positive HI titers of 1:8-1:32 are rarely seen within the first 6 months following acute infection.
- High-level HI titers (e.g., $\geq$1:256) may be present in up to 15% of the population and do not by themselves indicate acute infection.
- IgM antibodies can be detected only up to 4 weeks after rash onset. Positive titers indicate acute primary infection.
- Rubella-specific IgM is usually present in CRS infants and may persist for 6-12 months. This provides presumptive evidence of congenital infection.
- Rubella virus can be isolated from cerebrospinal fluid in approximately one-third of all infants.
- For CRS infant, observation of fetal anomalies as described in definition section
- Postnatal growth and development abnormalities dependent upon gestational age at onset of infection: early onset infection - cataracts, retarded height, weight; later onset infection - slow growth rates in preschool years with catch-up later on.

Assessment

- Maternal exposure to rubella
- R/O Rubella infection
- R/O Enteroviral infection
- R/O Measles
- R/O Parvovirus B19 disease

Plan

Diagnostic Tests   (See Figures 7.3-7.5, pp. 335-337).

- Diagnosis based on clinical evidence alone unreliable; serologic confirmation essential

- Serologic tests currently available include:

    - hemagglutination inhibition (HI) - IgG class antibody most commonly used for screening

    - complement fixation test

    - enzyme-linked immunosorbent assay (ELISA)

    - rubella specific IgM

    - immunofluorescence (e.g., IFA, FIA, FIAX)

    - passive hemagglutination (PHA)

- In a known immune patient with exposure to rubella there is no further testing required and no risk to the fetus.

- In a non-immune patient with suspected exposure or infection HI testing should be done 3-4 weeks after exposure or 10-14 days after rash onset in order to determine seroconversion and possible fetal risk. A $\geq$4-fold rise in HI titer is evidence of acute rubella infection. If the HI titer remains at <1:8 acute rubella infection has not occurred (ACOG, 1981).

- A patient with unknown rubella status presenting within 1 week after exposure to a rash illness should have an HI titer drawn and repeated in 3-4 weeks. A titer <1:8 in the first specimen followed by seroconversion is indicative of rubella infection (ACOG, 1981).

- A patient with unknown rubella status presenting 1-5 weeks after exposure to a rash illness or up to 3 weeks after rash onset should have an HI titer drawn. If HI titer is 1:8-1:32, redraw in 2 weeks and repeat titers on both sera. A $\geq$4-fold rise in titer is good evidence of acute rubella infection. If there is no significant change in titer obtain a complement fixation (CF) test on both sera. Absence of CF antibodies indicates no infection. A $\geq$4-fold rise in CF titer indicates rubella infection. In the case of an unchanged titer rubella-specific IgM should be obtained on both specimens. Absence of this antibody indicates no infection; presence indicates infection (ACOG, 1981).

- If a patient with unknown rubella status presents $\geq$5 weeks after exposure to a rash illness or $\geq$3 weeks after rash onset with an HI titer <1:8, this is indicative of no acute infection, rather, susceptibility. A titer of 1:8-1:32 would indicate previous rubella infection; unlikely to have been within the past 6 months. A titer >1:32 indicates previous infection, date indeterminate and risk to fetus unknown (ACOG, 1981).

Treatment/Management   (See also Diagnostic Tests)

- All pregnant patients should be screened for rubella immunity as soon as possible in pregnancy.

- Follow the guidelines outlined in the Diagnostic Test section to guide management of immune and non-immune patients with known or suspected exposure or infection.

Consultation

- Consultation is not required on a patient who is known to be rubella-immune.

- Consultation should be sought on a non-immune patient with known or suspected exposure or infection.

Patient Education

- A non-immune pregnant woman should be told to avoid exposure to school-age children with rash illnesses or known rubella.

- Counseling regarding the possible risk to the fetus is dependent upon the patient's immune status and the condition of known or suspected exposure or infection.

- Laboratory analyses, historical and clinical indices should be utilized to determine risk and guide counseling.

- First trimester maternal infection is associated with a 20-25% chance of CRS; a $\leq 1\%$ chance in the second and third trimesters.

- Clear evidence of first trimester infection would prompt discussion of elective pregnancy termination.

- The patient should be informed that if non-immune she will be vaccinated postpartum, usually in the hospital prior to discharge. Ensuing pregnancy should be avoided for at least 3 months post-vaccine.

Follow-up

- Non-immune patients should be vaccinated postpartum with the RA 27/3 live attenuated rubella vaccine. Ideally this should be done in the hospital prior to discharge.

- There is no contraindication to the breast feeding mother for the administration of the vaccine.

- Conception should be avoided for three months after the vaccine to avoid the negligible risk of CRS.

- Women opting to deliver at home should consider receiving the rubella vaccine shortly after delivery.

- Alert patient to possible side effects of the vaccine including fever, rash, and lymphadenopathy. These may occur 7-21 days after administration. Effects such as joint pain and arthritis may also occur but are rare.

- Document in problem list and progress notes.

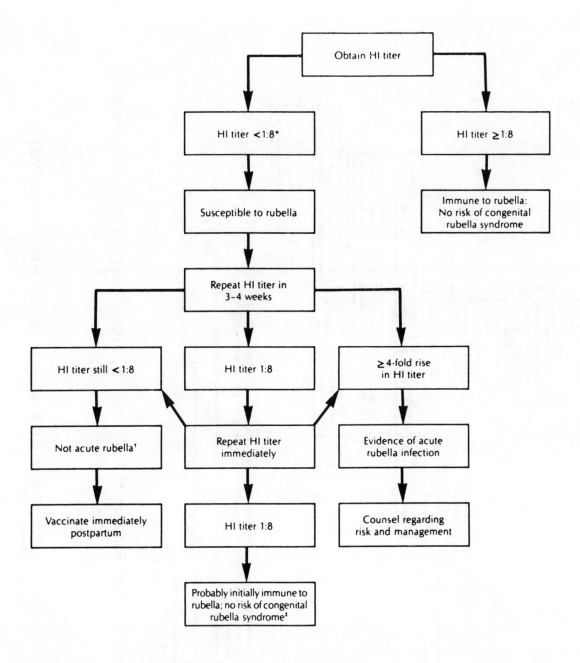

* An HI titer of 1:8 or less is used to indicate susceptibility. The actual susceptibility cutoff level may vary in different laboratories (eg, <1:10).

† The patient should be followed closely during the first trimester for rash illness or exposure to rubella. Another HI titer at the end of the first trimester is advisable, especially if rubella is present in the community.

‡ Over 99% of acute rubella infections will result in development and maintenance of HI titers of 1:32 or greater for at least 6 months after onset. Original HI titer of 1:8 or less is suspect.

Figure 7.3. Time Frame 1: Within 1 Week after Exposure to Rash Illness

SOURCE:

American College of Obstetricians and Gynecologists (1981). *Rubella: A clinical update* (Technical Bulletin No. 62). Washington, DC: Author. Reprinted with permission of Richard E. Hoffman, MD.

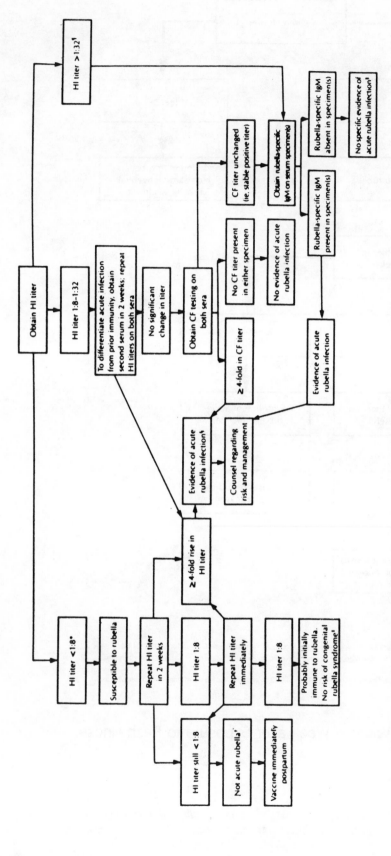

*   An acute titer of 1:8 or less is used to indicate susceptibility. The actual susceptibility cutoff level may vary in different laboratories (eg, <1:10).

†   The patient should be followed closely during the first trimester for rash illness or exposure to rubella. Another HI titer at the end of the first trimester is advisable, especially if rubella is present in the community.

‡   Over 99% of acute rubella infections will result in development and maintenance of HI titers of 1:32 or greater for at least 6 months after onset. Original HI titer of 1:8 or less is suspect.

§   In the absence of rash illness, if reinfection is a major consideration, a properly timed IgM antibody assay may help to differentiate primary from secondary infection.

‖   Absence of rubella-specific IgM may not exclude recent rubella infection.

¶   The physician may elect to proceed with a titer of 1:8–1:32.

Figure 7.4.   Time Frame 2: 1–5 Weeks after Exposure to Rash Illness or, if Rash Illness, up to 3 Weeks after Rash Onset

SOURCE:

American College of Obstetricians and Gynecologists (1981). *Rubella: A clinical update* (Technical Bulletin No. 62). Washington, DC: Author. Reprinted with permission of Richard E. Hoffman, MD.

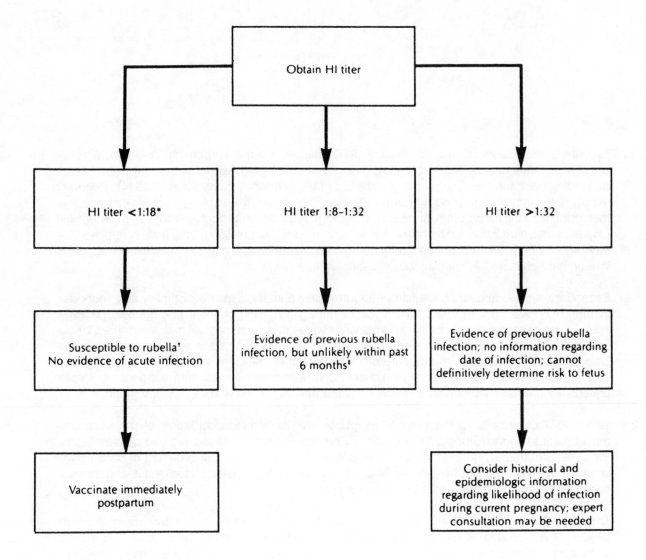

* An HI titer of 1:8 or less is used to indicate susceptibility. The actual susceptibility cutoff level may vary in different laboratories (eg, <1:10).

† The patient should be followed closely during the first trimester for rash illness or exposure to rubella. Another HI titer at the end of the first trimester is advisable, especially if rubella is present in the community.

‡ Over 99% of acute rubella infections will result in development and maintenance of HI titers of 1:32 or greater for at least 6 months after onset.

Figure 7.5. Time frame 3: Five Weeks or More after Exposure to Rash Illness, or 3 Weeks or More after Rash Onset or Single Titer from Pregnant Woman with Unknown Exposure and No Rash Illness.

SOURCE:

American College of Obstetricians and Gynecologists (1981). *Rubella: A clinical update* (Technical Bulletin No. 62). Washington, DC: Author. Reprinted with permission of Richard E. Hoffman, MD.

SYPHILIS

Winifred L. Star

Syphilis is a sexually transmitted disease (STD) caused by the Treponema pallidum, a motile spirochete. Risk of acquisition of the organism from an infected partner is thought to be 30-50% depending upon the morphology and distribution of the partner's lesions (Chapel, 1984). Following exposure the incubation period is from 10-90 days. The primary lesion of syphilis, the chancre, may then appear. This lesion often starts as a dull red macule which progresses to a papular eroded, ulcerated area with indurated margins. Associated regional lymphadenopathy usually appears 7-10 days later. About 5% of chancres are in non-genital locations and may not be clinically apparent. The primary chancre will spontaneously disappear in 2-6 weeks.

Secondary syphilis appears 6 weeks to 6 months after primary. (However primary and secondary syphilis may overlap with about 30% of cases having a healing chancre at diagnosis [McPhee, 1984]). The secondary stage is characterized by a widespread symmetrical macular or papular skin rash and generalized lymphadenopathy. Lesions on the palms and soles are common landmarks. Condylomata lata, wart-like infectious lesions may appear on the vulva, perineum or anus. The skin lesions of secondary syphilis usually resolve in 2-10 weeks with or without treatment. Untreated patients then enter a latent phase, which is for the majority of individuals, asymptomatic.

About 25% of patients in the early latent phase will have an exacerbation of the secondary mucotaneous lesions (Gibbs & Sweet, 1989). The latent phase is divided into two phases: early - one year's duration, and late - greater than one year's duration. About one-third of patients with latent disease develop late (tertiary) syphilis. Neuro/cardiovascular, musculoskeletal, and/or multi-organ system complications may occur in this stage.

Transplacental transmission of T. pallidum to a fetus may occur at any time during pregnancy; the degree of risk related to the quantity of spirochetes in the maternal bloodstream. Primary or secondary syphilitic mothers are more likely to transmit the infection (50% risk) than those in the latent or late phase of disease (40% & 10% risk respectively). Syphilis may cause preterm delivery, stillbirth, congenital infection, and/or neonatal death. Congenital syphilis is a multisystem disease ranging in severity with manifestations resembling secondary syphilis; often there is skeletal involvement (Main & Main, 1982). Most infants with early congenital syphilis are asymptomatic at birth. Active disease may not become evident until 10 days to 2 weeks of life. If left untreated (or incompletely treated) classic manifestations of late congenital syphilis will appear: Hutchington's teeth, eighth nerve deafness, and cardiovascular stigmata (Wendel, 1988; Gibbs & Sweet, 1989).

Increases in syphilis cases occurred in the U.S. in 1987 after a five year trend of decreasing incidence. The areas reporting the largest increases were California, Florida, and New York City. Heterosexuals have mostly been affected. The increase has prompted two major concerns: adverse effects on congenital syphilis control efforts, and increases in HIV acquisition (CDC, 1987).

Data Base

Subjective

- Positive sexual contact

- Symptoms of primary and/or secondary syphilis may include:

- oral and/or anogenital lesions, sores (chancres)
- skin lesion(s) or "rash"
- palmar erythema
- swollen lymph glands
- pain in long bones, muscles or joints
- patchy hair loss
- rectal pain, mucoid discharge, blood-streaked stool
- nausea, vomiting
- malaise
- low grade fever
- anorexia
- weight loss
- sore throat
- headache
- hearing loss
- photophobia, ocular pain, vision loss
- facial paralysis
- May have concomitant STD
- Previous history of syphilis or other STD

Objective

- Perform complete exam of cervical and inguinal lymph nodes, mouth, skin and hair, soles and palms, extremities, liver, spleen, external genitalia, vagina, cervix, anus,
  Note presence of: lymphadenopathy; hair loss (alopecia); diffuse maculopapular rash on palms or soles; presence of chancres in the mouth, vulvovaginal, cervical and/or anal area, or elsewhere; mucous patches (round, painless grey plaques on erythematous base) on lips, tongue, buccal mucosa, pharynx, tonsils, vaginal introitus; condyloma lata (cauliflower-like growths) in intertriginous areas
- Neurological exam as indicated
- Dark-field exam or serologic tests may be positive.
- Wet mounts may show evidence of vaginitis/cervicitis in presence of concomitant infection.
- Cervical cultures for gonorrhea and chlamydia may be positive.

Assessment

- Syphilis
- Positive VDRL or RPR, FTA-ABS or MHA-TP

Plan

Diagnostic tests

- Definitive diagnosis of early syphilis is based on dark field examinations and direct fluorescent antibody tests on lesions or tissue (CDC, 1989). To collect specimen for dark field exam gently abrade lesion then press glass slide onto the exudate. Cover with glass coverslip and transport directly to the lab. Diagnostic material may also be obtained from enlarged regional lymph nodes. Prep skin with antiseptic solution, then aspirate material using sterile 20-gauge needle attached to syringe.
NOTE: Dark field exam not routinely done; requires experienced microscopist. Consult with MD or practice protocols before performing.

- Presumptive diagnosis is based on two types of serologic tests:
  - nontreponemal
    - . Venereal Disease Research Laboratory (VDRL)
    - . rapid plasma reagin (RPR)
  - treponemal
    - . fluorescent treponemal antibody absorbed (FTA-ABS)
    - . microhemagglutination assay for antibody to T. pallidum (MHA-TP)

NOTE: Neither test alone sufficient for diagnosis. The former are used as screening tests with confirmation of positive results by the latter. Nontreponemal antibody tests are reported quantitatively, with titers rising and falling depending upon disease state and treatment. (A fourfold titer change equals a two-dilution change [e.g., from 1:16 to 1:4, or from 1:8 to 1:32]). Do not use the VDRL and RPR interchangeably for sequential testing; use one or the other (CDC, 1989). False positive nontreponemal serologic tests may occur in the following conditions: drug abuse, collagen-vascular disorders, malaria, leprosy, pneumonia, bacterial/viral infections, aging, pregnancy, lab error, and after vaccination/immunization (Noble, 1982; Wendel, 1988). Positive treponemal antibody tests remain so for life regardless of treatment and/or disease activity (CDC, 1989). In patients with early primary or incubating syphilis all of these tests may be negative.

- Neurosyphilis diagnosis can not be based on any single test. Cerebrospinal fluid (CSF) analysis is performed including cell count, protein, VDRL, and possibly FTA-ABS.

- Chlamydia and gonococcal cultures to be done to rule out concomitant STD.

- HIV-antibody test to be offered

- Wet mounts to be performed as indicated.

- Additional labs (e.g., CBC, sedimentation rate) as indicated

Treatment/Management

- Ideally all women should have syphilis screening at the first prenatal visit and again in the late third trimester if at high risk for STD.

- If the VDRL or RPR is reactive but the FTA-ABS or MHA-TP is negative and the patient is without clinical signs of disease, repeat the VDRL or RPR _and_ FTA-ABS or MHA-TP in 4-6 weeks. If the treponemal tests are still negative, then the patient has a biological false-positive test for syphilis and MD consultation is recommended for evaluation of autoimmune disorders.

- Suspicious lesions should be evaluated with dark field exam if the serologic tests are negative. Up to a 30% false negative rate of nontreponemal and treponemal testing has been documented in primary syphilis (Stewart, 1983).

- The treatments listed below are taken from the: Centers for Disease Control (1989). Sexually transmitted diseases treatment guidelines. *Morbidity and Mortality Weekly Report*, *38*(S-8), 5-13.

Primary, secondary, latent syphilis of less than 1 year's duration:

- Benzathine penicillin 2.4 million units IM, in one dose

Late latent syphilis of more than 1 year's duration:

- Benzathine penicillin 7.2 million units total, administered as 3 doses of 2.4 million units IM, given once a week x 3 weeks

- CSF analysis (to R/O neurosyphilis) to be performed in the following instances: neurologic signs, treatment failure, nontreponemal antibody titer $\geq$1:32, nonpenicillin therapy planned, positive HIV-antibody. See current CDC guidelines for drug regimens in neurosyphilis.

- Penicillin-allergic pregnant patients should be carefully assessed regarding the nature/validity of the allergy. Tetracycline/doxycycline are contraindicated in pregnancy and erythromycin is not likely to cure fetal infection. Therefore, pregnant women, if necessary, should receive skin testing and treated with penicillin, or referred for desensitization. Refer to CDC guidelines for these procedures.

- Sexual partners who have been exposed to syphilis within the preceding 90 days (or more if serologic testing is unavailable or follow-up uncertain) should be treated prophylactically as for early syphilis above.

Alternate regimens for penicillin-allergic nonpregnant individuals include:

- Doxycycline 100 mg po bid x 14 days or

- Tetracycline 500 mg po qid x 14 days or if these not tolerated

- Erythromycin 500 mg po qid x 14 days

Consultation

- Required in all cases of syphilis

- For biological false-positive nontreponemal tests

- When considering dark field examination

- For prescription as necessary

- Referral to MD in patients with suspicion/evidence of neurosyphilis

Patient Education

- Discuss etiology, transmission of disease, and potential fetal implications.

- Advise regarding importance of partner evaluation and treatment.

- IMPORTANT: Discuss the **Jarisch-Herxheimer reaction**. This is an acute febrile reaction which may be accompanied by headache, myalgias and other symptoms following any therapy for syphilis. Antipyretics may be taken. As preterm labor may ensue, patient to notify provider if contractions or change in fetal movements occur.

- Discuss safer sex practices for HIV/STD prevention, and recommend use of condoms with new/multiple/non-monogamous partner(s).

- Recommend careful "screening" of sexual partners for STD. Advise attention to partner signs/symptoms.

- Advise sexual abstinence until treatment completed and disease state cured.

- Follow-up is extremely important. Impress upon patient need for long-term serologic testing to ensure adequacy of therapy.

Follow-up

- If suspected as being high risk for syphilis/STD, order repeat VDRL or RPR in third trimester (32-34 weeks).

- The follow-up measures listed below are extrapolated from the 1989 CDC guidelines and are applicable during/after pregnancy:

  - Monthly VDRL or RPR titers should be done for the remainder of pregnancy if treated for syphilis. A 4-fold decline indicates adequate treatment.

  - If nontreponemal antibody titers have not declined 4-fold by 3 months in primary/secondary or by 6 months in early latent syphilis, or if signs/symptoms persist in the absence of reinfection, patients to have a CSF exam and be retreated appropriately.

  - Following pregnancy VDRL or RPR to be rechecked in 3, and 6 months after treatment for primary, secondary and early latent syphilis of less than 1 year's duration.

  - Additional VDRL or RPR to be done in 12 months if treated for late latent syphilis of more than 1 years duration. If titer increases >4-fold, an initially high titer ($\geq$1:32) fails to decrease, or patient has signs/symptoms of syphilis, evaluate for neurosyphilis and retreat appropriately.

  - Neurosyphilis patients should have a CSF exam every 6 months until normal. If cell count not decreased at 6 months or not normal by 2 years, consider retreatment.

- Patients may have persistent low level VDRL or RPR titers for life despite adequate treatment.

- In the presence of other STD (e.g., gonorrhea, chlamydia, condyloma, herpes) syphilis testing should be done. (Dual medication therapy for gonorrhea is probably effective for incubating syphilis.)

- Confidentiality morbidity and mortality report to be filed with Department of Public Health.

- Partner follow-up with own health care provider as indicated by his/her syphilis status

- Document in progress notes and problem list.

TOXOPLASMOSIS

Winifred L. Star

Toxoplasma gondii is one of the most widespread protozoan parasites existing in nature. The organism is found in all orders of mammals and birds. The lifecycle of toxoplasma occurs in three phases: trophozoite, tissue cyst, and oocyst. The trophozoite invades many kinds of mammal cells and is seen during the acute stage of infection. The tissue cyst forms within host cells and may contain thousands of organisms. Tissue cysts are found by the eighth day of infection and persist throughout the life of the host. Oocysts are present only in cats and are excreted in feces. Sporozoites formed in the oocysts are infective for man. Cats aquire toxoplasmosis by eating infected mice or other animals. Humans generally become infected by ingesting raw or poorly cooked meat of an infected animal or via contact with the feces of an infected cat. Transmission of infection can also occur through blood transfusions, organ transplants, or across the placenta.

About 15-40% of pregnant women have antibody to toxoplasma (Sever, 1990). If a woman is infected in pregnancy fetal involvement may occur. The incidence of congenital infection will depend upon the trimester in which maternal infection has occurred. The rate of fetal infection seems to be higher in the third trimester; however, the severity of fetal infection is greater if maternal disease occurs in the first trimester. Primary toxoplasmosis in pregnancy confers approximately a 30% chance of fetal infection. Most infants with congenital toxoplasmosis have only serologic abnormalities. However, more serious findings may include: intracerebral calcifications, chorioretinitis, hydrocephaly, micocephaly, abnormal spinal fluid, splenomegaly, jaundice, fever, lymphadenopathy, convulsions, and vomiting. Acute primary toxoplasmosis in pregnancy has been associated with abortion, prematurity, and growth retardation (Gibbs & Sweet, 1989).

Data Base

Subjective

- Subclinical disease usually

- Clinially apparent disease may resemble mononucleosis and is usually mild and self-limiting. Symptoms may include:

  - fever

  - malaise

  - myalgias

  - low-grade fever

  - headache

  - sore throat

  - non-tender cervical lymphadenopathy

  - maculopapular rash

  - ocular symptoms (more rare)

- Onset of symptoms generally occurs 1-2 weeks after infection and subsides over two weeks to several months.

Objective

- Observation of signs as above
- Atypical lymphocytosis
- Serologic techniques will confirm toxoplasmosis.
- Infant findings are described in the Definition section.

Assessment

- Toxoplasmosis
- R/O Mononucleosis
- R/O Viral Syndrome

Plan

Diagnostic Tests

- Due to the high incidence of antibody in the general population routine toxoplasmosis screening of pregnant women is not recommended (Gibbs & Sweet, 1989).
- Serologic techniques are used to confirm the diagnosis of toxoplasmosis. Reliability and interpretation of the tests, however, may make clinical application of results difficult. Testing should be limited to those patients with history and symptoms suggestive of toxoplasmosis (Sever, 1990).
- IgG antibodies can be detected by the indirect fluorescent antibody test, Sabin-Feldman dye test, indirect hemagglutination inhibition test, and complement fixation test.
- Two blood samples obtained three weeks apart (acute and convalescent titers) are generally required. A four-fold rise in titer is diagnostic of acute infection. Ideally paired sera should be tested.
- Acute infection IgG titers are generally >1:1000. The antibodies peak within 1-2 months of infection-onset and may persist for years.
- IgM antibodies appear within a week of infection-onset and last for several months to years. Krick and Remington (1978) advise the use of IgM indirect flourescent antibody test if IgG is positive. A negative IgM antibody with an IgG titer >1:1000 probably excludes the diagnosis of acute infection.
- In woman at high-risk of contracting toxoplasma (e.g., those with many cats) serial IgG titers may be performed q 1-2 months.
- Fetal blood IgM is positive after 22 weeks gestation but only 10-20% of infected fetuses may have IgM antibodies.

Treatment/Management

- Primary prevention is the key. See Patient Education section.
- There is no universal agreement on treatment in pregnancy to prevent fetal infection.
- If the diagnosis of acute toxoplasmosis is made give 25 mg of oral pyrimethamine daily plus 1 gram of oral sulfadiazine qid x 28 days. Additionally give 6 mg of folinic acid IM or po three times/week. Therapy may need to be continued for several months in severe cases (Sever, 1990).

NOTE: Pyrimethamine is not recommended in the first trimester because of possible teratogenicity. Sulfadiazine should be discontinued in the last few weeks of pregnancy.

- Symptomatic infants with congenital toxoplasmosis should be treated with a combination of sulfadiazine, pyrimethamine, and folinic acid.

Consultation

- Required in all cases
- MD management preferable

Patient Education

- Since disease prevention is key extensive teaching regarding toxoplasmosis is necessary.
- Advise that cats should be fed commercial cat food or well-cooked meat. Cats should not be allowed to hunt mice and, ideally, be kept indoors.
- A pregnant woman should avoid close contact with cats during the pregnancy. Handwashing is necessary after handling occurs especially before eating.
- Someone other than the pregnant woman should clean the litter box. Daily cleaning is recommended as the excreted organism becomes infectious after several days. Wipe the pan with household bleach and water, 1:10 dilution.
- Care should also be taken when working in a garden that cats have access to. Keep hands away from the face and wash them thoroughly when finished.
- Sandboxes for child-play are also a potential source of contamination. Keep covered when not in use and if the sand becomes contaminated with cat feces discard and replace it.
- Do not eat undercooked meat. Wash hands after touching meat that has not been cooked.
- Prevent flies and cockroaches from coming into contact with food since they are capable of carrying infected oocysts.

Follow-up

- Encourage compliance with prenatal care and good health maintenance.
- In high-risk cases the patient may be referred to a pediatrician prenatally to discuss care of the congenitally infected infant.
- Document in problem list and progress notes.

TUBERCULOSIS--PRIMARY IDENTIFICATION OF CARRIERS

Maureen T. Shannon

Tuberculosis (TB) is an infection caused by Mycobacterium tuberculosis bacilli which primarily affects the lungs but can also involve the kidneys, lymph system, genital tract, meninges and other systems of the body (Bush, 1986). Tuberculosis during pregnancy can have serious implications for the health of the patient and her newborn. Recent immigrants (e.g., Indochinese refugees, Hispanics) and urban indigent populations have been identified as being high risk groups for the development of this disease (Summers, 1987).

Data Base

Subjective

- Individual history of positive PPDs

- Household members with TB

- Member of a high risk group (e.g., Indochinese refugees, Hispanics, urban populations)

- Arrival in U.S.A. within last 2 years

- Symptoms of persistent cough, night sweats, bloody sputum, or fever

Objective

- Place PPD

- Induration 10 mm or greater is positive (regardless of previous BCG vaccination status)

- Test must be read within 48-72 hours of placement

Assessment

- PPD positive or negative

Plan

Diagnostic Tests

- PPD testing is recommended for all pregnant women and especially those in high-risk groups.

- If negative PPD, no further action is needed.

- If PPD is positive, consult with MD. The chest x-ray is the key examination for determining appropriate therapy. Ideally the chest x-ray should be ordered at the time the positive PPD is discovered. With shielding of the abdomen, a chest x-ray has a mean fetal dose of only 1-5 mrad (1/1000 the minimal dose implicated in teratogenicity, childhood leukemia, etc.). However, the chest x-ray with abdominal shielding may be deferred until the second trimester at discretion of provider or request of patient to minimize any theoretical risks (D. R. Field, personal communication, 1990).

- If chest x-ray is positive, refer to internal medicine.

- If chest x-ray is negative, document in chart and problem list. Refer to MD post-partum.

- If history of positive PPD, do not repeat PPD. Obtain chest x-ray after 20 weeks. Refer to MD post-partum.

- If history of positive PPD, with normal chest x-ray within last year, it is not necessary to repeat the chest x-ray. Document in chart.

Consultation

- Consult MD as necessary.

Patient Education

- Educate patient regarding PPDs and any need for referral to an MD or for further testing (e.g., chest x-ray).

Follow-up

- Document PPD status in progress notes and problem list.

VAGINITIS

Winifred L. Star

Vaginitis is any inflammation that involves the vagina. It may result from any event or process that disturbs the normal physiology, interferes with the nutritional status of the epithelium or alters the protective mechanisms normally present. This protocol will cover bacterial vaginosis, monilial and trichomonas vaginitis.

Bacterial vaginosis occurs as the result of an overgrowth of various anaerobic bacteria, a decrease in lactobacilli, and an altered vaginal pH. Commonly implicated bacteria include gardnerella, mobiluncus, bacteroides, peptococcus, and peptostreptococcus. Approximately 40% of women with this condition remain asymptomatic. Bacterial vaginosis is not considered to be solely an STD; there is evidence against exclusive sexual transmission (Bump & Buesching, 1988). Predisposing factors include: any condition which may result in increased (alkaline) vaginal pH (e.g., medication, douches, foreign body, semen, menstrual blood, stress ?) and sexual transmission via an infected male or female partner. BV has been implicated in preterm labor, postpartum endometritis, and pelvic inflammatory disease. Treatment in pregnancy of asymptomatic women is not routinely recommended unless complications arise.

Yeast are ubiquitous, unicellular fungal organisms present in the gastrointestinal tract, mouth, and vagina. Candida albicans is responsible for >90% of monilial (yeast) infections. Other species implicated include C. glabrata (torulopsis), and C. tropicalis. Yeast infections are estimated to affect 5-40% of the female population and are second to bacterial vaginosis as a cause of vaginitis. Predisposing factors to infection include: a glycogen-rich vaginal environment (as in pregnancy and diabetes); ingestion of excessive dairy products, simple sugars and/or alcohol; antibiotic therapy; steroid medication; endocrine and immunologic disorders; anemia and other medical conditions; stress and poor hygiene. Frequent recurrences may be a problem for some women. Sexual transmission of fungal organisms is uncommon, but may occur.

Trichomonas vaginalis is a motile protozoan which can infect the vagina via sexual intercourse. The organism may also infect the urethra and bladder. Trichomoniasis is considered the most prevalent non-viral sexually transmitted disease (STD). Approximately 35% of women with trichomonas have concomitant bacterial vaginosis and 40% have concomitant gonorrhea. Risk factors include multiple partners and a history of STD.

Data Base

Subjective (See also predisposing factors in Definition above)

- Patient may complain of: pruritus, irritation, excoriation, "rash", burning, abnormal vaginal discharge (i.e., color, odor, quantity, quality), abnormal bleeding, dysuria (internal or external), urgency, frequency, dyspareunia, lower abdominal pain, fever, swollen inguinal lymph glands.

- History of prior infection, concomitant STD

- Patient may report partner has symptoms of "rash", itching, dysuria, penile/vaginal discharge, history of STD.

Objective

- Vital signs as indicated

- Abdominal exam (including inguinal lymph nodes)

- Pelvic exam: May see any of the following:

    - BUS: abnormal discharge

    - External genitalia: erythema, edema, excoriation

    - Vagina: abnormal discharge (thin to thick white, yellow, grey, green, frothy, curdy, foul odor)

    - Cervix: abnormal discharge, erythema, edema, friability, "strawberry patches," cervical motion tenderness

    - Uterus: assess size, shape, consistency, mobility, tenderness

    - Adnexa: assess ovaries, abnormal masses, tenderness

    - Recto/vaginal: as indicated to assess masses, tenderness

- Additional exam as indicated (e.g., mouth, throat, cervical lymph nodes, skin, joints)

- Wet mounts: saline (NaCl) and potassium hydroxide (KOH) to be done. NaCl--assess presence of WBCs, trichomonads, clue cells, lactobacilli; KOH--assess presence of amine (fishy) odor, pseudohyphae, spores.

- Assess pH

- Pap smear may show inflammatory changes, atypia, yeast, clue cells, or trichomonads.

Assessment

- Bacterial vaginosis: thin, grey homogeneous discharge; positive amine odor. Vulvar involvement usually absent but may see mild erythema. Wet mounts: NaCl = clue cells, decreased lactobacilli, lack of or few WBCs; KOH = amine odor. pH = ≥ 5

- Yeast or monilial vaginitis: thin or thick/curdy white discharge with erythematous/excoriated vulvar involvement. Wet mounts: KOH = pseudophyphae; NaCl = WBCs, may see lactobacilli. pH = 3.8-4.2

- Trichomonas vaginitis: erythematous vulvovaginal area, frothy or homogeneous grey, green discharge with foul odor. Cervix may be friable or erythematous with "strawberry patches." Wet mounts: KOH = amine odor; NaCl = motile trichomonads, WBCs. pH = ≥ 5

- R/O Physiologic discharge

- R/O Cervicitis

- R/O Concomitant STD

- R/O Foreign body

- R/O Contact dermatitis

- R/O Allergic reaction

- R/O Cervical Intraepithelial Neoplasia (CIN)

- R/O Urinary tract infection

- R/O Underlying medical disorder

Plan

Diagnostic Tests

- Pap smear as indicated

- Wet mounts routinely performed

- Gonorrhea and chlamydia cultures mandatory

- RPR and other labs (e.g., CBC, sedimentation rate, urinalysis) as indicated

- Consider fasting blood sugar and HIV-antibody testing for multiple yeast recurrence.

- Routine vaginal cultures for specific organisms are not recommended unless patient has a significant history of recurrent infection.

Treatment/Management

See Vaginitis Treatment Modalities in Ob/Gyn, pp. 352-354.

Consultation

- For prescription as necessary

- For problematic infections

Patient Education

- Discuss normal and abnormal discharge, cause and transmission of infection, lifestyle behaviors which put client at risk, and methods to reduce risk/spread of infection as indicated.

- Provide guidelines on safer sex practices; encourage condom use with new/multiple/non-monogamous partners.

- Review/discuss vaginal health/hygiene: use of cotton underwear and loose clothing; proper wiping technique, white unscented toilet paper; avoidance of strong bath/laundry soap, feminine hygiene products and excessive douching. Best to wash vulvar area with water only, Aveeno, or other hypo-allergenic soap. "Pat" dry or use low setting hair dryer. Corn starch (not talcum powder) may be used in crural folds if excessive sweating a problem.

- For recurrent yeast may "sterilize" panties in microwave after laundering or soak in bleach overnight.

- Encourage good health maintenance: well balanced diet with avoidance of excessive simple sugars, dairy/yeast products, alcohol; adequate rest, exercise; stress reduction.

- Stress importance of completing full course of prescribed medication.

- Advise regarding side effects of metronidazole (e.g., GI upset, metallic taste in mouth, dark urine) and/or other medication. Warn against alcohol during treatment with metronidazole and for 24 hours thereafter.

- Advise of possibility of yeast vaginitis secondary to oral antibiotic and discuss indications for prophylactic therapy.

- Patient on oral contraceptive should be advised to use back-up birth control if on long-course antibiotic.

- Advise regarding desirability of abstinence during course of treatment for infection.

- In males not treated for bacterial vaginosis, condoms are advisable for 4-6 weeks.

Follow-up

- Patient to return as necessary if symptoms not improved with treatment.

- Sexual partner(s) to be referred to health care provider for evaluation and treatment as indicated. Depending upon site-specific protocol provider may offer prescription for male partner of patient with trichomoniasis, recurrent bacterial vaginosis, or certain cases of yeast vaginitis.

- Follow-up on cervical cultures and treat identified concomitant STD(s). Discuss importance of partner evaluation and treatment if STD identified. Advise patient return for follow-up cultures after treatment. See specific protocols.

- Refer patients with CIN for colposcopy.

- Address additional medical concerns as indicated.

- Document in progress notes and problem list.

VAGINITIS TREATMENT MODALITIES IN OB/GYN

Winifred L. Star

BACTERIAL VAGINOSIS

- Flagyl (metronidazole) 500 mg bid x 7 days

- Clindamycin 300 mg bid x 7 days
  NOTE: Flagyl not recommended in first trimester of pregnancy unless highly symptomatic; many authorities are comfortable with use in second and third trimesters as indicated (Mead & Eschenbach, 1989). CDC recommends clindamycin versus flagyl in pregnancy (CDC, 1989). During breastfeeding: pump breasts for 24 hours after administration of drug.

Alternative therapies

- Flagyl 2 gram stat dose (65-75% effective)

- Ampicillin or amoxicillin 500 mg qid x 7 days (50-65% effective)

- Clindamycin 2% cream intravaginally at hs x 7 days (on the horizon)

- Lactate gel (aci-gel) intravaginally x 7 days

- H_2O_2 douche (1-3% diluted half strengh) qd x 7 days (douching not recommended in pregnancy)

- Vinegar douche (2 Tbs./quart H_2O) qd x 7 days (douching not recommended in pregnancy)

Optional: yeast prophylaxis with long course antibiotic--see section on yeast vaginitis

Male:

Do not treat with first occurrence in female. Use flagyl as above if partner has recurrent infection.

YEAST VAGINITIS

- Mycelex-G, Gyne-Lotrimin (clotrimazole) 1% cream or 100 mg tablet

  - one vaginal cream or tablet application @ hs x 7 days

  - two vaginal tablets @ hs x 3 days

- Monistat-7 (miconazole nitrate) 2% cream or 100 mg suppository

  - one vaginal cream or suppository application @ hs x 7 days

- Monistat-3 (miconazole nitrate) 200 mg tablet

  - one vaginal tablet @ hs x 3 days

- Femstat (butoconazole nitrate) 2% cream

  - one vaginal cream application @ hs x 3 days

- Terazol-7 (terconazole) 0.4% cream, Terazol-3 80 mg tablet

  - one vaginal cream application @ hs x 7 days

  - one vaginal tablet @ hs x 3 days

- Mycelex-G, Gyne-Lotrimin (clotrimazole) 500 mg tablet

  - one vaginal tablet @ hs once

- Vagistat (tioconazole) 6.5% cream
  - one vaginal cream application @ hs once

  NOTE: Single and/or three day antifungal therapies may not be as effective in pregnancy.

Alternative therapies

- Boric acid powder in gelatin capsules: 600 mg/day x 7 days (may be followed by 600 mg twice/week x 3 weeks (contraindicated in pregnancy)

- Potassium sorbate 1-3% douche: douche qd or qod x 7 days (contraindicated in pregnancy)

- Vinegar, yogurt or Lactobacillus douches: 1-2 Tbs/I qt H_2O, douche once a day x 7 days (douching not recommended in pregnancy)

- Gentian violet 1%: painted on vulva and in vagina once/week x 3 weeks; use antifungal treatment x 1-3 weeks afterwards. May also use gentian violet tampons (Genapax): one in vagina qd or bid x 3-4 hrs/day for 12 days. Only effective treatment for *C. glabrata*. Do not use either solution or tampons in presence of vulvar excoriation or ulceration. Do not use in pregnancy.

- For recurrent yeast:
  - Vary amount, type, duration of antifungal agents:
    - Treat for minimum of 2 weeks regardless of drug chosen
    - Self-medicate @ hs x 3-7 days at symptom onset
    - Treat q hs x 5-7 days q month x 6-12 months (usually premenstrually)
  - Boric acid: 600 mg in gelatin capsules intravaginally 2-3 times/week (contraindicated in pregnancy)
  - Lactobacillus tablets: use intravaginally when yeast seems likely to occur
  - Nizoral (ketoconazole) 200-400 mg daily x 7-14 days initially; maintenance doses may be used x 6 months for significant recurrent yeast infections (contraindicated in pregnancy)
  - Treat male with antifungal agent to penis

Vulvitis

- Mild: use antifungal cream on affected area(s)
- Severe/extensive: use vaginal and topical fungicide
  - Monistst dual pack (3 vaginal tablets & vulvar cream)
  - Mycelex twin pack (1 vaginal tablet & vulvar cream)
- Pruritus:
  - Hydrocortisone 0.5-1% sparingly bid-tid to affected area(s)
  - Mycolog cream sparingly bid-tid to affected area(s). AVOID use of this fluorinated steroid for extended periods as skin atrophy may result.

TRICHOMONAS VAGINITIS

- Flagyl (metronidazole)

    - 2 gram stat dose

    - 500 mg bid x 7 days

If failure occurs with either regimen retreat with 500 mg bid x 7 days. In cases of repeated failure treat with 2 gm dose daily x 3-5 days (CDC, 1989).

NOTE: Flagyl not recommended in first trimester of pregnancy unless highly symptomatic; may be used in second and third trimester as indicated. Use single dose therapy versus longer course. During breastfeeding: single dose Flagyl; pump breasts for 24 hours after administration of drug.

Alternative drugs during Pregnancy:

- Vagisec Plus suppositories

    - one vaginal suppository bid x l4 days

- Mycelex, Gyne-lotrimin or Monistat cream or tablets

    - one vaginal application @ hs x 7-l4 days

Optional: yeast prophylaxis with long course Flagyl--see section on yeast vaginitis

Male: Treat with single dose Flagyl

Regarding Pap Smear:

- Do not treat trichomonas solely on the basis of a Pap smear report. Ideally recall the patient for re-evaluation of signs/symptoms. Perform a vaginal exam and wet mount to identify presence/absence of infection.

VARICELLA

Winifred L. Star

Varicella or chickenpox is caused by the varicella-zoster virus, one of the human herpes viruses. An attack of chickenpox is characterized by skin vesicles (most predominant on the trunk) and sensory nerve and ganglia involvement. A latent state exists in the nerve ganglia after disease resolution. This asymptomatic phase persists unless viral reactivation occurs. The reactivated state is known as herpes zoster or shingles, most common in the elderly or an immunocompromised host (Gershon, 1988).

Transmission is by direct vesicle/mucus membrane contact; respiratory transmission is less common. Varicella is almost exclusively a disease of childhood, however about 5-10% of children remain unaffected. Contagion lasts from approximately two days prior to onset of the rash to six days after it appears, or until the vesicles are dried. The incubation period is from 10-21 days. Twenty five percent of all adults with no history of chickenpox are susceptible (Boodley & Jaquis, 1989; Gershon, 1988). The incidence of maternal varicella is 5/10,000 pregnancies. Adult varicella runs a more virulent course with more frequent complications including potentially fatal pneumonia (Horstmann, 1982).

Congenital and neonatal chickenpox may develop from maternal transmission. In early pregnancy maternal varicella infection may result in spontaneous abortion or in the rare fetal congenital varicella syndrome. This is characterized by anomalies of the nervous system (paralysis, seizures, mental retardation), skeletal system (hypoplastic extremities) opthalmologic system (cataracts, chorioretinitis), gastrointestinal system (atresia) or genitourinary system (hydronephrosis). There have been fewer than 40 reported cases worldwide since 1947. In utero transmission of the virus is felt to occur in 25-40% of cases of maternal infection but <5% of fetuses will develop the syndrome (Boodley & Jaquis, 1989; Gershon, 1988; McGregor, Mark, Crawford, & Levin, 1987).

Maternal infection in later pregnancy may result in preterm labor. If maternal varicella occurs several weeks to six days prior to delivery the infant may be born with a chickenpox rash but in general does quite well. If maternal varicella occurs five days before delivery, 17-50% of infants will develop chickenpox and if left untreated 20% will die secondary to associated pneumonia (Boodley & Jaquis, 1989; Gershon, 1988; Horstmann, 1982). The earlier the maternal infection the more antibody is acquired by the fetus thus preventing or modifying fetal infection (Horstmann, 1982).

Data Base

Subjective

- Low grade fever

- Profuse pruritic rash on trunk, face, scalp

- Lesions which may involve the mouth, throat, conjunctiva

- Lesion progression within 48 hours from macules to papules to vesicles

- Crusted lesions lasting 1-3 weeks

- Dry cough or pleuritic chest pain (symptoms of pneumonia)

- Headache, drowsiness, convulsions, ataxia (symptoms of encephalitis)
- Bleeding from mucous membranes (hemorrhagic varicella)

Objective

- Lesion formation as described above
- Absence of chest findings on auscultation usually
- Chest x-ray demonstrating patchy opacities (pneumonitis)
- Thrombocytopenia (in hemorrhagic varicella)
- May see superinfection of skin lesions characterized by a dark red areola
- Fetal anomalies (as described in definition) may be demonstrated on ultrasound $\geq$16 weeks.
- Neonatal varicella rash may be present if mother exposed 5 days prior to delivery. Fever and pneumonia may also develop in these babies.

Assessment

- Varicella (chickenpox) infection
- R/O Herpes zoster (shingles)
- R/O Herpes simplex
- R/O Syphilis
- R/O Smallpox
- R/O Scabies/insect bites
- R/O Allergic reaction
- R/O Dermatitis

Plan

Diagnostic Tests

- Evidence of past infection can be determined by assaying varicella-zoster antibodies in serum utilizing either flourescent antibody to membrane antigen (FAMA), immune adherence hemoagglutination test (IAHA) or enzyme immunoassay (EIA).
- Compliment fixation test may also be used but is less sensitive.
- Recovery of virus particles from vesicles can also confirm the diagnosis.

Treatment/Management

- If patient has a known history of prior infection and has been exposed in pregnancy immunity is presumed and no further testing is necessary.
- If exposure was >96 hours ago and patient has no known history of varicella:
    - order a varicella test of immunity
    - if nonimmune advise of incubation/communicable period
    - advise postponement of prenatal office visits until period of communicability has passed
    - advise regarding symptomatic relief in event of infection (tylenol, calamine lotion etc.)

- If exposure was <96 hours ago and patient has no prior/unsure history:

  - establish varicella immunity utilizing one of the above described laboratory tests

  - if immune no further testing/treatment is necessary

  - if nonimmune offer passive immunization with varicella-zoster immune glogulin (VZIG); usual adult dose is 5 vials or 625 units IM (1 vial/10kg body weight)

- NOTE: No active immunization against varicella is available in the U.S. at the present time. FDA approval is forthcoming.

- Established maternal varicella infections may be treated with antiviral drugs. Intravenous acyclovir (Zovirax) has been used in cases of life-threatening disease with pneumonia.

- There is no treatment for congenital varicella syndrome. Ultrasound may identify anomalies if pregnancy termination is being considered.

- Infants exposed to maternal infection 5 days prior to birth should be given VZIG 125 units as soon as possible postdelivery. Antiviral therapy with acyclovir may be utilized in very sick infants.

Consultation

- MD consultation is advised in instances where mother is exposed to varicella and is nonimmune.

Patient Education

- See also Treatment/Management section.

- Advise women who are nonimmune to varicella to avoid contact with chickenpox and shingles and to report exposure promptly.

- If a nonimmune gravida has been exposed to varicella discuss the diagnostic testing involved to determine maternal antibodies. Stress the importance of timing in this situation (i.e., VZIG must be administered within 96 hours of exposure).

- If an injection fee is charged the patient should be informed that the present cost of VZIG is $75.00. Advise the patient of possible reactions to the injection: local pain and swelling; constitutional symptoms; anaphylaxis, rarely.

- It should be emphasized that passive immunization is aimed at prevention of maternal/fetal varicella infection.

- Discuss the incidence of congenital varicella syndrome and emphasize that this is not a common complication. Patient education of this disorder may also be done by the MD involved in the patient's care.

Follow-up

- Referral to pychosocial support services may be indicated in cases where it is known that the patient will deliver an infant with congenital varicella syndrome.

- Document in progress notes and problem list.

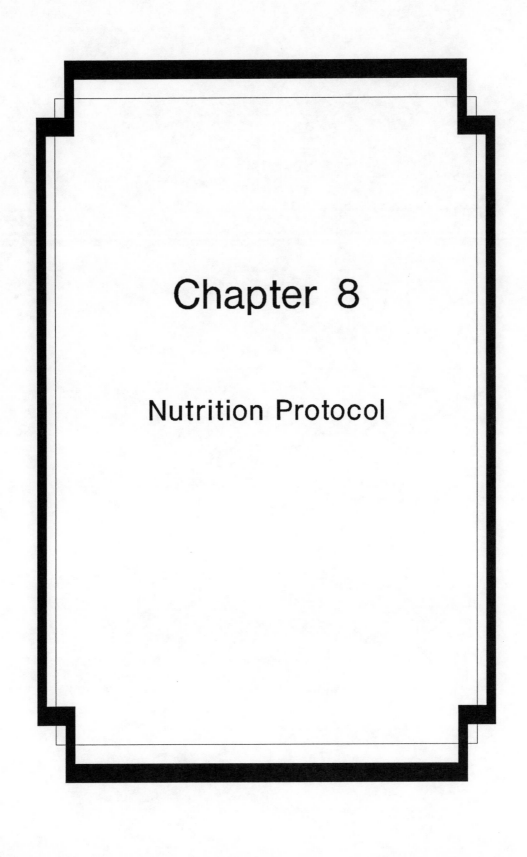

Chapter 8

Nutrition Protocol

NUTRITION PROTOCOL

Yolanda Gutierrez

The purpose of this protocol is to provide the opportunity for nurse practitioners/nurse-midwives and other health professionals to offer meaningful diet counseling to pregnant women and their families, taking into consideration nutritional, economic, social, and ethnic variables.

Objectives

- To provide health professionals with skills to identify nutritional needs and factors that place the patient in a special category of nutritional risk.

- To participate in the process of the <u>complete nutritional assessment</u>.
    - Health history and physical exam, nutritionally oriented
    - Anthropometric measurements, weight and height
    - Laboratory tests
    - Dietary history and evaluation

Minimum Skills

In order to identify the relationship of food intake and nutritive quality to the kind of health problem reported, a series of minimum skills should be mastered in order to meet the specific objectives listed above. These skills include:

- Knowledge of and rationale for the increased nutritional needs during pregnancy and lactation

- Knowledge of the nutritive value of food and the major food sources of nutrients which are likely to be deficient in American diets

- Knowledge of food groups and recommended servings of these foods according to the patient's needs

- Ability to take an adequate diet history

- Ability to assess dietary needs

- Ability to use clinical judgment for the recommendation of vitamin and mineral supplements other than routine prenatal vitamins

- Ability to plan nutritional care based on medical and nutritional aspects of care

- Ability to implement and follow up on a patient's nutritional care plan

- Ability to prepare adequately for instruction (i.e., with educational handouts, referrals, and audiovisual materials)

- Ability to present information clearly and effectively

- Assertiveness in contacting and competence in discussing nutritional care with the physician/nutritionist or other health personnel (the health team approach)

- Ability to evaluate effectiveness of teaching (e.g., patient's intended behavior for improvement or changes in diet)

- Ability to document nutrition intervention in medical records

The reader is encouraged to acquire access to at least three major publications pertinent to maternal nutrition for assistance in acquiring these skills.

- National Academy of Sciences (1990). *Maternal nutrition*. Washington, DC: National Academy Press.

- National Academy of Sciences, National Research Council (1989, October). *Recommended dietary allowances* (10th ed.). Washington, DC: National Academy Press.

- California Department of Health Services, (1989). *Nutrition during pregnancy and the postpartum period: A manual for health care professionals*. Sacramento, CA: Author.

- Gutierrez, Y. (1990a). Maternal and infant nutrition in the fourth trimester. In K. A. May (Ed.), *Comprehensive maternity nursing*. Philadelphia: J. B. Lippincott Co.

- Gutierrez, Y. (1990b). Nutritional aspects of pregnancy. In K. A. May (Ed.), *Comprehensive maternity nursing*. Philadelphia: J. B. Lippincott Co.

NUTRITIONAL RISK FACTORS
(California Department of Health Services, 1989)

Factors at the Onset of Pregnancy

- Prepregnant weight at first prenatal visit of less than 90% or greater than 135% of standard weight

- Adolescent less than l5 years of age or less than 4 years post-menarche

- Two or more pregnancies during the past two years

- Multiple pregnancy

- History of poor obstetric or fetal outcome (e.g., pregnancy complications, perinatal loss, or low birthweight infant), economic deprivation

- Food faddism with ingestion of bizarre or nutritionally restrictive diet; megavitamin therapy

- Heavy smoking, drug addiction, or alcoholism

- Therapeutic diet for chronic systemic disease (e.g., diabetes, cardiac disease, kidney disease, etc.)

- Vegetarian diet

- Food allergies or intolerances

- Oral contraception predating pregnancy

- Breastfeeding

Factors During Pregnancy

- Excessive weight gain during pregnancy

  - 1st trimester, greater than 10 lbs*

- 2nd trimester, greater than 2 lbs/week*

- 3rd trimester, greater than 2 lbs/week*

- Inadequate weight gain or loss during pregnancy

  - 1st trimester gain less than 4 lbs; gain of <2.2 lbs (1 kg)/month in any month during 2nd or 3rd trimester

  - weight loss of >5 lbs during 1st trimester

  - weight less than pregravid weight at 14 weeks gestation

  - any weight loss in 2nd or 3rd trimester

  NOTE: Adequate weight gain is 10 lbs by 20 weeks and close to 1 lb/week thereafter until term. Weight reduction regimens should never be used during pregnancy.

- Low or deficient Hb/Hct

- Hyperemesis gravidarum

- Pre-eclampsia or eclampsia

- Pica

- Failure of uterine/fetal growth

*In the absence of edema, pre-pregnant underweight status or adolescent.

Social factors

- Income inadequate for food purchase

- Inadequate cooking and storage facilities

- Eligibility for food assistance

- Cultural and/or religious influences compromising nutritional status

- Any activity which would increase daily caloric needs (e.g., heavy physical activity, athletic performance)

- Lack of control over food purchasing and preparation

- Lack of knowledge of sound nutritional practice

PREGNANCY NUTRITIONAL GUIDELINES

During pregnancy, the mother must meet her own nutritional needs, in addition to the needs of the growing fetus. Although this growth process means that requirements for all nutrients are increased during pregnancy, some nutrients are of particular importance in pregnancy.

Additional calories are needed during pregnancy to support increased tissue synthesis by the mother and fetus and the additional metabolic cost incurred by this new tissue. Adequate intake of calories for energy is necessary for optimal protein utilization and tissue growth.

The generally accepted figure for the total energy cost of pregnancy is 80,000 kcal. When this figure is divided over the length of pregnancy, it averages out to an additional 300 calories per day above nonpregnant needs. Because caloric requirements are difficult to predict and vary widely among pregnant women, factors such as maternal age, activity, height, prepregnant weight, health, and stage of pregnancy must be considered. Because of differences in these parameters, individual caloric needs should be calculated by allowing a minimum of 36 kcal per kilogram of pregnant body weight. The pregnant adolescent's energy needs may be as high as 50 kcal/kg/day, depending on her daily activity levels and growth rate (National Academy of Sciences, National Research Council, 1989).

Additional protein is needed in increased amounts during pregnancy to provide sufficient amino acids for fetal development, for blood volume expansion, and for growth of maternal breast and uterine tissues. The current recommended dietary allowances (RDA) for protein intake is an additional 10 grams protein per day over nonpregnant needs. It is important to remember that adequate protein intake without adequate calories should be avoided; if caloric intake is below the required amount, protein will be used for maternal energy needs rather than for its primary function of tissue building and maintenance.

Generally, requirements for all vitamins are increased during pregnancy. The accelerated energy and protein metabolism require increased amounts of vitamins for tissue synthesis and energy production. Vitamins requiring special attention in pregnancy are iron and folic acid (folacin). The recommendations to pregnant women about these vitamins should stress that the needs during pregnancy are increased and the intake in most diets is low.

The 1989 MCH Daily Good Guide (see Table 8.1, *Daily Food Guide*, p. 378) has been developed to ensure an intake of at least 80% of the RDA for pregnant and lactating women of average height (64 inches) and average weight (120 pounds prepregnant). The current MCH Daily Food Guide is based on computerized analyses of sample menus. Consequently, the recommended number of servings from each group are actually the minimum during pregnancy and lactation. If the guide is followed, and if it is recognized that each food group has more nourishing and less nourishing choices within it, it will ensure an intake of at least 80% of the RDAs. This tool is the most practical and best available for the nurse in evaluating how adequate the pregnant and lactating women's diets are. After the 24-hour recall has been completed, the food intake reported by the woman is then compared to the recommended servings of the Daily Food Guide for the pregnant/lactating woman. If the woman is postpartum and non-lactating, the column in the guide labeled Postpartum/Non-lactating can be used.

Consider the following factors when comparing a patient's diet to the Daily Food Guide.

- **Calories**. Depending on the choice of foods within each group, the calorie intake based on the Daily Food Guide can range from 2000 to 3000 calories for the pregnant and lactating woman. Therefore, in order to consume adequate calories (most pregnant women need at least 2300), this can be obtained from increased servings of the food groups. But if foods not listed are eaten or methods of food preparation increase the calories from fats, the patient should be encouraged to make nutritious selections.

- **Protein**. Each serving recommended on the Daily Food Guide supplies approximately 7 grams of protein, 1.2 mg of iron (supplementation needed), and 0.9 mg of zinc. However, light poultry, meat, fish, and tofu are lower in zinc than other foods in this group. In general, the Daily Food Guide provides about 150% of the RDA for protein. It is important to understand that the RDA level of protein must be exceeded in order to insure an adequate intake of B_6, iron, and zinc in the diet.

- **Calcium**. Each serving of the milk group supplies approximately 275 to 300 mg of calcium. Milk is also a good source of vitamin D. For some women, this food group serves as primary sources of protein in the diet. If the recommended number of servings from this group is inadequate, the calcium intake is likely to be inadequate.

- **Folacin**. Each serving of dark green vegetables contributes significant amounts of folacin and magnesium; average is 75 μg/serving of folacin and 30 mg/serving of magnesium.

- **Vitamin C-rich Foods**. Each serving supplies about 60 mg of vitamin C. In addition, most foods from this group are good sources of folacin and vitamin A. Those foods that are particularly rich in vitamin A provide more than 2750 IU per serving. They include such foods as cantaloupe, mango, papaya, greens, bok choy, and spinach.

- **Breads and Cereals**. This group is divided into two parts: whole grains and enriched products. Whole grain breads, cereals, and pastas provide significantly more magnesium, zinc, vitamins E, B_6, and folacin, and fiber than enriched products. It is recommended that at least half of the bread and cereal servings eaten daily be made from whole grains (California Department of Health Services, 1989).

SCREENING INDICES

Weight

Recommended weight gain during pregnancy will vary depending on pregravid weight status. It must be remembered that desirable body weight is an abstract rather than an absolute concept. Height/weight tables may not be representative for some segments of the population (such as lower socioeconomic groups and specific ethnic groups); they ignore other risk factors (such as smoking), they do not measure degree of fatness or fat distribution, and they have relied on an ill-defined concept of "frame size." Nutrition is a multi-faceted issue, as is client assessment, especially in the area of weight management. Health care professionals should use height/weight tables with caution and in conjunction with other parameters to assist in assessment of nutritional status.

Desirable Body Weight (DBW) Calculations

For women 5' = 100 lbs, add 5 lbs per inch,
e.g., 5'4" = 120 lbs $\pm$ 10 lbs for individual variations
(See Table 8.2, *Desirable Weight for Height: For Women 25 Years or Older*, p. 379)

Calculations to Determine % of Standard Weight

Example: 5'4" = 120 lbs DBW.

If 5'4" = 100 lbs $\dfrac{100 \text{ lbs (actual weight)}}{120 \text{ lbs (desired weight or DBW)}}$ x 100 = 83%,

If 5'4" = 150 lbs $\dfrac{150 \text{ lbs (actual weight)}}{120 \text{ lbs (desired weight or DBW)}}$ x 100 = 125%,

Weight Gain During Pregnancy

- Desirable weight gain recommendations during pregnancy are based on pregravid weight.

Classifications of Pregravid Weight for Height (California Department of Health Services, 1989)

- Underweight: $\leq$90% DBW

- Desirable: 91 - 120% DBW

- Moderately overweight: 121 - 135% DBW

- Very overweight: >135% DBW

Total Weight Gain Recommendations in Relation to Pregravid Weight (California Department of Health Services, 1989)

- Underweight: 28 - 36 lbs
- Desirable: 24 - 32 lbs
- Moderately overweight: 24 - 32 lbs
- Very overweight: 20 - 24 lbs (individualize)
- Twins: 40 lbs or more

Note: Modifications in weight gain may be needed for special risk categories, such as women who smoke, teens, multiple gestation, etc. For twin pregnancies, these are general guidelines only. The optimal weight gain for these individuals will depend on a variety of factors. Therefore individualized nutrition counseling is important to interpret the significance of weight gain patterns. See Table 8.3, *Provisional Weight Gain Recommendations for Twin Pregnancies*, p. 380 for recommended weight gain in twin pregnancies.

Prenatal Weight Gain Grid

The recommended rate of weight gain depicted on the grid (see Table 8.4, *Prenatal Weight Gain Grid*, p. 381) reflects a gradual and progressive increase in weight and was derived from the weight gain grid published by the National Academy of Sciences in 1970. It has been in common use since that time. This grid provides a visual comparison of the woman's actual weight gain with the recommended pattern, which will differ according to her pregravid weight.

The upper line of the grid corresponds to the upper end of the recommended range of weight gain for underweight women; the middle line is the midpoint of the recommended range for normal or overweight women; and the lower line represents the lower end of the recommended range for very overweight women. The weight gain pattern in the table may vary for adolescents, smokers, women with multiple pregnancies, or women with poor weight gain in early pregnancy.

Optimum prenatal care includes routine use of the Prenatal Weight Gain Grid, which is not only an effective tool for patient education but for clinical evaluation as well.

Plan

Based on the client's subjective and objective data obtained to establish a nutritional assessment, the nurse practitioner/midwife proceeds to initiate the individualized plan of care for the client.

Diagnostic Tests

- Hemoglobin and hematocrit
- Serum iron/TIBC
- Red blood cell count
- Serum ferritin
- Glucose screen
- Urinalysis
- Additional lab(s) as indicated

Treatment/Management

- Monitor weight (pre-pregnant and interval weight gain); record patient's height, and calculate DBW

- Complete 24o diet recall

- Review patient's medical, OB, and social history

- Review medication intake

- Review laboratory results

Patient Education

- Weight gain rationale (desirable pattern of gain and components of weight gain during pregnancy)

- Instruct patient regarding use of Daily Food Guide (see Table 8.1, p. 378).

- Recommended modifications

    - Dietary modifications for nutritionally-related health problems (e.g., hypertension)

    - Physical activity

    - Recommendations regarding ingestion of coffee, alcohol, drugs and cigarettes

- Review educational materials

- Special Considerations

    - Use of vitamin/mineral supplements including iron

    - Pica

    - Lactose intolerance

    - Vegetarian diets

    - Religious/cultural influences

    - Food allergies

    - Remedies for nausea, vomiting, heartburn, constipation

    - Preparation for breastfeeding

    - Infant nutrition guidelines

    - Food assistance programs

    - Eating disorders (e.g., anorexia, bulimia)

Follow-up

- Document in progress notes:

    - Content of the counseling session

    - The type of nutrition education received
      Example: basic nutrition and review of food groups, or high-risk patient receiving more aggressive nutritional intervention (i.e., diet modification)

    - The specific behavioral objectives for the patient

    - Materials used or given

- Patient's response to counseling
- The inability or refusal of the patient to attend or participate in nutrition counseling and education
- Progress of the patient and future plans
- Evaluation of patient's success
  - Demonstrated improvements in physiological or biochemical indicators of health
  - Behavior intentions; answers to the following questions:
    - What does the patient intend to eat tomorrow for breakfast?
    - What snacks does she think she will have tomorrow?
    - Does she intend to buy special foods tomorrow?
    - What foods does she intend to add for lunch/dinner, and why is she choosing these foods?
    - Does she intend to walk or exercise tomorrow?

DIETARY MODIFICATIONS FOR NUTRITIONALLY RELATED HEALTH PROBLEMS

Hypertension

The dietary factors that have been implicated with varying degrees of certainty in the pathogenesis of hypertension include:

- Sodium (excessive)
- Energy balance (obesity)
- Magnesium (inadequate intakes)
- Calcium (inadequate intakes)
- Alcohol (excessive)
- Polyunsaturated fats (inadequate intakes)

A large body of evidence suggests that dietary sodium plays a particularly important role in the development of hypertension. There is, however, also evidence to suggest that sodium is not very important. The truth probably falls somewhere in between; that is, for some people sodium may be very important while for others it is not.

Data on the role of other dietary factors is suggestive, but at best preliminary. Obesity clearly is a risk factor for hypertension. Few would argue that weight loss is an effective treatment modality for most obese hypertensive patients. There should be no weight loss for pregnant women.

Current indications for the treatment of mild hypertension remain controversial. The present recommendations on the dietary treatment of hypertension include:

- Decrease dietary sodium (processed foods and added salt, only moderate during pregnancy).
- Monitor weight for pregnant obese women (avoid excessive gains, follow adequate recommendations, increase exercise, behavior modification).

368

- Increase potassium (increase fruits, vegetables and juices).

- Increase dietary fiber (increase whole grains, fruits and vegetables).

- Increase proportion of unsaturated fat (decrease animal fat).

- Recommend no alcohol intake during pregnancy.

Gestational Diabetes (Adapted from Gunderson, 1990)

Tight control of blood glucose levels is required during pregnancy because the growing fetus can be adversely affected by abnormal maternal blood glucose levels. The need for strict "normoglycemia" necessitates a nutrition care plan that may be more limited in food choices than available to the nonpregnant diabetic population. Many women who develop gestational diabetes would like to avoid insulin therapy if possible. For these women, careful selection of foods and types of carbohydrate is essential. The majority of gestational diabetic women can be controlled by diet alone (about 80%). All meal patterns must be individualized by the registered dietician for each woman and adjusted depending on the blood glucose and urinary ketone tests. The American Dietetic Association (ADA) exchanges are utilized for the education of the pregnant diabetic woman. However, there are different degrees of glucose intolerance. One woman may be able to tolerate milk at breakfast, while another may not. Some of the ADA selections, such as cold breakfast cereals, fruit juices, and processed foods, may not achieve tight blood glucose control for certain patients. The following outline provides some general information about the types of modifications in meal patterns and food selections necessary for gestational diabetes.

Eating Pattern

- Plan <u>six small meals</u> a day or 3 meals and 3 snacks.

- Space meals and snacks at regular intervals, about 2 to 3 hours apart.

- Schedule meals and snacks at approximately the <u>same time</u> each day. Skipping meals or snacks is discouraged because it may result in weight loss, urinary ketone excretion or overeating later in the day.

- Recommend inclusion of a protein rich food at each meal and the bedtime snack such as cheese, meat, fish, eggs or poultry.

Morning Meal Composition

- Relatively small meal; lower carbohydrate content.

- Exclude foods containing primarily simple sugars such as fruit, fruit juice and milk.

- Exclude highly processed dry breakfast cereals such as Product 19, Cornflakes, Kix, Total, Nutragrain, etc.

- Recommend whole grain breads, tortillas, or hot cereals such as old-fashioned oatmeal, non-instant Malt-O-Meal, or oatbran.

- Recommend a protein rich food at the morning meal such as cheese, meat, eggs, poultry, or dried beans.

- It may be possible to add milk to the meal if blood sugar tests after the meal are normal (<140 mg/dl one hour postprandial or post-meal peak)

Types of Foods to Recommend

- High fiber and complex carbohydrate rich foods such as whole grain breads, corn tortillas, and whole grain pasta are helpful.

- Other high fiber foods such as hot cereals (oatmeal and oatbran) and dried beans and legumes are particularly good choices because of the soluble fiber content that slows the blood glucose rise.

- Fresh fruits and vegetables are nutrient rich. Frozen varieties may also be used. Canned fruits and vegetables are less desirable because of possible added sugar, losses in nutrient content and lower fiber content.

- Encourage patients to read labels carefully on all packaged or canned foods for hidden simple sugars (dextrose, sucrose, honey, molasses, fructose, corn syrup, brown sugar, maple syrup, modified food starch).

- Free foods: counsel patients to eat as much of the following foods as desired (lettuce, mustard, herbs, mushrooms, chiles, lemon juice, radish, garlic, broth, vinegar, herb tea, etc.).

Types of Foods Not Recommended

- Convenience foods generally result in a more rapid rise in blood glucose than fresh or less-processed foods. Encourage patients to avoid the following products: canned soups, instant potatoes, instant noodles or cereals, frozen dinners or entrees, packaged stuffing mix or fast foods such as hamburgers or pizza. These foods are also usually high in fat and sodium which can contribute to excess weight gain or unexplained rises in blood sugar levels.

Sugary Foods and Concentrated Sweets

- Beverages such as fruit juices, juice drinks, soft drinks, Kool-Aid, nectars, and Hi-C should not be used. Flavored mineral waters and sodas with added juice may also contain added sugars.

- Desserts and other sweets such as cookies, cakes, candy, pies, chocolate, table sugar, jams, and jellies should not be eaten.

- Other foods with hidden sugars such as chocolate milk, granola, soymilk, applesauce, yogurt, commercially prepared spaghetti sauce, teriyaki sauce, and canned fruits are not good choices.

- Read labels on all products to check for hidden sugar content from sucrose, fructose, dextrose, honey, corn syrup, molasses, corn sweeteners, and cornstarch.

Strategies to Avoid Excess Weight Gain

- Food Preparation: Remove all visible fat. For example, cut off the fat from beef and the skin from poultry.

- Cooking Methods: Baked, broiled, steamed, boiled, or barbecued foods are preferred to reduce the fat used in cooking. Frying foods in large amounts of oil is not recommended. Less fat may be used by cooking with nonstick pans or PAM instead of oil, margarine, or butter.

- Types of Foods: Lean cuts of meat such as roast beef, turkey, ham, or chicken may be used more often, and luncheon meat, sausage, or hot dogs used less often. Kcals can be

decreased easily by using nonfat or lowfat dairy products such as skim milk cheeses (mozzarella, ricotta, cottage cheese) and lowfat plain yogurt or milk.

- <u>Added Fats</u>: Identify sources of added fat in the diet and moderate their use (e.g., butter, margarine, mayonnaise, salad dressings, cream, sour cream, cream cheese, bacon, olives, nuts, avocados, etc.

Exercise Recommendations

- Blood glucose control may be improved with regular exercise. Recommend <u>walking</u> at least 10-15 minutes after each meal. Pregnant women should check with their health care provider about the types of exercise and the amount allowed.

Restricted Activity (Adapted from Abrams, 1985a)

Nurse practitioners/nurse-midwives and other health professionals must be sensitive about the eating difficulties when the patient must restrict her activity during pregnancy.

- Some women not only have a normal appetite, but the combination of less activity and boredom of lying in bed all day can increase food cravings and intake so that too much weight gain occurs.

- Some women find that the combination of constant bedrest along with anxiety about "Will my baby be all right?" decreases appetite and weight gain.

- Some women find that inactivity can cause constipation which is uncomfortable and may also make eating seem less appealing.

Advice for Excessive Appetite/High Weight Gain

- Eating at regular times
- Eating more low caloric, high nutrient foods (e.g., raw vegetables, fruit, low or non-fat milk, low fat yogurt, diluted juices)
- Write down what she eats. Try to identify when and what she could delete throughout the day (e.g., cookies)
- Including the intake of low caloric but nutritious snacks (e.g., plain yogurt/fruit, hardboiled eggs, celery, peanut butter, fruit juice popsicles, unbuttered popcorn and mineral water)
- Referring to the nutritionist for advice on diet

Advice for Poor Appetite/Low Weight Gain

- Eating small frequent meals and not going too long without food (3 hours or more)
- Eating at regular times
- Choosing foods that give the most nutrition for the calories (e.g., milk, hard-boiled eggs, milk shake, yogurt)
- Drinking fluids between rather than during meals
- Write down what she eats. Have her identify when and what she could add throughout the day (e.g., peanuts, trail mix, milkshake)
- Scheduling visitors at mealtime for company
- Referring to the nutritionist for advice on diet
- Including the intake of high caloric but nutritious snacks

Examples:

Milk Shake

Blend together:		or try:
3/4 cup	Milk	Ice cream blended with orange juice
1 cup	Ice cream	Peanut butter & jelly on whole wheat bread
1 Tbsp	Chocolate syrup	Pudding & custard
1/4	Ripe banana	Dry roasted nuts
1/3 cup	Dry milk	Shakes with varied ingredients

Advice for Constipation

- All the advice in Constipation protocol

- Because of restricted activity, no regular exercise is advised.

- May be helpful to try 2-3 Tbsp/day of unprocessed bran - can be used on cereals, as coating for baked chicken, on soups, etc.

- If dietary measures are not producing results, a stool softener may be recommended.

Advice for Food Preparation and Availability

- Plan a list of foods that require little or no preparation

   Examples:
   - eggs (hard boiled)   - canned fruits
   - yogurt   - peaches
   - nuts   - pears
   - peanut butter   - mandarin/oranges
   - cheese/cottage cheese   - whole grain breads
   - small cans of fruit juice

- Keep a pitcher of water or fluids by the bed. Advisable to drink at least 4-6 cups of liquids per day.

- Keep a thermos by the bed; use for soups, milks, or shakes.

- Keep a positive attitude and a happy atmosphere. Remind the patient that it is especially important what she eats now. These are critical growing periods for the baby and essential nutrients are needed now especially if the baby comes early.

VITAMIN/MINERAL SUPPLEMENTS

Although the need for vitamins and minerals is increased during pregnancy, a well balanced diet based on the Daily Food Guide for Pregnancy can provide all the nutrients for optimal maternal and fetal health with the exception of iron and possibly folic acid. However, vitamin/mineral supplementation is a common self-care practice.

The California Department of Health Services and the National Academy of Sciences, who have established the Recommended Dietary Allowances (RDA), recommend that all pregnant women receive daily supplements of at least 0.4-0.8 mcg folic acid and 30-60 mg elemental iron. Most prenatal supplements contain a variety of vitamins and minerals in addition to the recommended levels of folic acid and iron. Certain nutrient interactions, as well as other factors, need to be considered when choosing an appropriate prenatal supplement.

- Nutritional supplements should complement a healthy diet. See Tables 8.5-8.7, *Dietary Sources of Iron, Folacin, Calcium*, pp. 382-384.

- Characteristics of the ideal prenatal supplement

    - Contains a wide range of vitamins and minerals (particularly vitamins B6 and D, folic acid, pantothenic acid, calcium, magnesium, iron and zinc)

    - Contains folic acid at the level of 0.4-0.8 mcg per daily dose

    - Contains iron at the level of 30-60 mg per daily dose--see Anemia protocol for iron supplementation

    - Does not contain high levels of calcium and magnesium and does not contain calcium in the form of calcium phosphate

    - Contains vitamin E and zinc at, or near, the Recommended Dietary Allowance levels (15 IU and 20 mg respectively)

    - Contains 4-10 mg of vitamin B6 per daily dose

    - Be reasonably priced and readily available

Recommended Prenatal Vitamin/Mineral Supplements

On the basis of the requirements listed above, four available preparations are recommended:

- Prenatal (Bronson)..........................no prescription needed
- Prenatal (Great Earth).......................no prescription needed
- Materna 1-60 (Lederle)......................prescription required
- Natalins Rx (Mead-Johnson).................prescription required

The Bronson prenatal supplement is the least expensive and requires no prescription. It is available by mail order (Bronson Pharmaceuticals, 4526 Rinetti Lane, La Canada, CA 91011-0628). Prescription is required if the Prenatal Supplement contains 1 mg of folic acid.

Calcium Supplements

Calcium supplements may be recommended during pregnancy for women unwilling or unable to ingest sufficient calcium from milk products or other nondairy calcium-rich foods. The amount of calcium required from supplements depends on the diet. If more than 250-300 mg of supplemental calcium is required daily, it is recommended that the dosage be split into 250-300 mg increments and that each be taken with a meal or snack to enhance absorption. Daily supplementation with more than a gram (1,000 mg) of calcium is not recommended. Excessive calcium supplementation has been demonstrated to have mixed effects of calcium on iron and zinc absorption and retention.

The amount of elemental calcium in common calcium supplements is (Windholz, 1976):

Supplements	Calcium
Calcium carbonate	40%
Calcium citrate	24%
Calcium lactate	14%
Calcium gluconate	9%

Some calcium supplements list their contents only in grains. A grain equals approximately 65 mg; thus a 10 grain tablet supplies 650 mg. If the 10 grain tablet contains calcium lactate, which is 14% elemental calcium, each tablet would provide approximately 91 mg of elemental calcium (14% of

650 mg equals 91 mg) (California Department of Health Services, 1989). The forms of calcium listed above are recommended because of their absorption. Calcium phosphate is not recommended because this form of calcium is poorly absorbed and interferes with iron absorption. Because stomach acidity normally decreases somewhat in pregnancy, it has been demonstrated that calcium citrate is far better absorbed.

Management of Women Who Require Calcium Supplementation

Lactase deficiency may make milk products unacceptable to some women. Symptoms of lactase deficiency include gas, intestinal pain, cramps, and possibly vomiting or diarrhea as a result of ingesting lactose from milk products. Two-thirds of the world's population experiences some degree of lactase deficiency after early childhood (Newcomer & McGill, 1984). Most Hispanics, Black Americans, Asians, and Native Americans are lactase deficient to some degree, but may still be able to digest limited amounts of lactose. There is also evidence for a physiological "adaptation" in pregnancy to improve the efficiency of lactose absorption (Villar, Kestler, Castillo, & Solomons, 1987). Therefore, a woman can be encouraged to consume small amounts of milk (½ cup) or other milk products several times a day rather than a large amount at any one time. It has also been found that milk products are better tolerated by lactase-deficient individuals when eaten in combination with other foods.

Women unable to tolerate any quantity of milk can substitute naturally aged hard cheeses or fermented milk products, such as yogurt. These foods have negligible lactose content and thus may be better tolerated. Yogurt also has the advantage of containing some of the enzyme lactase, which can help digest lactose from other foods ingested at the same meal (Kolars, Levitt, Aouji, & Savaiano, 1984). However, the lactase activity of yogurt cultures varies among brands (Wytock, 1988). Various other products are available for use by lactase-deficient persons. For example, milk containing predigested lactose (such as Lact-Aid) may be tolerated very well. The enzyme lactase is also sold commercially and can be added to regular milk to predigest the lactose.

Because calcium requirements increase during pregnancy and lactation, lactase deficiency may not present a significant problem if nonmilk products are tolerated. All women consuming less than the recommended number of servings of milk products should substitute foods from the nondairy calcium-rich foods such as sardines, tofu, broccoli, turnip greens, kale, or mustard greens. Foods from the protein foods group may also have to be increased to compensate for the protein and other nutrients usually contributed by milk products. In cases where too few servings of milk products or nondairy calcium-rich foods are consumed, supplementation with calcium and possibly vitamin D may be necessary.

POSTPARTUM NUTRITIONAL GUIDELINES

The nutritional quality of a woman's diet remains very important during the postpartum period, regardless of whether she chooses to breastfeed or bottlefeed her baby. In either case, she is recovering from the physiological stresses of pregnancy and delivery, as well as coping with the additional work and demands of the new baby. Dietary modifications begun during pregnancy can be extended into the interconceptional period, and should focus on maintaining health and reducing the risk of chronic disease. Consequently, the postpartum woman should be encouraged to continue do the following:

- Continue to follow the Dietary Guidelines

- Gradually lose the weight gained during pregnancy

- Continue a daily prenatal supplement containing 30-60 mg of elemental iron for 2-3 months

- Minimize use of harmful substances (alcohol, cigarettes, drugs), particularly if breastfeeding

- Drink when thirsty (approximately 2-3 quarts of liquids daily if breastfeeding)

Constipation may be a problem for a few weeks after delivery. Women should be encouraged to drink plenty of fluids (at least six 8-ounce glasses daily) and eat foods rich in fiber, such as whole grains, legumes, vegetables, and fruits. Exercise, such as walking, will also be helpful. Excessive flatulence is common after a cesarean section. It can be lessened by decreasing the intake of known offenders, which vary among individuals. The most common offenders are legumes, onions, cabbage, and wheat. Eating small, frequent meals, and taking frequent walks may also be helpful.

Breastfeeding

Breastfeeding is currently favored over formula feeding in the United States. Advances in the field of infant feeding and nutrition have revealed that breastfeeding has many advantages, both nutritional and immunologic.

<u>Maternal Nutrition During Lactation</u>

The breastfeeding woman must produce an adequate volume of milk that meets her baby's nutritional needs. A woman's caloric, fluid, protein, vitamin, and mineral requirements are increased during the breastfeeding period. Lactating women produce an average of 600 - 800 ml of milk daily, but it takes several weeks for most mother-infant pairs to reach this quantity. Therefore, an extra 300 - 500 calories/day above the usual intake will be needed during lactation (National Academy of Sciences, 1990). Further caloric increases are indicated for women in whom gestation weight gain is subnormal, weight during lactation falls below standards for height and age, lactation continues for longer than 3 - 4 months, or more than one infant is being nursed.

Protein requirements are increased during lactation to 65 gm per day during the first six months and 62 gm during the second six months of lactation. See Table 8.1, *Daily Food Guide*, p. 378 for recommended servings of the different food groups.

<u>Fluid Requirements</u>

The breastfeeding mother should drink to satisfy thirst (approximately 2 - 3 quarts of liquid daily). This fluid is essential to provide the liquid volume for the breast milk and to meet the mother's normal needs. There are no data to support the assumption that increasing fluid beyond the recommended intake will increase milk volume. In order to insure an adequate fluid intake, breastfeeding mothers can be encouraged to drink a beverage (preferably water, juice, or milk) each time they nurse the baby.

It is best to avoid excessive coffee, tea, and caffeine-containing soft drinks because the caffeine in these beverages has a diuretic effect. Although only a small amount (1%) of the caffeine a mother ingests passes into her milk, caffeine does reach the infant and it can accumulate over time. Thus, a mother who drinks more than 6 - 8 cups of any caffeine-containing beverage in a day might expect her infant to demonstrate "coffee nerves" (Worthington-Roberts & Williams, 1989).

Tips for Feeding a Baby (Adapted from Abrams, 1985b)

- Breast milk or formula is sufficient for the first 4 to 6 months of life for most babies.

- Many babies show signs of readiness for solid food by the age of 6 months. When the baby is ready for baby food:

  - Introduce the simplest foods first.

- Add only one new food at a time (no mixtures) and wait 5 to 7 days to see how the baby adjusts to that food. If the baby shows an allergic reaction, discontinue that food and discuss the reaction with the baby's health care provider.

- At first, offer small amounts (1 Tbsp or less) of food from a spoon. Make the food thin and smooth by mixing it with a little breast milk or formula.

- Allergy symptoms are vomiting, diarrhea, colic, skin rash, eczema, wheezing, and runny nose. Usually symptoms occur 2 to 3 days after introduction of the food.

- Foods most likely to cause allergies are cow's milk, egg white, wheat, peanuts, corn, soybeans, citrus, strawberries, tomatoes, chocolate, and fish.

- As the baby grows older, vary the textures of the foods provided. A 6-month old needs strained (very thin) food; by 8 months most babies do well with mashed, lumpy foods; by 10 months give the baby bits of tender, well-cooked foods to feed himself or herself.

- For homemade baby food, the client will need some inexpensive kitchen equipment. Refer her to a nutritionist for information on making baby food. Store-bought baby food is nutritious if you follow these suggestions:

  - Buy only single foods (there is as much protein in 1 jar of strained chicken as in 4 jars of chicken and noodles).

  - Read labels to avoid sugars, salt, and starches.

  - Check the date on the top of the jar for freshness and make sure the vacuum poptop has not been broken.

  - Do not feed your baby directly from the jar unless she or he can eat the entire portion in one sitting; refrigerated leftovers eaten later can cause food poisoning.

- Bottle feeding is for water, formula, or breast milk **only.**

  - No solids (cereals, etc.) should be put in bottles; feed solids with a spoon.

  - Kool-aid, sodas, and even juices can give a baby cavities when fed from a bottle. Juices should be fed from a cup. Kool-aid and sodas should be avoided: they provide only empty calories.

  - Always hold the baby when giving a bottle. "Propping" the bottle can cause problems such as choking, cavities, and ear infections.

- Never force the baby to finish food or milk she or he doesn't want. Overfeeding can lead to weight problems.

- Do not give the baby the following foods during the first year or two of life: nuts, raw carrots, popcorn, seeds and other foods that might cause choking, or honey in any form (honey can cause food poisoning).

FOOD ASSISTANCE PROGRAMS

Women, Infants and Children (WIC) is a food assistance program funded by USDA and administered by the California State Department of Health. First, it provides food assistance and nutrition education for pregnant and postpartum women and infants. Secondly, it involves ongoing health care because all applicants must be screened by a health care provider. Low-income women, infants and children (varies according to funding levels) who have been identified as being at nutritional risk are eligible. Participants receive a monthly coupon book that may be redeemed at any grocery store for the approved items (infant formula, juice, eggs, milk, cereal, cheese).

<u>Commodity Supplemental Food Program</u> is administered by the Economic Opportunity Council. Low-income women (pregnant and one-year postpartum), infants and children (up to 72 months) are eligible. Participants receive a monthly package including a combination of the following: iron-fortified formula, juice, cereal, eggs, milk, vegetables, meat, beans, mashed potatoes, and peanut butter. Applicants may be enrolled by the nutritionist or community health worker.

<u>Extended Food and Nutrition Education Program</u> (EFNEP) is a nutrition education program administered by the USDA. Community aides, trained in nutrition, visit families with children to educate them regarding nutritious low-cost foods.

RELATIONSHIPS BETWEEN DIET AND HEALTH

- Obesity increases the risk for coronary heart disease, non-insulin-dependent diabetes, and hypertension. Obesity also increases the risk of gall bladder disease, degenerative joint disease, and some types of cancer (e.g., breast, endometrial).

- Frequent consumption of highly cariogenic foods (those containing fermentable, orally-retentive carbohydrates), especially between meals, can nullify some of the preventive benefits of adequate fluoride intake and promote dental caries.

- Excessive sodium and inadequate potassium intake have been associated with high blood pressure. A possible role for dietary calcium and magnesium in the regulation of blood pressure has also been suggested.

- Total fat, saturated fat, and cholesterol intake are contributing risk factors for heart disease.

- Low dietary fiber may contribute to the symptoms of chronic constipation, diverticulosis, and some types of irritable bowel syndrome.

- Dietary fat has been associated epidemiologically with some types of cancer (e.g., breast, colon).

- Poor nutritional status may enhance susceptibility or impair response to infections.

- Inadequate intakes of calcium and/or vitamin D may put women at risk for osteoporosis later in life.

- Inadequate intake of iron predisposes premenopausal women to iron-deficiency anemia.

In addition to the above relationships between diet and common diseases, some birth control methods may affect nutritional status. Oral contraceptives tend to alter the metabolism of certain nutrients, and the intrauterine device (IUD) may cause greater-than-usual menstrual losses, increasing the need for iron (Committee on Diet and Health, Food and Nutrition Board, 1989; U.S. Department of Health and Human Services, 1988).

To help all pre-pregnant, pregnant, postpartum, and lactating women achieve optimal nutritional status, nutritional services should be available from health care professionals who are trained to provide the best quality of care, who are well informed, and who keep up-to-date with well-documented publications. Health care professionals should be prepared to alert women that excessive or inappropriate consumption of some nutrients and food substances contributes to adverse health conditions. The table on nutritional contents of selected fast foods can be used to assist the nurse practitioner/midwife in illustrating the high fat/sodium contents of most fast foods. See Table 8.8, *Nutritional Contents of Selected Fast Foods*, pp. 385-386.

Table 8.1

Daily Food Guide

Food Group	One Serving Equals		Recommended Minimum Servings	
			Nonpregnant/ Nonlactating Woman	Pregnant/ Lactating
PROTEIN FOODS Excellent sources of protein, vitamin B-6, iron, and zinc. Animal protein supplies vitamin B-12. Vegetable protein is a good source of folic acid, magnesium, and fiber.	**Animal Protein:** 1 oz. cooked lean meat, fish, poultry, or seafood 1 egg 2 hot dogs 2 slices luncheon meat 2 oz. or 3 links sausage 2 fish sticks	**Vegetable Protein:** 1/2 cup cooked dry beans 1 egg 3 oz. tofu 1 oz. or 1/4 cup peanuts, pumpkin, or sunflower seeds 1 1/2 oz. or 1/3 cup other nuts 2 tbsp. peanut butter	6 Have at least 1-2 servings from vegetable protein	8
MILK PRODUCTS Excellent sources of protein and calcium. In addition, milk products are good sources of vitamins A, B-12, riboflavin, and zinc. Fortified fluid milk contains 100 IU of vitamin D per cup.	1 cup milk or yogurt 1 cup milkshake 1 1/2 cups cream soups (made with milk) 1 1/2 oz. or 1/3 cup grated bricktype cheese (like cheddar or jack)	1 1/2 slices presliced American cheese 4 tbsp. parmesan 2 cups cottage cheese 1 cup pudding or custard 1 1/2 cups ice cream or frozen yogurt	2 (3 for teens)	4
BREADS, CEREALS, GRAINS All provide carbohydrates and some protein, as well as thiamin, riboflavin, niacin, and iron. Whole grains provide additional vitamin B-6, folic acid, vitamin E, magnesium, zinc, and fiber.	1 slice bread 1 dinner roll 1/2 bun, bagel, English muffin or pita 1 small tortilla 3/4 cup dry cereal 1/2 cup granola	1/2 cup cooked cereal, noodles, or rice 4 tbsp. wheat germ 1 4-inch pancake or waffle 1 muffin 8 medium crackers 4 graham cracker squares	6 Have at least 4 servings from whole-grain products	6
VITAMIN C-RICH FRUITS AND VEGETABLES Excellent sources of vitamin C and fiber. They also supply vitamins A, B-6, and folic acid.	6 oz. orange, grapefruit, tomato, vegetable juice cocktail, or fruit juice enriched with Vitamin C 1 orange, kiwi, mango 1/2 grapefruit cantaloupe 1/4 papaya 2 tangerines, tomatoes	1/2 cup strawberries, broccoli, Brussels sprouts, cabbage, cauliflower, snow peas, sweet peppers, or tomato puree 2 tbsp. fresh or 1/2 cup cooked hot peppers	1	2
VITAMIN A-RICH FRUITS AND VEGETABLES Excellent sources of beta carotene and vitamin A. Most are good sources of fiber. The dark green vegetables also supply good amounts of vitamin B-6, folic acid, and magnesium.	6 oz. apricot nectar or vegetable juice cocktail 3 raw or 1/4 cup dried apricots 1/4 cantaloupe or mango 1/2 papaya 1 small or 1/2 cup sliced carrots	1/2 cup greens (beet, chard, collards, dandelion, kale, mustard, spinach) 1/2 cup pumpkin, sweet potato or winter squash 2 tbsp. raw or cooked hot peppers 2 tomatoes	1	1
OTHER FRUITS AND VEGETABLES Provide carbohydrates and fiber, as well as smaller amounts of other essential vitamins and minerals.	6 oz. fruit juice 1 medium or 1/2 cup sliced fruit (apple, banana, berries, cherries, grapes, peach, pear) 1/2 cup pineapple or watermelon 1/4 cup dried fruit	1/2 cup sliced vegetable (asparagus, beets, green beans, celery, corn, eggplant, mushrooms, onion, peas, potato, summer squash) 1/2 artichoke 1 cup lettuce	3	3

SOURCE:

California Department of Health Services, (1989). *Nutrition during pregnancy and the post-partum period: A manual for health care professionals.* Sacramento, CA: Author.

Table 8.2

Desirable Weight for Height: For Women 25 Years or Older*

Height (in)	Desirable Weight Range (lbs)	Midpoint of Desirable Weight Range (lbs)	Less than 90% of Midpoint of Desirable Weight Range (lbs)	Greater than 120% of Midpoint of Desirable Weight Range (lbs)	Greater than 135% of Midpoint of Desirable Weight Range (lbs)
58	92-121	106	94	128	144
59	95-124	109	97	132	148
60	98-127	112	100	136	152
61	101-130	115	102	139	156
62	104-134	119	106	144	162
63	107-138	122	109	148	166
64	110-142	126	112	152	171
65	114-146	130	116	157	177
66	118-150	134	119	162	182
67	122-154	138	123	167	188
68	126-159	142	126	172	193
69	130-164	147	131	178	200
70	134-169	151	134	183	205

*Height without shoes; weight without clothes

SOURCE:

Adapted from: California Department of Health Services (1989). *Nutrition during pregnancy and the post-partum period: A manual for health care professionals.* Sacramento, CA: Author.

Table 8.3

Provisional Weight Gain Recommendations for Twin Pregnancies (based on singleton pregnancies and observations in twins)

	Singleton	Twin
Overall Total Range:	**20 to 35 lbs**	Expected Range- **40 to 60 lbs** (optimal level not known)
Total Weight Gain by Pregravid Weight for Height	**Underweight** 30 lbs or more **Desirable** 24 to 35 lbs **Overweight** **20 to 24 lbs**	**Underweight** OR **Desirable**: upper end to mid-portion of range **Overweight**: gain at mid- to lower end of range
Rate of Weight Gain Expected:	0.5 to 1.25 lbs/wk	1.25 to 2.0 lbs/wk

SOURCE:

San Francisco Department of Public Health (1989). *Perinatal nutrition protocols*. San Francisco: Author.

Table 8.4

Prenatal Weight Gain Grid

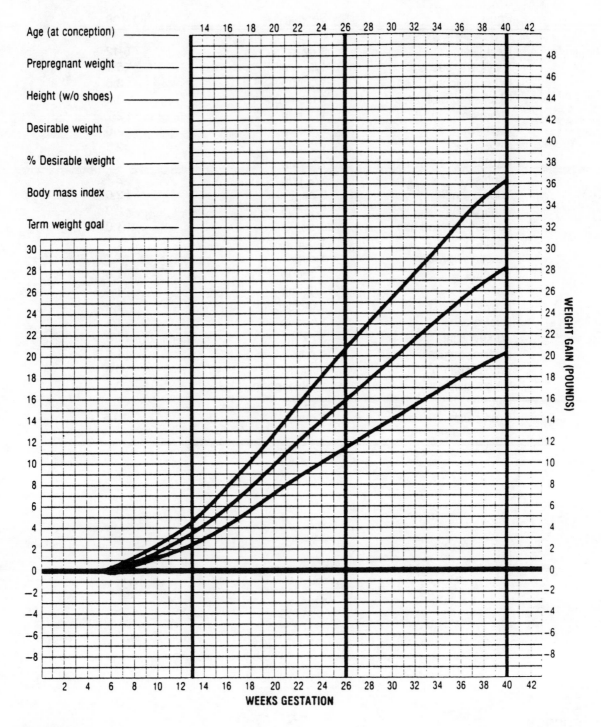

SOURCE:

California Department of Health Services (1989). *Nutrition during pregnancy and the post-partum period: A manual for health care professionals.* Sacramento, CA: Author.

Table 8.5

Dietary Sources of Iron

Food	Serving	Mg Iron
Beef liver	3 oz	7.5-12
Sunflower seeds	1/2 cup	5.1
Dried apricots	1/2 cup	3.6
Blackstrap molasses	1 tablespoon	3.2
Almonds	1/2 cup	2.7
Cashews	1/2 cup	2.6
Soybeans	1/2 cup	2.5
Raisins	1/2 cup	2.5
Lentils	1/2 cup	2.1
Turkey, dark	3 oz	2.0
Lima beans	1/2 cup	2.0
haddock or cod fish	6 oz	1.0
Spinach	1 cup	1.7
Brussels sprouts	1 cup	1.7
Peanuts	1/2 cup	1.6
Peas	1/2 cup	1.4
Brewer's yeast	1 tablespoon	1.4
Beet greens	1/2 cup	1.4
Turkey, light	3 oz	1.0
Endive, escarole	1 cup	1.0
Whole grain bread	1 slice	0.8
Wheat germ	1 tablespoon	0.5
Duck	3 oz	2.0
Prune juice	1 cup	10.5

SOURCE:

Adapted from: California Department of Health Services (1989). *Nutrition during pregnancy and the post-partum period: A manual for health care professionals.* Sacramento, CA: Author.

Table 8.6

Dietary Sources of Folacin

Rich Sources	Greater than 75 mcg per serving
Asparagus	6 stalks or 1/2 cup cooked
Beans: garbanzo, kidney, navy, pinto	1/2 cup cooked
Lentils	1/2 cup cooked
Lettuce: romaine	1 cup raw
Orange juice	6 oz
Spinach	1 cup raw or 1/2 cup cooked
Yeast, nutritional	2 tablespoons

Good Sources	From 35-75 mcg per serving
Avocado	1/2 medium
Beans:baked, pork and beans	1/2 cup cooked
Bean sprouts	1 cup raw
Beets, fresh	1/2 cup cooked
Broccoli	1/2 cup cooked
Brussels sprouts	1/2 cup cooked
Cabbage	1 cup raw
Collards	1/2 cup cooked
Corn	1/2 cup cooked
Falafel (garbanzo croquettes)	3 patties
Humus (garbanzo-sesame dip)	1/2 cup
Lettuce: bibb, Boston, endive	1 cup raw
Liver	1 oz cooked
Mustard greens	1/2 cup cooked
Orange	1 medium
Peanuts	1/4 cup
Peas, green	1/2 cup cooked
Peas, split	1/2 cup cooked
Pineapple juice	6 oz
Sesame butter (tahini)	3 tablespoons
Soybean kernels, roasted	2 ½ tablespoons
Sunflower seeds	1 oz or 1/4 cup
Tomato juice	6 oz
Vegetable juice cocktail	6 oz

SOURCE:

Adapted from: California Department of Health Services (1989). *Nutrition during pregnancy and the post-partum period: A manual for health care professionals.* Sacramento, CA: Author.

Table 8.7

Dietary Sources of Calcium

Dairy Products		Mg Calcium
Milk, whole	1 cup	288
Milk, low-fat (2%)	1 cup	297
Milk, skim	1 cup	298
Buttermilk	1 cup	296
Yogurt (low-fat)	1 cup	270
Nonfat milk powder	¼ cup	367
Fish		
Fish canned with bones	3 oz	345
Oysters	1 cup	226
Shrimp	1 cup	147
Tofu (soy curd)*	4 oz	150
Sesame Seeds		
Ground or meal	¼ cup	270
Vegetables **		
Collard greens	1 cup	360
Dandelion greens	1 cup	150
Okra	1 cup	150
Bok choy	1 cup	250
Kale	1 cup	200
Mustard greens	1 cup	180
Broccoli	1 stalk	267
Turnip greens	1 cup	267

* Fortified soymilk, which is acceptable, can offer the same calcium content as milk.
** Vegetables and grains may contain relatively high levels of calcium, but the mineral is bound by oxalates or phytates, and hence not well absorbed. The above vegetables offer unbound calcium.

SOURCE:

Adapted from: California Department of Health Services (1989). *Nutrition during pregnancy and the post-partum period: A manual for health care professionals.* Sacramento, CA: Author.

Table 8.8

Nutritional Contents of Selected Fast Foods

	Calories	Fat (pats)	Fat (grams)	Sodium (Percent of calories)	Sodium (mg)
McDONALD'S					
Hamburger	255	2.6	10	35	520
Chicken McNuggets	314	5.0	19	54	525
Filet-O-Fish	432	6.6	25	52	781
Big Mac	563	8.7	33	53	1,010
Sausage Biscuit	582	10.4	39	61	1,380
ROY ROGERS					
Plain Potato	211	0	0	0	65
Potato w/oleo	274	1.9	7.2	24	161
Roast Beef Sandwich	317	2.7	10	29	785
Crescent Roll	287	4.7	18	56	547
Potato w/Broccoli 'n Cheese	376	4.8	18.2	43	523
Crescent Sandwich w/Sausage	449	7.7	29	59	1,289
Crescent Sandwich w/Ham	442	7.5	28	58	1,192
WENDY'S					
Pasta Salad (1/2 cup)	134	1.6	6	40	400
Chicken Sandwich on wheat bun	320	2.6	10	28	500
Taco Salad	390	4.8	18	40	1,100
Broccoli & Cheese Potato Cheese	500	6.6	25	45	430
Stuffed Potato	590	9.0	34	52	450
HARDEE'S					
Chef's Salad	272	4.2	16	53	517
Chicken Fillet Sandwich	510	6.9	26	46	360
Shrimp Salad	362	7.7	29	72	941
Bacon Cheeseburger	686	11.1	42	55	1,074
ARBY'S					
Roasted Chicken Breast (no bun)	254	1.9	7.2	25	930
Broccoli & Cheese Potato	540	5.8	22	37	480
Mushroom & Cheese Potato	510	5.8	22	39	640
(Fried) Chick Breast Sandwich	584	7.4	28	43	1,323
Sausage & Egg Croissant	530	9.3	35	59	745

Table 8.8 (continued)

	Calories	Fat (pats)	Fat (grams)	Sodium (Percent of calories)	Sodium (mg)
LONG JOHN SILVER'S					
Baked Fish w/sauce	151	0.5	1.9	12	361
Mixed Vegetables	54	0.5	1.9	33	570
Corn on the Cob	176	1.1	4	20	0
Coleslaw	182	4.0	15	74	367
Fish w/batter (2 pc)	404	6.4	24	53	1,346
BURGER KING					
Veal Parmigiana	580	7.1	27	42	805
Bacon Double Cheeseburger	600	9.3	35	53	985
Specialty Chicken Sandwich	690	11.1	42	55	775
JACK IN THE BOX					
Shrimp Salad (no dressing)	115	0.3	1.1	8	460
Taco Salad	377	6.3	24	57	1,436
Chicken Supreme Sandwich	601	9.5	36	54	1,582
KENTUCKY FRIED CHICKEN					
Breast (original Recipe)	199	3.1	12	53	558
Extra Crispy Dark Dinner*	765	14.2	54	63	1,480

*Includes drumstick, thigh, mashed potatoes, gravy, coleslaw, and roll

SOURCE:

Adapted from: Center for Science in the Public Interest (1985). *Nutrition Action Magazine.* Bonnie Liebman and the Editors.

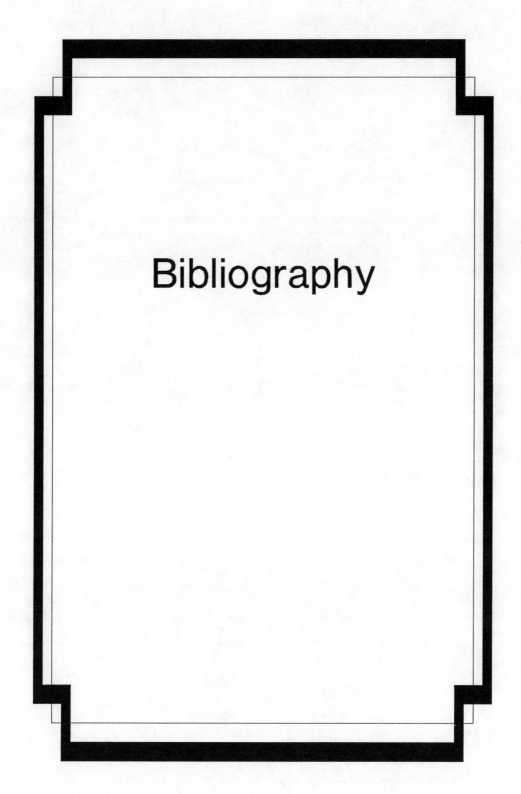

Bibliography

CHAPTER 1

INITIAL PRENATAL VISIT

American College of Obstetricians and Gynecologists (ACOG) (1990). *Scope of services for uncomplicated obstetric care* (Committee Opinion No. 79). Washington, DC: Author.

Cunningham, F. G., MacDonald, P. C., & Gant, N. F. (1989). *Williams obstetrics* (18th ed., pp. 257-275). Norwalk, CT: Appleton & Lange.

Varney, H. (1987). *Nurse-midwifery* (2nd ed., pp. 75-91). Boston: Blackwell Scientific.

Whitley, N. (1985). *A manual of clinical obstetrics* (pp. 6-184). Philadelphia: J. B. Lippincott.

RETURN PRENATAL VISITS

American College of Obstetricians and Gynecologists (ACOG) (1990). *Scope of services for uncomplicated obstetric care* (Committee Opinion No. 79). Washington, DC: Author.

Cunningham, F. G., MacDonald, P. C., & Gant, N. F. (1989). *Williams obstetrics* (18th ed., pp. 257-275). Norwalk, CT: Appleton & Lange.

Varney, H. (1987). *Nurse-midwifery* (2nd ed., pp. 75-91). Boston: Blackwell Scientific.

Whitley, N. (1985). *A manual of clinical obstetrics* (pp. 1-7). Philadelphia: J. B. Lippincott.

POSTPARTUM VISIT

Affonso, D. D. (1987). Assessment of maternal postpartum adaptation. *Public Health Nursing, 4*(1), 9-20.

Cunningham, F. G., MacDonald, P. C., & Gant, N. F. (1989). *Williams obstetrics* (18th ed.). Norwalk, CT: Appleton & Lange.

Novy, M. J. (1987). The normal puerperium. In M. L. Pernoll & R. C. Benson (Eds.), *Current obstetric and gynecologic diagnosis and treatment 1987* (pp. 216-245). Norwalk, CT: Appleton & Lange.

Reik, L. (1988). Headaches in pregnancy. *Seminars in neurology, 8*(3), 187-192.

Tulman, L., & Fawcett, J. (1988). Return of functional ability after childbirth. *Nursing Research, 37*(2), 77-81.

Varney, H. (1987). *Nurse-midwifery* (pp. 475-515). Boston: Blackwell Scientific.

Weber, J. (1988). *Nurses' handbook of health assessment (pp. 289-299). Philadelphia: J. B. Lippincott.*

Willson, J. R. (1987). The puerperium. In J. R. Willson & E. R. Carrington (Eds.), *Obstetrics and gynecology* (8th ed., pp. 598-607). St. Louis: C. V. Mosby.

CHAPTER 2

ALPHA-FETOPROTEIN SCREENING

Burton, B. K. (1988). Elevated maternal serum alpha-fetoprotein (MSAFP): Interpretation and follow-up. *Clinical Obstetrics and Gynecology, 31*(2), 293-305.

Drugan, A., Dvorin, E., Koppitch, F. C., Greb, A., Krivchenia, E. L., & Evans, M. I. (1989). Counseling for low maternal serum alpha-fetoprotein should emphasize all chromosome anomalies, not just Down's syndrome! *Obstetrics & Gynecology, 73*(2), 271-274.

Knight, G. J., Palomaki, G. E., & Haddow, J. E. (1988). Use of maternal serum alpha-fetoprotein measurements to screen for Down's syndrome. *Clinical Obstetrics and Gynecology, 31*(2), 306-327.

Main, D. M., & Mennuti, M. T. (1986). Neural tube defects: Issues in prenatal diagnosis and counseling. *Obstetrics & Gynecology, 67*(1), 1-16.

Robinson, L., Grau, P., & Crandall, B. F. (1989). Pregnancy outcomes after increasing maternal serum alpha-fetoprotein levels. *Obstetrics & Gynecology, 74*(1), 17-20.

AMNIOCENTESIS

American College of Obstetricians and Gynecologists (ACOG) (1987). *Antenatal diagnosis of genetic disorders* (Technical Bulletin No. 108). Washington DC: Author.

Brandenburg, H., Pipers, L., & Wladimiroff, J. W. (1989). Rhesus sensitization after midtrimester genetic amniocentesis. *American Journal of Medical Genetics, 32*, 225-226.

Evans, M. I., Drugen, A., Koppitch, F. C., Zador, I. E., Sacks, A. J., & Sokol, R. J. (1989). Genetic diagnosis in the first trimester: The norm for the 1990's. *American Journal of Obstetrics and Gynecology, 160*(6), 1332-1339.

Evans, M. I., Koppich F. C., Nemitz, B., Quigg, M. H., & Zador, I. E. (1988). Early genetic amniocentesis and chorionic villi sampling. *Journal of Reproductive Medicine, 33*(5), 450-452.

Gold R. B., Goyert, G. L., Schwartz, D. B., Evans, M. I., & Seabolt, L. A. (1989). Conservative management of second-trimester post amniocentesis fluid leakage. *Obstetrics and Gynecology, 74*(5), 745-747.

Johnson A., & Godmilow L. (1988). Genetic amniocentesis at 14 weeks or less. *Clinical Obstetrics and Gynecology, 31*(2), 345-352.

Knuppel, R. A., & Drukker, J. E. (1986). *High-risk pregnancy: A team approach.* Philadelphia, PA: W.B. Saunders.

Robinson, G. E., Garner, D. M., Olmstead, M. P., Shime, J., Hutton, E. M., & Crawford, B. M. (1988). Anxiety reduction after chorionic villus sampling and genetic amniocentesis. *American Journal of Obstetrics and Gynecology, 159*(4), 953-956.

Sjögren, B., & Uddenberg, N. (1989). Prenatal diagnosis and psychological distress: Amniocentesis or chorionic villus biopsy? *Prenatal Diagnosis, 9*, 477-487.

Spencer, J. W., & Cox, D. V. (1988). A comparison of chorionic villi sampling and amniocentesis: acceptability of procedure and maternal attachment to pregnancy. *Obstetrics and Gynecology, 72*(5), 714-718.

Tabor, A. (1988). Genetic amniocentesis--indications and risks. *Danish Medical Bulletin, 35*(6), 520-537.

CHORIONIC VILLUS SAMPLING

American College of Obstetricians and Gynecologists (ACOG) (1987). *Antenatal diagnosis of genetic disorders* (Technical Bulletin No. 108). Washington DC: Author.

Blakemore, K. J. (1988). Prenatal diagnosis by chorionic villus sampling. *Obstetrics and Gynecology Clinics of North America, 15*(2), 179-213.

Jackson, L. G., & Wapner, R. J. (1987). Risks of chorionic villus sampling. *Baillière's Clinical Obstetrics and Gynaecology, 1*(3), 513-531.

Rhoads, G. G., Jackson, L. G., Schlesselman, S. E., De La Cruz, F. F., Desnick, R. J., Golbus, M. S., Ledbetter, D. H., Lubs, H. A., Mahoney, M. J., Pergament E., Simpson, J. L., Carpenter, R. J., Elias, S., Ginsberg, N. A., Goldberg, J. D., Hobbins, J. C., Lynch, L., Shiono, P. H., Wapner, R. J., & Zachary, J. M. (1989). The safety and efficacy of chorionic villus sampling for early prenatal diagnosis of cytogenetic abnormalities. *New England Journal of Medicine, 320*(10), 609-617.

Robinson, G. E., Garner, D. M., Olmsted, M. P., Shime, J., Hutton, E. M., & Crawford, B. M. (1988). Anxiety reduction after chorionic villus sampling and genetic amniocentesis. *American Journal of Obstetrics and Gynecology, 159*(4), 953-956.

Sjögren, B., & Uddenberg, N. (1989). Prenatal diagnosis and psychological distress: Amniocentesis or chorionic villus biopsy? *Prenatal Diagnosis, 9,* 477-487.

Spencer, J. W., & Cox, D. V. (1988). A comparison of chorionic villi sampling and amniocentesis: Acceptability of procedure and maternal attachment to pregnancy. *Obstetrics and Gynecology, 72*(5), 714-718.

Wapner, R. J., & Jackson, L. (1988). Chorionic villus sampling. *Clinical Obstetrics and Gynecology, 31*(2), 328-344.

ANTEPARTUM FETAL SURVEILLANCE

American College of Obstetricians and Gynecologists (ACOG) (1987). *Antepartum fetal surveillance* (Technical Bulletin No. 107). Washington, DC: Author.

American College of Obstetricians and Gynecologists (ACOG) (1988). *Antepartum fetal surveillance* (Technical Bulletin No. 116). Washington, DC: Author.

American Institute of Ultrasound in Medicine, Bioeffects Committee (1988). Bioeffects considerations for the safety of diagnostic ultrasound. *Journal of Ultrasound Medicine, 7*(9 suppl.), S1-38.

Brar, H. S., Platt, L. D., & Devore, G. R. (1987). The biophysical profile. *Clinical Obstetrics and Gynecology, 30*(4), 936-947.

Chamberlain, P. F., Manning, F. A., Morrison, I., Harman, C. R., & Lange, I. R. (1984). Ultrasound evaluation of amniotic fluid volumes. I. The relationship of marginal and decreased amniotic fluid volumes and perinatal outcome. *American Journal of Obstetrics and Gynecology, 150*(3), 245-249.

Clark, S. L. (1990). How a modified NST improves fetal surveillance. *Contemporary Ob/Gyn, 35*(5), 45-48.

Dunn, P. A., Weiner, S., & Ludomirski, A. (1988). Percutaneous umbilical blood sampling. *JOGNN, 17*(5), 308-313.

Field, D. R. (1989). Changing patterns in antepartum surveillance. In J.T. Parer (Ed.), *Antepartum and intrapartum management*. Philadelphia: Lea and Febinger.

Freeman, R. K. (1987). Antepartum case management. *Clinical Obstetrics and Gynecology, 30*(4), 1007-1014.

Gabbe, S. G., Freeman, R. K., & Goebelsman, U. W. E. (1978). Evaluation of the contraction stress test before 33 weeks' gestation. *Obstetrics and Gynecology, 52*(6), 649-652.

Gagnon, R., Hunse, C. & Patrick, J. (1988). Fetal responses to vibratory acoustic stimulation: Influence of basal heart rate. *American Journal of Obstetrics and Gynecology, 159*(4), 835-839.

Goodman, L. D., Visser, F. G., & Dawes, G. S. (1984). Effects of maternal smoking on fetal trunk movements, fetal breathing movements and fetal heart rate. *British Journal of Obstetrics and Gynaecology, 91*(7), 657-661.

Huddleston, J. F., & Quinlan, R. W. (1987). Clinical utility of the contraction stress test. *Clinical Obstetrics and Gynecology, 30*(4), 912-920.

Huddleston, J. F., Sutliff, J. B., & Robinson, D. (1984). Contraction stress test by intermittent nipple stimulation. *Obstetrics and Gynecology, 63*(5), 669-673.

Keegan, K. A. (1987). The Nonstress Test. *Clinical Obstetrics and Gynecology, 30*(4), 921-935.

Ludomirski, A., & Weiner, S. (1988). Percutaneous fetal umbilical blood sampling. *Clinical Obstetrics and Gynecology, 31*(1), 19-26.

Manning, F. A., Morrison, I., Lange, I.R., & Harman, C. (1982). Antepartum determination of fetal health: Composite biophysical profile scoring. *Clinics in Perinatology, 9*(2), 285-296.

Manning, F. A., Morrison, I., Lange, I. R., Harman, C. R., & Chamberlain, P.F. (1985). Fetal assessment based on fetal biophysical scoring: Experience in 12,620 referred high-risk pregnancies. *American Journal of Obstetrics and Gynecology, 151*(3), 343-350.

Modica, M. M., & Timor-Trisch, I.E. (1988). Transvaginal sonography provides a sharper view into the pelvis. *JOGNN, 17*(2), 89-95.

Moore, T. R., & Piacquadio, K. (1989). A prospective evaluation of fetal movement screening to reduce the incidence of antepartum fetal death. *American Journal of Obstetrics and Gynecology, 160*(5), 1075-1080.

National Institute of Health Consensus Development Panel (1984). Diagnostic ultrasound imaging in pregnancy. *National Institutes of Health Consensus Development, Conference Consensus Statement, 5*(1), 1-6.

Neldman, S. (1980). Fetal movements as an indicator of fetal wellbeing. *The Lancet, 1*(8180), 1222-1224.

Paine, L. L., Johnson, T. R. B., & Alexander, G. R., (1988). Auscultated fetal heart rate accelerations, III. Use of vibratory acoustic stimulation. *American Journal of Obstetrics and Gynecology, 159*(5), 1163-1167.

Patrick, J., Campbell, K., Carmichael, L., & Probert, C. (1982). Influence of maternal heart rate and gross body movements on the daily pattern of fetal heart rate near term. *American Journal of Obstetrics and Gynecology, 144*(5), 533-538.

Pearson, J. F., & Weaver, J. B. (1976). Fetal activity and fetal well-being: An evaluation. *British Medical Journal, 1*(6020), 1305-1307.

Platt, L. C., DeVore, G. R., Schulman, H., & Wladimiroff, J. (1989). Assessing the fetus with Doppler ultrasound. *Contemporary Ob/Gyn, 33*(1), 168-199.

Polzin, G. B., Blakemore, K. J., Petrie, R. H., & Amom, E. (1988). Fetal vibro-acoustic stimulation: Magnitude and duration of fetal heart rate accelerations as a marker of fetal health. *Obstetrics & Gynecology, 72*(4), 621-626.

Porto, M. (1987). Comparing and contrasting methods of fetal surveillance. *Clinical Obstetrics and Gynecology, 30*(4), 956-967.

Rayburn, W. F. (1987). Monitoring fetal body movement. *Clinical Obstetrics and Gynecology, 3*(4), 899-910.

Rayburn, W. F., & McKean, H. E. (1980). Maternal perception of fetal movement and perinatal outcome. *Obstetrics and Gynecology, 56*(2), 161-164.

Sadovsky, E., & Polishuk, W. (1977). Fetal movements in utero. *Obstetrics and Gynecology, 50*(1), 49-55.

Schifrin, B. S., & Clement, D. (1990). Why fetal monitoring remains a good idea. *Contemporary Ob/Gyn, 35*(2), 70-86.

Seeds, J. W. (1988). PUBS: important new aid for prenatal diagnosis. *Contemporary Ob/Gyn, 31*(2), 117-133.

Timor-Trisch, I. E., & Rottem, S. (1988). High-frequency transvaginal sonography: new diagnostic boom. *Contemporary Ob/Gyn, 31*(4), 111-133.

Vintzileos, A. M., Campbell, W. A., Ingardia, C. J., & Nochimson, D. J. (1983). The fetal biophysical profile and its predictive value. *Obstetrics and Gynecology, 62*(3), 271-278.

Vintzileos, A. M., Campbell, W. A., Nochimson, D. J., & Weinbaum, P. J. (1987). The use and misuse of the fetal biophysical profile. *American Journal of Obstetrics and Gynecology, 156*(3), 527-533.

Watson, P. T., Young, W. P., & Hegge, F. N. (1987). Doppler measurements of maternal and fetal blood flow. *Clinical Obstetrics and Gynecology, 30*(4), 948-955.

CHAPTER 3

COMMON DISCOMFORTS

Ameli, F. M. (1986). Current concepts in the management of varicose veins. *The Canadian Journal of Surgery, 29*(1), 21-23.

Bowen, J. D., & Larson, E. B. (1989). Understanding the dizzy patient: A challenge to primary care physicians. *The Journal of Family Practice, 29*(1), 30-32.

Briggs, G. G., Freeman, R. K., & Yaffe, S. J. (1986). *Drugs in pregnancy and lactation* (2nd ed.). Baltimore: Williams & Wilkins.

Brucker, M. C. (1987). Management of common minor discomforts in pregnancy, Part I: Managing upper respiratory infections in pregnancy. *Journal of Nurse-Midwifery, 32*(6), 349-356.

Brucker, M. C. (1988). Management of common minor discomforts in pregnancy. Part III: Managing gastrointestinal problems in pregnancy. *Journal of Nurse-Midwifery, 33*(2), 67-73.

Centers for Disease Control (1984). Influenza--United States. *Morbidity and Mortality Weekly Report, 33*, 252.

Coalition for Medical Rights of Women (1987). *Natural remedies for pregnancy discomforts* (rev. ed.). Campbell, CA: Education Programs Associates.

Cunningham, F. G., MacDonald, P. C., & Gant, N. F. (1989). *Williams obstetrics* (18th ed.). Norwalk, CT. Appleton & Lange.

Dennison, A. R., Whiston, R. J., Rooney, S., & Morris, D. L. (1989). The management of hemorrhoids. *The American Journal of Gastroenterology, 84*(5), 475-481.

Dilorio, C. (1985). First trimester nausea in pregnant teenagers: Incidence, characteristics, intervention. *Nursing Research, 34*(6), 372-374.

Dilorio, C. (1988). The management of nausea and vomiting in pregnancy. *The Nurse Practitioner, 13*(5), 23-28.

Dilorio, C., & van Lier, D. J. (1989). Nausea and vomiting in pregnancy. In E. M. Tornquist, M. T. Champagne, L. A. Copp, & R. A. Wiese (Eds.), *Key aspects of comfort: Management of pain, fatigue and nausea* (pp. 259-266). New York: Springer.

Dundee, J. W., Sourial, F. B. R., Ghaly, R. G., & Bell, P. F. (1988). P6 acupressure reduces morning sickness. *Journal of the Royal Society of Medicine, 81*, 456-457.

Ehudin-Pagano, E., Paluzzi, P. A., Ivory, L. C., & McCartney, M. (1987). The use of herbs in nurse-midwifery practice. *Journal of Nurse-Midwifery, 32*(4), 260-262.

Friedlander, M. A. (1987). Fluid retention: Evaluation and use of diuretics. *Clinical Obstetrics and Gynecology, 30*(2), 431-442.

Fuller, J., & Schaller-Ayres, J. (1990). *Health assessment: A nursing approach.* Grand Rapids: Lippincott.

Guyton, A. C. (1986). *Textbook of medical physiology* (7th ed.). Philadelphia: W. B. Saunders.

Incaudo, G. A. (1987). Diagnosis and treatment of rhinitis during pregnancy and lactation. *Clinical Reviews in Allergy, 5*(4), 325-337.

Jarnfelt-Samsioe, A. (1987). Nausea and vomiting in pregnancy: A review. *Obstetrical and Gynecological Survey, 41*(7), 422-427.

Jenkins, M. L., & Shelton, B. J. (1989). The effectiveness of self-care actions in reducing "morning sickness." In E. M. Tornquist, M. T. Champagne, L. A. Copp, & R. A. Wiese (Eds.), *Key aspects of comfort: Management of pain, fatigue and nausea* (pp. 267-272). New York: Springer.

Johnson & Johnson Products (1979). Nosebleed. In *First aid guide* (p. 21). New Brunswick, NJ: Author.

Jones, J. M., Cox, A. R., Levy, E. Y., & Thompson, C. E. (1984). *Women's health management: Guidelines for nurse practitioners.* Reston, VA: Reston Publishing.

Laros, R. K. (1987). Diseases of the respiratory system, the circulatory system, and the blood during pregnancy. In J. R. Willson & E. R. Carrington (Eds.), *Obstetrics and gynecology* (8th ed., pp. 313-325). St. Louis: C. V. Mosby.

Leff, E. (1987). Hemorrhoids: Current approaches to an ancient problem. *Postgraduate Medicine, 82*(7), 95-101.

Mabry, R. L. (1986). Rhinitis of pregnancy. *Southern Medical Journal, 79*(8), 965-971.

Martignoni, E., Sances, G., & Nappi, G. (1987). Significance of hormonal changes in migraine and cluster headache. *Gynecological Endocrinology, 1*(3), 295-319.

McLoughlin, I. J. (1987). The picas. *British Journal of Hospital Medicine, 37*(4), 286-290.

Morrison, J. C., & Palmer, S. M. (1987). General medical disorders during pregnancy. In M. L. Pernoll & R. C. Benson (Eds.), *Current obstetric and gynecologic diagnosis and treatment* (6th ed., pp. 386-402). Norwalk, CT: Appleton & Lange.

Neeson, J. D., & Stockdale, C. R. (1981). *The practitioner's handbook of ambulatory Ob/Gyn.* New York: John Wiley & Sons.

Noble, P. W., Lavee, A. E., & Jacobs, M. M. (1988). Respiratory diseases in pregnancy. *Obstetrics and Gynecology Clinics of North America, 15*(2), 391-428.

Nuwayhid, B. (1986). Medical complications of pregnancy. In N. F. Hacker & J. G. Moore (Eds.), *Essentials of obstetrics and gynecology* (pp. 142-164). Philadelphia: W. B. Saunders.

Physician's desk reference (43rd ed.) (1989). Oradell, NJ: Medical Economics.

Poole, C. J. (1986). Fatigue during the first trimester of pregnancy. *JOGNN, 15*(5), 375-379.

Reik, L. (1988). Headaches in pregnancy. *Seminars in Neurology, 8*(3), 187-192.

Sammons, L. N. (1986). Maternal anxiety, somatic symptoms, marital adjustment, and family relationships in second pregnancy (Doctoral dissertation, University of California, San Francisco, 1985). *Dissertation Abstracts International, 46,* 3785B.

Scherer, J. C. (1985). *Lippincott's nurses' drug manual.* Philadelphia: J. B. Lippincott.

Seller, R. H. (1986). *Differential diagnosis of common complaints.* Philadelphia: W. B. Saunders.

Smith, L. E. (1987). Hemorrhoids: A review of current techniques and management. *Gastroenterology Clinics of North America, 16*(1). 79-91.

Streitfeld, H. (1986). Morning sickness in pregnancy. *Parents' Press, 7*(6), 9-11.

Taylor, C. M., & Pernoll, M. L. (1987). Normal pregnancy and prenatal care. In M. L. Pernoll & R. C. Benson (Eds.), *Current obstetric and gynecologic diagnosis and treatment* (pp. 161-177). Norwalk, CT: Appleton & Lange.

Thomas, C. L. (Ed.) (1989). *Taber's cyclopedic medical dictionary* (16th ed.). Philadelphia: F. A. Davis.

Varney, H. (1987). *Nurse-midwifery* (2nd ed.). Boston: Blackwell Scientific.

Vintzileos, A. M., Deaton, J. L., & Campbell, W. A. (1986). What to give the patient who has hay fever or cold. *Contemporary Ob/Gyn, 27*(4), 198-208.

Worthington-Roberts, B. S. (1989). Maternal nutrition and the outcome of pregnancy. In B. S. Worthington-Roberts & S. R. Williams (Ed.), *Nutrition in pregnancy and lactation* (4th ed., pp. 47-140). St. Louis: Times Mirror/Mosby.

CHAPTER 4

BACTERIURIA - ASYMPTOMATIC

Biswas, M., & Perloff, D. (1987). Cardiac, hematologic, pulmonary, and renal and urinary tract disorders in pregnancy. In M. L. Pernoll & R. C. Benson (Eds.), *Current obstetric and gynecologic diagnosis and treatment, 1987* (6th ed., pp. 379-380). Norwalk, CT: Appleton & Lange.

Davison, J. M., & Lindheimer, M. D. (1989). Renal disorders. In R. K. Creasy & R. Resnik (Eds.), *Maternal-fetal medicine* (2nd ed., pp. 825-826). Philadelphia: W. B. Saunders.

Gilstrap, L. C., & Cox, S. M. (1987). An aggressive approach to UTI during pregnancy. *Contemporary Ob/Gyn, 30*(5), 23-28.

McNeeley, S. G. (1988). Treatment of urinary tract infections during pregnancy. *Clinical Obstetrics and Gynecology, 31*(2), 480-487.

Pauerstein, C. J. (1987). *Clinical obstetrics* (pp. 677-690). New York: John Wiley & Sons.

Robertson, A. W., & Duff, P. (1988). The nitrite and leukocyte esterase tests for the evaluation of asymptomatic bacteriuria in obstetric patients. *Obstetrics and Gynecology, 71*(6), 878-881.

BATTERED WOMAN/PERINATAL DOMESTIC VIOLENCE

American College of Obstetricians and Gynecologists (ACOG) (1989). *The battered woman* (Technical Bulletin No. 124). Washington, DC: Author.

Bojanowski, C., Hill, K., & Martin, D. (1988). Assessment of the pregnant trauma patient. *Dimensions of Critical Care Nursing, 7*(6), 356-363.

Chez, R. A. (1989). Battered pregnant women. *Genesis, 11*(1), 15-16.

Helton, A. S. (1986). Battering during pregnancy. *American Journal of Nursing, 86*(8), 910-913.

Helton, A. S. (1987). *Protocol of care for the battered woman*. White Plains, NY: March of Dimes Birth Defects Foundation.

Helton, A., McFarlane, J., & Anderson, E. (1987). Prevention of battering during pregnancy: Focus on behavioral change. *Public Health Nursing, 4*(3), 166-174.

Hillard, P.J. (1985). Physical abuse in pregnancy. *Obstetrics and Gynecology, 66*, 185-190.

Sammons, L. N. (1981). Battered and pregnant. *MCN-The American Journal of Maternal-Child Nursing, 6*(4), 246-250.

Viken, R. M. (1982). Family violence: Aids to recognition. *Postgraduate Medicine, 71*(15), 115-122.

Walker, L. E. (1984). *The battered woman syndrome*. New York: Springer.

BLEEDING

Cunningham, F. G., MacDonald, P. C., & Gant, N. F. (1989). *Williams obstetrics* (18th ed., pp. 489-498, 701-716). Norwalk, CT. Appleton & Lange.

Gottesfeld, K. R. (1983a). Placenta previa. In J. T. Queenan & J. C. Hobbins (Eds.), *Protocols for high-risk pregnancies* (pp. 218-222). Oradell: Medical Economics.

Gottesfeld, K. R. (1983b). Placental abruption. In J. T. Queenan & J. C. Hobbins (Eds.), *Protocols for high-risk pregnancies* (pp. 223-226). Oradell: Medical Economics.

Neeson, J. D., & Stockdale, C. R. (1981). *The practitioner's handbook of ambulatory Ob/Gyn*. New York: John Wiley & Sons.

Wible-Kant, J., & Beer, A. E. (1983). Antepartum Rh immune globulin. *Clinics in Perinatology, 10*(2), 343-355.

Willson, J. R. (1983a). Bleeding during late pregnancy. In J. R. Willson, E. R. Carrington, & W. J. Ledger (Eds.), *Obstetrics and gynecology* (7th ed., pp. 356-371). St. Louis: C. V. Mosby.

Willson, J. R. (1983b). Spontaneous and induced abortion. In J. R. Willson, E. R. Carrington, & W. J. Ledger (Eds.), *Obstetrics and gynecology* (7th ed., pp. 187-204). St. Louis: C. V. Mosby.

BREAST MASS

American Cancer Society (1988). A fact sheet on mammography. San Francisco: American Cancer Society, San Francisco Unit.

American College of Obstetricians and Gynecologists (ACOG) (1983). *Epidemiology and diagnosis of breast disease* (Technical Bulletin No. 17). Washington, DC: Author.

Borten, M. (1987). Breast mass. In E. A. Freidman, D. B. Acker, & B. P. Sachs (Eds.), *Obstetrical decision making* (2nd ed., p. 106). Toronto: B. C. Dicker.

Ellerhorst-Ryan, J. M., Turba, E. P., & Stahl, D. L. (1988). Evaluating benign breast disease. *The Nurse Practitioner, 13*(9), 13-28.

Feller, W. F. (1988, June 15). Steps in evaluation of a breast mass. *Contemporary Ob/Gyn, 32*(Special Issue), 11-27.

CYSTITIS

Balgobin, B. (1987). Bacteriuria. In E. A. Friedman, D. B. Acker, & B. P. Sachs (Eds.), *Obstetrical decision making* (2nd ed., pp.164-165). Toronto: B. C. Decker.

Davison, J. M., & Lindheimer, M. D. (1989). Renal disorders. In R.K. Creasy & R. Resnik (Eds.), *Maternal-fetal medicine: Principles and practice* (2nd ed., pp. 824-827). Philadelphia: W.B. Saunders.

Fowler, J. E. (1989). *Urinary tract infection and inflammation* (pp. 196-198). Chicago: Yearbook Medical Publishers.

McNeeley, S. G. (1988). Treatment of urinary tract infections during pregnancy. *Clinical Obstetrics and Gynecology, 31*(2), 480-487.

Pauerstein, C. J. (1987). Renal disease. In C. J. Pauerstein (Ed.), *Clinical obstetrics* (pp. 677-680). New York: John Wiley & Sons.

Robertson, A. W., & Duff, P. (1988). The nitrite and leukocyte esterase tests for the evaluation of asymptomatic bacteriuria in obstetric patients. *Obstetrics and Gynecology, 71*(6), 878-881.

DEPRESSION--POSTPARTUM

Affonso, D. D., & Domino, G. (1984). Postpartum depression: A review. *Birth, 11*(4), 231-235.

Daw, J. L. (1988). Postpartum depression. *Southern Medical Journal, 81*(2), 207-209.

Dreyfus, J. K. (1987). The prevalence of depression in women in an ambulatory care setting. *The Nurse Practitioner, 12*(4), 34-50.

Goodwin, J. M., Kleiner, G. J., & Saks, B. R. (1986). Managing pregnancy-related depression. *Patient Care, 20*(3), 101-114.

Martell, L. (1990). Postpartum depression as a family problem. *MCN-The American Journal of Maternal-Child Nursing, 15.* 90-93.

O'Hara, M. W. (1987). Post-partum "blues," depression, and psychosis: A review. *Journal of Psychosomatic Obstetrics and Gynaecology*, 7, 205-227.

Theesen, K., Alderson, M., & Hill, W. (1989). Caring for the depressed obstetric patient. *Contemporary Ob/Gyn*, 33(2), 123-139.

ECTOPIC PREGNANCY

de Crespigny, L. (1987). The value of ultrasound in ectopic pregnancy. *Clinical Obstetrics and Gynecology*, 30(1), 136-147.

Dorfman, S. F. (1987). Epidemiology of ectopic pregnancy. *Clinical Obstetrics and Gynecology*, 30(1), 173-180.

Fedele, L., Acaia, B., Parazzini, F., Ricciardiello, O., & Candiani, G. B. (1989). Ectopic pregnancy and recurrent spontaneous abortion: Two associated reproductive failures. *Obstetrics and Gynecology*, 73(2), 206-208.

Osguthorpe, N. C. (1987). Ectopic pregnancy. *JOGNN*, 16(1), 36-41.

Rivlin, M. (1986). Ectopic pregnancy. In M. E. Rivlin, J. C. Morrison, & G. W. Bates (Eds.), *Manual of clinical problems in obstetrics and gynecology* (2nd ed., pp. 8-12). Boston: Little, Brown & Company.

Russell, J. B. (1987). The etiology of ectopic pregnancy. *Clinical Obstetrics and Gynecology*, 30(1), 181-190.

Shapiro, B. S. (1987). The nonsurgical management of ectopic pregnancy. *Clinical Obstetrics and Gynecology*, 30(1), 230-235.

Sopelak, V. M., & Bates, G. W. (1987). Role of transmigration and abnormal embryogenesis in ectopic pregnancy. *Clinical Obstetrics and Gynecology*, 30(1), 236-244.

Weckstein, I. N. (1987). Clinical diagnosis of ectopic pregnancy. *Clinical Obstetrics and Gynecology*, 30(1), 236-244.

Wible-Kant, J., & Beer, A. E. (1983). Antepartum Rh immune globulin. *Clinics in Perinatology*, 10(2), 343-355.

ENDOMETRITIS--POSTPARTUM

Briggs, G. G., Freeman, R. K., & Yaffe, S. J. (1986). *Drugs in pregnancy and lactation* (2nd ed.). Baltimore: Williams & Wilkins.

Cox, S. M., & Gilstrap, L. C. (1989). Postpartum endometritis. *Obstetrics and Gynecology Clinics of North America*, 16(2), 363-371.

Cunningham, F. G., MacDonald, P. C., & Gant, N. F. (1989). *Williams obstetrics* (18th ed., pp. 461-476). Norwalk, CT: Appleton & Lange.

Fortunato, S. J., & Dodson, M. G. (1988). Therpeutic considerations in postpartum endometritis. *The Journal of Reproductive Medicine*, 33(1, Supp.), 101-106.

Gibbs, R. S. (1989). Severe infections in pregnancy. *Medical Clinics of North America, 73*(3), 713-721.

Ledger, W. J. (1987). Obstetric and gynecologic infections. In J. R. Willson & E. R. Carrington (Eds.), *Obstetrics and gynecology* (18th ed., pp. 577-597). St. Louis: C. V. Mosby.

Novy, M. J. (1987). The normal puerperium. In M. L. Pernoll & R. C. Benson (Eds.), *Current obstetric and gynecologic diagnosis and treatment 1987* (6th ed., pp. 216-245). Norwalk, CT: Appleton & Lange.

Soper, D. E. (1988). Postpartum endometritis: Pathophysiology and prevention. *Journal of Reproductive Medicine, 33*(1, supp.), 97-100.

GESTATIONAL DIABETES MELLITUS

American College of Obstetricians and Gynecologists (ACOG) (1986). *Management of diabetes mellitus in pregnancy* (Technical Bulletin No. 92). Washington, DC: Author.

Berry, J. L., & Gabbe, S. G. (1986). Diabetes mellitus in pregnancy. In R. A. Knuppel & J. E. Drukker (Eds.), *High risk pregnancy: A team approach*. Philadelphia: W.B. Saunders.

Coustan, D. R. & Carpenter, M. W. (1985). Detection and treatment of gestational diabetes. *Clinical Obstetrics and Gynecology, 28*(3), 507-515.

Coustan, D. R., Widness, J. A., Carpenter, M. W., Rotondo, J., Pratt, D. C., & Oh, W. (1986). Should the fifty-gram, one-hour plasma glucose screening test for gestational diabetes be administered in the fasting or fed state? *American Journal of Obstetrics and Gynecology, 154*(5), 1031-1035.

Diabetes (1985). Summary and recommendations of the Second International Workshop Conference on gestational diabetes mellitus. *Diabetes, 34*(2), 123-126.

Gabbe, S. G., & Landon, M. B. (1987). Diabetes mellitus. In C. J. Pauerstein (Ed.), *Clinical obstetrics*. New York: John Wiley & Sons.

Harris, I., Hadden, W. C., Knowler, W. C., & Bennett, P. H. (1985). International criteria for the diagnosis of diabetes and impaired glucose tolerance. *Diabetes Care, 8,* 562-567.

Hollingsworth, D. R. (1985). Maternal metabolism in normal pregnancy and pregnancy complicated by diabetes. *Clinical Obstetrics and Gynecology, 28*(3), 457-472.

Kitzmiller, J. L., Gavin, L. A., Gin, G. D., Iverson, M., Gunderson, E., Farley, P., Cohen, H., & Sheerer, L. J. (1988). Managing diabetes and pregnancy. *Current Problems in Obstetrics, Gynecology, and Fertility, 11*(4), July/August, 107-167.

National Diabetes Data Group (NDDG) (1979). Classification and diagnosis of diabetes mellitus and other categories of glucose intolerance. *Diabetes, 28,* 1039-1057.

Nelson, D. M. (1984). Diabetes and pregnancy. In F. Arias (Ed.), *High risk pregnancy and delivery* (pp. 121-147). St. Louis: C. V. Mosby.

O'Sullivan, J. B., & Mahan, C. M. (1964). Criteria for the oral glucose tolerence test in pregnancy. *Diabetes, 13,* 278.

O'Sullivan, J. B., Mahan, C. M., & Charles, D. (1973). Screening criteria for high risk gestational diabetic patients. *Obstetrics and Gynecology, 116*, 895.

Reed, B. D. (1988). Gestational diabetes mellitus. *Primary Care, 15*(2), 371-387.

Sweet Success (1988). California Diabetes and Pregnancy Program: Guidelines for Care. Maternal and Child Health Branch, Department of Health Services.

GESTATIONAL TROPHOBLASTIC NEOPLASIA

Celeste, S. M., & Smith, M. D. (1986). Gestational trophoblastic neoplasms. *Journal of Obstetric, Gynecologic, and Neonatal Nursing, 15*(1), 11-16.

Cunningham, F. G., MacDonald, P. C., & Gant, N. F. (1989). *Williams obstetrics* (18th ed., pp. 540-553). Norwalk, CT: Appleton & Lange.

Neeson, J. D., & Stockdale, C. R. (1981). *The practitioner's handbook of ambulatory Ob/Gyn.* New York: John Wiley & Sons.

HYPERTENSIVE DISORDERS OF PREGNANCY

Abrams, R. S. (1989). *Handbook of medical problems during pregnancy* (pp. 91-111). Norwalk, CT: Appleton & Lange.

Ales, K. L., Norton, M. E., & Druzin, M. L. (1989). Early prediction of antepartum hypertension. *Obstetrics and Gynecology, 73*(6), 928-933.

American College of Obstetricians and Gynecologists (ACOG) (1986). *Management of pre-eclampsia* (Technical Bulletin No. 91). Washington, DC: Author.

Cunningham, F. G., MacDonald, P.C., & Gant, N. F. (1989). *Williams obstetrics* (18th ed., pp. 653-694). Norwalk, CT: Appleton & Lange.

Gavette, L., & Roberts, J. (1987). Use of mean arterial pressure (MAP-2) to predict pregnancy-induced hypertension in adolescents. *Journal of Nurse-Midwifery, 32*(6), 357-364.

Kirshon, B., & Cotton, D. (1989). Heading off problems in pre-eclampsia management. *Contemporary Ob/Gyn, 33*(special issue June 15, 1989), 163-170.

Sibai, B. M. (1988). Preeclampsia-eclampsia maternal and perinatal outcomes. *Contemporary Ob/Gyn, 32*(6), 109-118.

Sibai, B. M., & Moretti, M. M. (1988). PIH: Still common and still dangerous. *Contemporary Ob/Gyn, 31*(2), 57-70.

Sibai, B. M., Taslimi, M. M., El-Nazar, A., Amon, E., Mabie, B. C., & Ryan, G. M. (1986). Maternal-perinatal outcome associated with the syndrome of hemolysis, elevated liver enzymes, and low platelets in severe pre-eclampsia-eclampsia. *American Journal of Obstetrics & Gynecology, 155*(3), 501-509.

Weinstein, L. (1986). The HELLP syndrome: A severe consequence of hypertension in pregnancy. *Journal of Perinatology, 6*(4), 316-320.

INTRAUTERINE GROWTH RETARDATION/SMALL FOR GESTATIONAL AGE

Brar, H. S., & Rutherford, S. E. (1988). Classification of intrauterine growth retardation. *Seminars in Perinatology, 12*(1), 2-10.

Chiswick, M. L. (1985). Intrauterine growth retardation. *British Medical Journal, 291,* 845-848.

Hobbins, J. C., Berkowitz, R. L., Manning, F. A., & Medearis, A. L. (1988). Assessing fetal growth. *Contemporary Ob/Gyn, 32*(6), 121-140.

Mintz, M. C., & Landon, M. B. (1988). Sonographic diagnosis of fetal growth disorders. *Clinical Obstetrics and Gynecology, 31*(1), 44-52.

Simpson, G. F., & Creasy, R. K. (1984). Obstetric management of the growth retarded baby. *Clinics in Obstetrics and Gynecology, 11*(2), 481-497.

KETONURIA

Corbett, J. (1987). *Laboratory test and diagnostic procedures with nursing diagnosis* (2nd ed.). Norwalk, CT: Appleton & Lange.

Varney, H. (1987). *Nurse-midwifery* (2nd ed.). Boston, MA: Blackwell Scientific.

MALPRESENTATION OF THE FETUS

Cunningham, F. G., MacDonald, P. C., & Gant, N. F. (1989). *Williams obstetrics* (18th ed., pp. 349-362). Norwalk, CT: Appleton & Lange.

Dyson, D. C., Ferguson, J. E., & Hensleigh, P. (1986). Antepartum external cephalic version under tocolysis. *Obstetrics and Gynecology, 67*(1), 63-68.

Morrison, J. C., Myatt, R. E., Martin, J. N., Meeks, G. R., Martin, R. W., Bucovaz, E. T., & Wiser, W. L. (1986). External cephalic version of the breech presentation under tocolysis. *American Journal of Obstetrics and Gynecology, 154*(4), 900-903.

Whitley, N. (1985). *A manual of clinical obstetrics.* Philadelphia: J. B. Lippincott.

MASTITIS

Briggs, G. G., Freeman, R. K., & Yaffee, S. J. (1986). *Drugs in pregnancy and lactation* (2nd ed.). Baltimore: Williams & Wilkins.

Cunningham, F. G., MacDonald, P. C., & Gant, N. F. (1989). *Williams obstetrics* (18th ed., pp. 477-488). Norwalk, CT: Appleton & Lange.

Kapernick, P. S. (1987). Postpartum hemorrhage and the abnormal puerperium. In M. L. Pernoll & R. C. Benson (Eds.), *Current obstetric and gynecologic diagnosis and treatment* (pp. 524-540). Norwalk, CT: Appleton & Lange.

Lawrence, R. A. (1985). *Breast-feeding: A guide for the medical professional* (2nd ed.). St. Louis: C. V. Mosby.

Love, S. M., Schnitt, S. J., Connolly, J. L., & Shirley, R. L. (1987). Benign breast disorders. In J. R. Harris, S. Hellman, I. C. Henderson, & D. W. Kinne (Eds.), *Breast disease*. Philadelphia: J. B. Lippincott.

Neifert, M. R., & Seacat, J. M. (1986). Medical management of successful breast-feeding. *Pediatric Clinics of North America, 30*(4), 743-762.

Ogle, K. S., & Davis, M. (1988). Mastitis in lactating women. *The Journal of Family Practice, 26*(2), 139-144.

Thomsen, A. C., Espersen, T., & Maigaard, S. (1984). Course and treatment of milk stases, noninfections inflammation of the breast, and infectious mastitis in nursing women. *American Journal of Obstetrics and Gynecology, 149*, 492-495.

MITRAL VALVE PROLAPSE

Abrams, R. S. (1989). *Handbook of medical problems during pregnancy* (pp. 113-135). Norwalk, CT: Appleton & Lange.

Arias, F. (1988). When the pregnant patient has mitral valve prolapse. *Contemporary Ob/Gyn, 32*(5), 84-90.

Gottlieb, S. H. (1987). Mitral valve prolapse: From syndrome to disease. *American Journal of Cardiology, 60*, 53J-58J.

Jeresaty, R. M. (1985). Mitral valve prolapse - an update. *JAMA, 254*(6), 793-795.

Rivlin, M. E. (1986). Cardiac disease in pregnancy. In M. E. Rivlin, J. C. Morrison, & G. W. Bates (Eds.), *Manual of clinical problems in obstetrics & gynecology* (2nd ed., pp. 55-58). Boston: Little, Brown & Company.

MULTIPLE GESTATION

Ahn, M. O., & Phelan, J. P. (1988). Multiple pregnancy: Antepartum management. *Clinics in Perinatology, 15*(1), 55-69.

Alvarez, M., & Berkowitz, R. (1990). Multifetal gestation. *Obstetrics and Gynecology, 33*(1), 79-87.

Cunningham, F. G., MacDonald, P. C., & Gant, N. F. (1989). *Williams obstetrics* (18th ed., pp. 629-652). Norwalk, CT: Appleton & Lange.

Halfar, M. M. (1987). Collaborative management of twins. *Journal of Nurse-Midwifery, 32*(3), 140-148.

Hunter, L. P. (1989). Twin gestation: Antepartum management. *The Journal of Perinatal and Neonatal Nursing, 3*(1), 1-13.

Hollenbach, K. A., & Hickok, D. E. (1990). Epidemiology and diagnosis of twin gestation. *Clinical Obstetrics and Gynecology, 33*(1), 3-9.

Jones, J. M., Sbarra, A. J., & Cetrulo, C. L. (1990). Antepartum management of twin gestation. *Clinical Obstetrics and Gynecology, 33*(1), 32-41.

Nageotte, M. P. (1990). Prevention and treatment of preterm labor in twin gestation. *Clinical Obstetrics and Gynecology, 33*(1), 61-68.

Neifert, M., & Thorpe, J. (1990). Twins: Family adjustment, parenting, and infant feeding in the fourth trimester. *Obstetrics and Gynecology, 33*(1), 102-115.

Neilson, J. P., & Mutambira, M. (1989). Coitus, twin pregnancy, and preterm labor. *American Journal of Obstetrics and Gynecology, 160*(2), 416-418.

Scerbo, J. C., Rattan, P., & Drukker, J. (1986). Twins and other multiple gestations. In R. A. Knuppel & J. E. Drukker (Eds.), *High-risk pregnancy: A team approach* (pp. 335-361). Philadelphia: W. B. Saunders.

Sollid, D. T., Evans, B. T., McClowry, S. G., & Garrett, A. (1989). Breastfeeding multiples. *The Journal of Perinatal and Neonatal Nursing, 3*, 46-63.

Yeast, J. D. (1990). Maternal physiologic adaptation to twin gestation. *Clinical Obstetrics and Gynecology, 33*(1), 10-17.

OLIGOHYDRAMNIOS

Beischer, N. A., & MacKay, E. V. (1986). *Obstetrics and the newborn* (2nd ed.). Philadelphia: W. B. Saunders.

Chamberlain, P. F., Manning, F. A., Morrison, I., Harman, C. R., & Lange, I. R. (1984). Ultrasound evaluation and amniotic fluid volumes. I. The relationship of marginal and decreased amniotic fluid volumes and perinatal outcome. *American Journal of Obstetrics and Gynecology, 150*(3), 245-249.

Rutherford, S. E., Phelan, J. P., Smith, C. V., & Jacobs, N. (1987). The four-quadrant assessment of amniotic fluid volume: An adjunct to antepartum fetal heart rate testing. *Obstetrics and Gynecology, 70*(3, Part 1), 353-356.

Steele, B. T., Paes, B., Towell, M. E., & Hunter, J. S. (1988). Fetal renal failure associated with intrauterine growth retardation. *American Journal of Obstetrics and Gynecology, 159*(5), 1200-1202.

PAP SMEAR--ABNORMAL

National Cancer Institute Workshop (1989). The 1988 Bethesda system of reporting cervical/vaginal cytological diagnoses. *JAMA, 262*(7), 931-934.

Nelson, J. H., Averette, H. E., & Richart, R. M. (1984). Dysplasia, carcinoma *in situ*, and early invasive cervical carcinoma. *CA-A Cancer Journal for Clinicians, 34*(6), 306-327.

POLYHYDRAMNIOS

Beischer, N. A., & MacKay, E. V. (1986). *Obstetrics and the newborn* (2nd ed., pp. 178-181). Philadelphia: W. B. Saunders.

Cardwell, M. (1987). Polyhydramnios: A review. *Obstetrical and Gynecologic Survey, 42*(10), 612-617.

Cunningham, F. G., MacDonald, P. C., & Gant, N. F. (1989). *Williams obstetrics* (18th ed.). Norwalk, CT: Appleton & Lange.

Kirshon, B. (1989). Fetal urine output in hydramnios. *Obstetrics and Gynecology, 73*(2), 240-242.

POSTDATE PREGNANCY

Eden, R. (1989). Standards of care for the postdate pregnancy. *Contemporary Ob/Gyn, 34*(2), 39-55.

Freeman, R. K. (1986). Problems of postdate pregnancy. *Contemporary Ob/Gyn, 28*(4), 73-81.

Hendricksen, A. (1985). Prolonged pregnancy: A literature review. *Journal of Nurse-Midwifery, 30*(1), 33-42.

Lagrew, D. C., & Freeman, R. K. (1986). Management of postdate pregnancy. *American Journal of Obstetrics and Gynecology, 154*(1), 8-13.

Nichols, C. W. (1985). Postdate pregnancy part II: Clinical implications. *Journal of Nurse-Midwifery, 31*(5), 259-268.

PREMATURE RUPTURE OF MEMBRANES

American College of Obstetricians and Gynecologists (ACOG) (1988). *Premature rupture of membranes* (Technical Bulletin No. 115). Washington, D.C.: Author.

Garite, T. J. (1982). What's the best care in preterm labor? *Contemporary Ob/Gyn, 19*(2), 178-187.

Garite, T. J., (1985). Premature rupture of membranes: The enigma of the obstetrician. *American Journal of Obstetrics and Gynecology, 151*(8), 1001-1005.

Gibbs, R. S., & Sweet, R. L. (1989). Clinical disorders. In R. K. Creasy & R. Resnik (Eds.), *Maternal-fetal medicine* (2nd ed., pp. 656-662). Philadelphia: W. B. Saunders.

Golde, S. (1983). Use of obstetrical perineal pads in collection of amnionic fluid in patients with rupture of membranes. *American Journal of Obstetrics and Gynecology, 146*(6), 710-712.

Pauerstein, C. J. (1987). *Clinical obstetrics* (pp. 367-381). New York: John Wiley and Sons.

Yonekura, M. L. (1989, June). *Premature rupture of the fetal membranes: Strategies for management*. Paper presented at the Kaiser Permanente Medical Care Program, National Ob/Gyn Conference, Kauai, Hawaii.

PRETERM BIRTH PREVENTION

Arias, F. (1984). Preterm labor. In F. Arias (Ed.), *High risk pregnancy and delivery* (pp. 37-62). St. Louis, MO: C. V. Mosby.

Creasy, R. K. (1989). Preterm labor and delivery. In R. K. Creasy & R. Resnik (Eds.), *Maternal-fetal medicine* (2nd ed., pp. 477-504). Philadelphia: W.B. Saunders.

Hamilton, M. P. R., Abdalla, H. I., & Whitfield, C. R. (1985). Significance of raised maternal serum alpha-fetoprotein in singleton pregnancies with normally formed fetuses. *Obstetrics and Gynecology, 65*(4), 465-470.

Iams, J. D., & Creasy, R. K. (1988). Prevention of preterm birth. *Clinical Obstetrics and Gynecology, 31*(3), 599-615.

Iams, J. D., Johnson, F. F., & O'Shaughnessy, R. W. (1988). A prospective random trial of home uterine activity monitoring in pregnancies at increased risk of preterm labor. *American Journal of Obstetrics and Gynecology, 159*(3), 595-603.

Katz, M., Gill, P. J., & Newman, R. B. (1986). Detection of preterm labor by ambulatory monitoring of uterine activity: A preliminary report. *Obstetrics and Gynecology, 68*(6), 773-778.

Katz, M., & Scheerer, L. J. (1988). Ambulatory monitoring of uterine contractions. *Clinical Obstetrics and Gynecology, 31*(3), 616-634.

Laros, R. (1988). *Preterm labor screen.* San Francisco: University of California.

Lipshitz, J., & Brown, R. L. (1986). Preterm labor. In R. A. Knuppel & J. E. Drukker (Eds.), *High risk pregnancy: A team approach* (pp. 303-324). Philadelphia: W. B. Saunders.

Lubbe, W. F., & Wiggins, G. C. (1985). Lupus anticoagulant and pregnancy. *American Journal of Obstetrics and Gynecology, 153*(3), 322-327.

Main, D. M. (1988). The epidemiology of preterm birth. *Clinical Obstetrics and Gynecology, 31*(3), 521-532.

McGregor, J. A. (1987). Preventing preterm birth caused by infection. *Contemporary Ob/Gyn, 29*(4), 33-42.

Parisi, V. M. (1988). Cervical incompetence and preterm labor. *Clinical Obstetrics and Gynecology, 31*(3), 585-598.

Pernoll, M. L. (1987). Untimely termination of pregnancy. In M. L. Pernoll & R. C. Benson (Eds.), *Current obstetric & gynecologic treatment 1987* (pp. 303-310). Norwalk, CT: Appleton & Lange.

Romero, R., & Mazor, M. (1988). Infection and preterm labor. *Clinical Obstetrics and Gynecology, 312*(3), 553-584.

PROTEINURIA

Beischer, N. A., & Mackay, E. V. (1986). *Obstetrics and the newborn.* Philadelphia: W. B. Saunders.

Corbett, J. (1987). *Laboratory tests and diagnostic procedures with nursing diagnosis* (2nd ed.). Norwalk: CT: Appleton & Lange.

PYELONEPHRITIS

Gibbs, R. S., & Sweet, R. L. (1989). Clinical disorders. In R. K. Creasy & R. Resnik (Eds.), *Maternal-fetal medicine: Principles and practice* (2nd ed., pp. 662-667). Philadelphia: W. B. Saunders.

McNeeley, S. G. (1988). Treatment of urinary tract infections during pregnancy. *Clinical Obstetrics and Gynecology, 31*(2), 480-487.

Pauerstein, C. J. (1987). *Clinical obstetrics* (pp. 679-680, 756-757). New York: John Wiley and Sons.

VanDorsten, J. P. (1986). Pyelonephritis in pregnancy: A guide to prevention, diagnosis, and treatment. *The Female Patient, 11*, 100-107.

RADIATION EXPOSURE

Brent, R. (1987). Ionizing radiation. *Contemporary Ob/Gyn, 30*(2), 20-29.

Brent, R. (1980a). Radiation teratogenesis. *Teratology, 21*, 281-298.

Brent, R. (1980b). X-ray, microwave, and ultrasound: The real and unreal hazards. *Pediatric Annals, 9*(12), 43-47.

Drugan, A., & Evans, M. (1988). Exposure of the pregnant patient to ionizing radiation. *Contemporary Ob/Gyn, 32*(4), 16-21.

Jankowski, C. (1986). Radiation and pregnancy: Putting the risks in proportion. *American Journal of Nursing*, pp. 260-265.

Maulik, D. (1989). Biologic effects of ultrasound. *Clinical Obstetrics and Gynecology, 32*(4), 645-659.

Medical News (1976). *Journal of the American Medical Association, 236*(20), 2269-2279.

National Council on Radiation Protection and Measurements (1977a). *Medical radiation exposure of pregnant and potential pregnant women* (NCRP Report No. 54). Washington, DC: U.S. Government Printing Office.

National Council on Radiation Protection and Measurement (1977b). *Review on NCRP radiation dose limit for embryo and fetus in occupationally exposed women* (NCRP Report No. 53). Washington, DC: U.S. Government Printing Office.

SIZE/DATES DISCREPANCY

Nichols, C. W. (1985). Clinical management for size/dates discrepancy. *Journal of Nurse-Midwifery, 30*(1), 15-24.

Varney, H. (1987). *Nurse-midwifery* (2nd ed., pp. 192-195). Boston: Blackwell Scientific.

SUBINVOLUTION

Andrew, A. C., Bulmer, J. N., Wells, M., Morrison, L., & Buckley, C. H. (1989). Subinvolution of the uteroplacental arteries in the human placental bed. *Histopathology, 15*, 395-405.

Cunningham, F. G., MacDonald, P. C., & Gant, N. F. (1989). *Williams obstetrics* (18th ed., p. 481). Norwalk, CT: Appleton & Lange.

Novy, M. J. (1987). The normal puerperium. In M. L. Pernoll & R. C. Benson (Eds.), *Current obstetric and gynecologic diagnosis and treatment 1987* (pp. 216-245). Norwalk, CT: Appleton & Lange.

Thomas, C. L. (Ed.) (1989). *Taber's cyclopedic medical dictionary* (16th ed.). Philadelphia: F. A. Davis.

Willson, J. R. (1987). The puerperium. In J. R. Willson & E. R. Carrington (Eds.), *Obstetrics and gynecology* (7th ed., pp. 187-204). St. Louis: C. V. Mosby.

SUBSTANCE ABUSE

American College of Obstetricians and Gynecologists (ACOG) (1986). *Drug abuse and pregnancy* (Technical Bulletin No. 96). Washington, DC: Author.

Bushong, M. (1989, Spring). Perinatal substance abuse. *Mid-coastal California perinatal outreach program newsletter*, pp. 1-7.

Chasnoff, I. J. (1986a). Alcohol use in pregnancy. In I. J. Chasnoff (Ed.), *Drug use in pregnancy: Mother and child* (pp. 75-80). Norwell, MA: MTP Press.

Chasnoff, I. J. (1986b). Consequences of intrauterine exposure to opiate and nonopiate drugs. In I. J. Chasnoff (Ed.), *Drug use in pregnancy: Mother and child* (pp. 52-63). Norwell, MA: MTP Press.

Chasnoff, I. J. (1987). Perinatal effects of cocaine. *Contemporary Ob/Gyn, 29*(5), 163-179.

Chisum, G. M. (1986). Recognition and initial management of the pregnant substance-abusing woman. In I. J. Chasnoff (Ed.), *Drug use in pregnancy: Mother and child* (pp. 17-22). Norwell, MA: MTP Press.

Dombrowski, M. P., & Sokol, R. J. (1990). Cocaine and abruption. *Contemporary Ob/Gyn, 35*(4), 13-19.

Fried, P. A. (1986). Marijuana and human pregnancy. In I. J. Chasnoff (Ed.), *Drug use in pregnancy: Mother and child* (pp. 64-74). Norwell, MA: MTP Press.

Jessup, M., & Green, J. (1987). Treatment of the pregnant alcohol-dependent woman. *Journal of Psychoactive Drugs, 19*(2), 193-203.

Jessup, M., & Roth, R. (1988). Clinical and legal perspectives on prenatal drug and alcohol use: Guidelines for individual and community response. *Medicine and Law, 7*, 377-389.

Keith, L, Donald, W. Rosner, M., Mitchell, M., & Bianchi, J. (1986). Obstetric aspects of perinatal addiction. In I. J. Chasnoff (Ed.), *Drug use in pregnancy: Mother and child* (pp. 23-41). Norwell, MA: MTP Press.

Novy, M. J. (1987). The normal puerperium. In M. L. Pernoll & R. C. Benson (Eds.), *Current obstetric and gynecologic diagnosis and treatment 1987* (pp. 216-245). Norwalk, CT: Appleton & Lange.

Obstetric Advisory Committee of the Perinatal Advisory Council of Los Angeles Communities (1988). Perinatal protocol: Maternal substance use and neonatal drug withdrawal. *Journal of Perinatology, 8*(4), 387-392.

Puentes, A. J. (1990). *Maternal/fetal/neonatal effects of substances commonly abused by pregnant women.* Santa Clara County Substance Abuse Services, San Jose, California.

Ronkin, S., FitzSimmons, J., Wapner, R., & Finnegan, L. (1988). Protecting mother and fetus from narcotic abuse. *Contemporary Ob/Gyn, 31*(3), 178-187.

Tennant, F. (1988). The rapid eye test to detect drug abuse. *Postgraduate Medicine, 84*(1), 108-114.

University of California, San Francisco Medical Center, Perinatal Substance Abuse Protocol Committee (UCSFMC) (1989). *Protocol for perinatal patients with chemical dependency.* San Francisco: Author.

THYROID DISEASE

Abrams, R. S. (1989). *Handbook of medical problems during pregnancy* (pp. 23-25). Norwalk, CT: Appleton & Lange.

Affonso, D. D., Andreyko, J., & Mills, K. (1987). Postpartum thyroiditis: A new challenge in nurse-midwifery. *Journal of Nurse-Midwifery, 32*(5), 308-316.

Cunningham, F. G., MacDonald, P. C., & Gant, N. F. (1989). *Williams obstetrics* (18th ed., pp. 153-154, 822-825). Norwalk, CT: Appleton & Lange.

Mestman, J. H. (1985). Thyroid disease in pregnancy. *Clinics in Perinatology, 12*(3), 651-667.

Palmer, S. M. (1986). Thyroid disease in pregnancy. In M. E. Rivlin, J. C. Morrison, & G. W. Bates (Eds.), *Manual of clinical problems in obstetrics and gynecology* (2nd ed., pp. 64-68). Boston: Little, Brown and Company.

TRIAL OF LABOR/VAGINAL BIRTH AFTER CESAREAN SECTION

American College of Obstetricians and Gynecologists (ACOG) (1988). *Guidelines for vaginal delivery after a previous cesarean birth* (Committee Opinion No. 64). Washington, DC: Author.

Clark, S. L. (1988). Rupture of the scarred uterus. *Obstetrics and Gynecology Clinics of North America, 15*(4), 737-744.

Hangsleben, K. L., Taylor, M. A., & Lynn, N. M. (1989). VBAC program in a nurse-midwifery program. *Journal of Nurse-Midwifery, 34*(4), 179-184.

Haq, C. L. (1988). Vaginal birth after cesarean delivery. *American Family Physician, 37*(6), 167-171.

Martin, J. N., Morrison, J. C., & Wiser, W. L. (1988). Vaginal birth after cesarean section: The demise of routine repeat abdominal delivery. *Obstetrics and Gynecology Clinics of North America, 15*(4), 719-735.

CHAPTER 5

ABO INCOMPATIBILITY/IRREGULAR ANTIBODIES

American College of Obstetricians and Gynecologists (ACOG) (1986). *Management of isoimmunization in pregnancy* (Technical Bulletin Number 90). Washington, DC: Author.

Barss, V. A., Frigoletto, F. D., & Konugres, A. (1988). The cost of irregular antibody screening. *American Journal of Obstetrics and Gynecology, 159*, 428.

Cook, L. N. (1982). ABO hemolytic disease. *Clinical Obstetrics and Gynecology, 25*(2), 333-339.

Durfee, R. B. (1987). Obstetric complications of pregnancy. In M. L. Pernoll & R. C. Benson (Eds.), *Current obstetrics and gynecology diagnosis and treatment 1987* (6th ed., pp. 255-278). Norwalk, CT: Appleton & Lange.

Weinstein, L. (1982). Irregular antibodies causing hemolytic disease of the newborn: A continuing problem. *Clinical Obstetrics and Gynecology, 25*(2), 321-329.

ALPHA THALASSEMIA

Irwin Memorial Blood Center (1990). *The relative risks of blood transfusion: Autologous vs community vs directed donors*. San Francisco: Author.

Laros, R. K., & Golbus, M. S. (1977). Prenatal diagnosis of thalassemia trait. *University of Michigan Medical Center Journal, 43*(23).

Paterson, K. A. (1986). In J. D. Neeson & K. A. May (Eds.), *Comprehensive maternity nursing* (p. 502). Philadelphia: J. B. Lippincott Co.

Wintrobe, M. (1981). *Clinical hematology* (8th ed.). Philadelphia: Lea & Febiger.

ANEMIA

Anderson, H. M. (1989). Maternal hematologic disorders. In R.K. Creasy & R. Resnik (Eds.), *Maternal-fetal medicine: Principles and practice* (2nd ed., pp. 892-896). Philadelphi: W. B. Saunders.

Biswas, M., & Perloff, D. (1987). Cardiac, hematologic, pulmonary, and renal and urinary tract disorders in pregnancy. In M. L. Pernoll & R. C. Benson (Eds.), *Current obstetric and gynecologic diagnosis and treatment 1987* (6th ed., p. 369). Norwalk, CT: Appleton & Lange.

Dimperio, D. (1988). *Prenatal nutrition: Clinical guidelines for nurses*. White Plains: March of Dimes Birth Defects Foundation.

Harvey, A. (1980). *The principles and practice of medicine* (20th ed., pp, 476-522). New York: Appleton-Century-Crofts.

Laros, R. K., & Golbus, M. S. (1977). Prenatal diagnosis of thalassemia trait. *University of Michigan Medical Center Journal, 43*(23).

Lubkin, I. (1982). Evaluating iron deficiency anemia. *The Nurse Practitioner, 7*(9), 34-38.

National Academy of Sciences, National Research Council (1989, October). *Recommended dietary allowances* (10th ed.). Washington, DC: National Academy Press.

Patterson, K. A. (1986). In J. D. Neeson & K. A. May (Eds.), *Comprehensive maternity nursing* (p. 502). Philadelphia: J. B. Lippincott.

Reich, P. R. (1984). *Hematology* (2nd ed.). Boston: Little, Brown & Co.

BETA THALASSEMIA

Bunn, H. F., Forget, B. G., & Ranney, H. M. (1977). *Human hemoglobinopathies*. Philadelphia: W.B. Saunders.

GLUCOSE-6-PHOSPHATE DEHYDROGENASE DEFICIENCY

Cunningham, F. G., MacDonald, P. C., & Gant, N. F. (1989). *Williams obstetrics* (18th ed., pp. 785, 791). Norwalk, CT: Appleton & Lange.

Fischbach, F. (1988). *A manual of laboratory diagnostic tests* (3rd, ed., pp. 54-56). Philadelphia: J. B. Lippincott.

Rh ISOIMMUNIZATION

American College of Obstetricians and Gynecologists (ACOG) (1984). *Prevention of RHO(D) isoimmunization* (Technical Bulletin No. 79). Washington, DC: Author.

American College of Obstetricians and Gynecologists (ACOG) (1986). *Management of isoimmunization in pregnancy* (Technical Bulletin No. 90). Washington, DC: Author.

Fleischer, A. A. (1989). Rh disease. *Journal of Perinatology, 9*(2), 224-228.

Hammer, R. M., Bower, E. J., & Messina, L. J. (1984). The prenatal use of Rho(D) immune globulin. *Maternal Child Nursing, 9*, 29-31.

Lloyd, T. (1987). Rh-factor incompatibility: A primer for prevention. *Journal of Nurse-Midwifery, 32*(5), 299-307.

Rote, N. S. (1982). Pathophysiology of Rh isoimmunization. *Clinical Obstetrics and Gynecology, 25*(2), 243-253.

Sutton, G. P., Jay, A., Lim, Y. S., Noland, J. E., & Boral L. J. (1988). The use of Rh immune globulin: A review. *Indiana Medicine, 81*(4), 321-322.

CHAPTER 6

Abrams, R. S. (1989). *Handbook of medical problems during pregnancy* (pp. 91-111). Norwalk, CT: Appleton & Lange.

Braverman, I. M. (1988). The skin in pregnancy. In G. N. Burrow & T. F. Ferris (Ed.), *Medical complications during pregnancy* (3rd ed., pp. 526-539). Philadelphia: W. B. Saunders Company.

Lamberg, S. I. (1986). *Dermatology in primary care* (pp. 334-340). Philadelphia: W. B. Saunders Company.

Sodhi, V. K., & Sausker, W. F. (1988). Dermatoses of pregnancy. *American Family Physician, 37*(1), 131-138.

CHAPTER 7

CHLAMYDIA

American College of Obstetricians and Gynecologists (ACOG) (1985). *Gonorrhea and chlamydial infections* (Technical Bulletin No. 89). Washington, D.C.: Author.

Centers for Disease Control (CDC) (1989). Sexually transmitted diseases treatment guidelines. *Morbidity and Mortality Weekly Report, 38*(S-8), 27-29.

Centers for Disease Control (CDC) (1985). 1985 STD treatment guidelines. *Morbidity a n d Mortality Weekly Report, 34*(4S), 77S-79S.

Gibbs, R. S., & Sweet, R. L. (1989). Clinical disorders. In R. K. Creasy & R. Resnik (Eds.), *Maternal-fetal medicine* (2nd ed., pp. 708-713). Philadelphia: W.B. Saunders.

Rettig, P. J. (1988). Perinatal infections with chlamydia trachomatis. *Clinics in Perinatology, 15*(2), 321-351.

CONDYLOMATA ACUMINATA

Buscema, J., Naghashfar, Z., Sawada, E., Daniel, R., Woodruff, D., & Shah K. (1988). The predominance of human papillomavirus type 16 in vulvar neoplasia. *Obstetrics & Gynecology, 71*(4), 601-605.

Buck, H. W., & The Task Force on Human Papillomavirus (1989). *Genital human papillomavirus disease: Diagnosis, management and prevention*. Rockville, MD: American College Health Association.

Enterline, J. A., & Leonardo, J. P. (1989). Condylomata acuminata (venereal warts). *The Nurse Practitioner, 14*(4), 8-26.

Ferenczy, A. (1989). HPV-associated lesions in pregnancy and their clinical implication. *Clinical Obstetrics and Gynecology, 32*(1), 191-199.

Gissmann, L. (1989). Linking HPV to cancer. *Clinical Obstetrics and Gynecology, 32*(1), 141-147.

Horn, J. (1989). Genital human papillomavirus infection: New challenges from an old culprit. *STD Bulletin, 9*(3), 3-10.

Krebs, H. (1989). Genital HPV Infection in Men. *Obstetrics and Gynecology, 73*(3), 180-190.

Reid, R., & Campion, M. J. (1989). HPV-associated lesions of the cervix: Biology and colposcopic features. *Clinical Obstetrics and Gynecology, 32*(1), 157-179.

Richart, R., Becker, T. M., Ferenczy, A. M., Reid, R., & Townsend, D. E. (1989). HPV DNA: Quicker ways to discern viral types. *Contemporary Ob/Gyn, 33*(4), 112-133.

Richart, R. M., Barrasso, R., & Ferenczy, A. (1988). Examining male partners of women who have abnormal smears. *Contemporary Ob/Gyn, 31*(4), 157-172.

Schneider, S., (1988). HPV infection in women and their male partners. *Contemporary Ob/Gyn*, *32*,(5), 131-144.

Stone, K., (1989). Epidemiologic aspects of genital HPV infection. *Clinical Obstetrics and Gynecology*, *32*(1), 112-116.

Swartz, D., Greenberg, M., Daoud, Y., & Reid, R. (1988). Genital condylomas in pregnancy: Use of trichloroacetic acid and laser therapy. *American Journal of Obstetrics and Gynecology*, *158*(6), 1407-1416.

CYTOMEGALOVIRUS

Amstey, M. S. (1988). Treatment and prevention of viral infections (HSV, CMV, HPV, HBV). *Clinical Obstetrics and Gynecology*, *31*(2), 501-509.

Gibbs, R. S., & Sweet, R. L. (1989). Clinical disorders. In R. K. Creasy & R. Resnik (Eds.), *Maternal-fetal medicine* (2nd ed., pp. 683-686). Philadelphia: W.B. Saunders.

GENITAL HERPES SIMPLEX VIRAL INFECTIONS

Arvin, A. M., Hensleigh, P. A., Prober, C. G., Au, D. S., Yasukawa, L. L., Wittek, A. E., Palumbo, P. E., Paryani, S. G., & Yeager, A. S. (1986). Failure of antepartum maternal cultures to predict the infant's risk of exposure to herpes simplex virus at delivery. *The New England Journal of Medicine*, *315*(13), 796-800.

Bleich, L. (1987). Nongenital herpes simplex virus: Obstetrical significance. *Journal of Nurse-Midwifery*, *32*(6), 339-348.

Brown, Z. A., Berry, S., & Vontner, L. A. (1986). Genital herpes virus infections complicating pregnancy: Natural history and peripartum management. *The Journal of Reproductive Medicine*, *31*(5), 420-425.

Connell, E. B., & Tatum, H. J. (1985). *Sexually transmitted diseases and treatment* (pp. 41-46). Durant, OK: Creative Infomatics.

Cunningham, F. G., MacDonald, P. C., & Gant, N. F. (1989). *Williams obstetrics* (18th ed.). Norwalk, CT: Appleton & Lange.

Freij, B. J., & Sever, J. L. (1988). Herpesvirus infections in pregnancy: Risks to embryo, fetus, and neonate. *Clinics in perinatology*, *15*(2), 203-231.

Maslow, A. S., & Bobitt, J. R. (1988). Herpes in pregnancy: Exploring clinical options. *Contemporary Ob/Gyn*, *32*(4), 44-61.

Stagno, S., & Whitley, R. J. (1985). Herpes virus infections of pregnancy. *The New England Journal of Medicine*, *313*(21), 1327-1330.

Straus, S. E., Rooney, J. F., Sever, J. L., Seidlin, M., Nusinoff-Lehrman, S., & Cremer, K. (1985). Herpes simplex virus infection: Biology, treatment and prevention. *Annals of Internal Medicine*, *103*(3), 404-408.

GONORRHEA

American College of Obstetricians and Gynecologists (ACOG) (1985). *Gonorrhea and chlamydial infections* (Technical Bulletin No. 89). Washington, D.C.: Author.

Centers for Disease Control (CDC) (1989). Sexually transmitted disease guidelines. *Morbidity and Mortality Weekly Report, 38*(S-8), 21-27.

Centers for Disease Control (CDC) (1987). Antibiotic-resistant strains of Neisseria gonorrhoeae. *Morbidity and Mortality Weekly Report, 36*(5S), 1S-18S.

City and County of San Francisco (1989). *Medical alert - PPNG in San Francisco.* San Francisco: Department of Public Health.

Fogel, C. I. F. (1988). Gonorrhea: Not a new problem but a serious one. *Nursing Clinics of North America, 23*(4) 885-897.

Gibbs, R. S. & Sweet, R. (1989). Clinical disorders. In R. K. Creasy & R. Resnik (Eds.), *Maternal-fetal medicine: Priniciples and practice* (2nd ed., pp.704-707). Philadelphia: W. B. Saunders.

Spence, M. R. (1988). The treatment of gonorrhea, syphilis, chancroid, lymphogranuloma venereum, and granuloma inguinale. *Clinical Obstetrics and Gynecology, 31*(2), 453-465.

Wilson, D. (1988). An overview of sexually transmissable diseases in the perinatal period. *Journal of Nurse-Midwifery, 33*(3), 115-128.

GROUP B STREPTOCOCCUS

Boyer, K. M., & Gotoff, S. P. (1988). Antimicrobial prophylaxis of neonatal group B streptoccal sepsis. *Clinics in Perinatology, 15*(4), 831-851.

Brady, K., Duff, P., Schilhab, J. C., & Herd, M. (1989). Reliability of a rapid fixation test for detecting group B streptococci in the genital tract of parturients at term. *Obstetrics and Gynecology, 73*(4), 678-681.

Dinsmoor, M. J. (1990). Group B streptococcus still poses a challenge. *Contemporary Ob/Gyn, 35*(5), 93-104.

Eschenbach, D. A. (1985). Contending with the problem of chlamydial infection. *Contemporary Ob/Gyn, 25*(2), 125-136.

Gibbs, R. S. & Sweet, R. L. (1989). Clinical disorders. In R. C. Creasy & R. Resnik (Eds.), *Maternal-fetal medicine: Principles and practice* (2nd ed., pp. 678-681). Philadelphia: W.B. Saunders.

Gotoff, S. P. (1988). Prophylaxis for early-onset group B strep. *Contemporary Ob/Gyn, 32*(5), 25-40.

Watts, D. H., & Eschenbach, D. A. (1988). Treatment of chlamydia, mycoplasma, and group B streptococcal infections. *Clinical Obstetrics and Gynecology, 31*(2), 435-568.

HEPATITIS B

Boehme, T. L. (1985). Hepatitis B: The nurse midwife's role in management and prevention. *Journal of Nurse Midwifery, 30*(2), 79-87.

Centers for Disease Control (CDC) (1988). Prevention of perinatal transmission of hepatitis B virus: Prenatal screening of all pregnant women for hepatitis B surface antigen. *Morbidity and Mortality Weekly Report, 37*(2), 341-346.

Clark, D., & Kao, H. (1983). Meaningful markers for hepatitis Dx. and Px. *Contemporary Ob/Gyn* (Special Issue), *21*, 31-50.

Edwards, M. S. (1988). Hepatitis B serology-helps in interpretation. *Pediatric Clinics of North America, 35*(3), 503-511.

Klein, M. E. (1988). Hepatitis B virus: Perinatal management. *Journal of Perinatal Neonatal Nursing, 1*(4), 12-23.

Pastorek II, J. G. (1989). Hepatitis B screening during pregnancy. *Contemporary Ob/Gyn, 34*(5), 36-48.

Schreeder, M. (1988). Viral hepatitis. *Primary Care, 15*(1), 157-171.

Sweet, R. L., & Gibbs, R. S. (1985). *Infectious diseases of the female genital tract* (p. 195). Baltimore: Williams & Wilkins.

HUMAN IMMUNODEFICIENCY VIRUS INFECTION SCREENING

American Academy of Pediatrics (1988). *Report of the committee on infectious diseases* (21st ed., pp. 91-115). Elk Grove Village, IL: Author.

Buckingham, S. L., & Rehm, S. J. (1987). AIDS and women at risk. *Health and Social Work, 12*(1), 5-11.

Castro, K. G., Hardy, A. M., & Curran, J. W. (1986). The acquired immunodeficiency syndrome: Epidemiology and risk factors for transmission. *Medical Clinics of North America, 70*(3), 635-649.

Centers for Disease Control (CDC) (1990, April). *HIV/AIDS surveillance report*, pp. 1-18.

Feinkind, L., & Minkoff, H. L. (1988). HIV in pregnancy. *Clinics in Perinatology, 15*(2), 189-202.

Johnson, M. A., & Webster, A. (1989). Human immunodeficiency virus infection in women. *British Journal of Obstetrics & Gynecology, 96*, 129-132.

Koonin, L. M., Ellerbrock, T. V., Atrash, H. K., et al. [AUTHORS] (1989). Pregnancy-associated deaths due to AIDS in the United States. *JAMA, 261*(9), 1306-1309.

Landesman, S. H. (1989). Human immunodeficiency virus infection in women: An overview. *Seminars in Perinatology, 13*(1), 2-6.

Lapointe, N., Michaud, J., Pekovic, D., Chausseau, J. P., & Dupuy, J. M. (1985). Transplacental transmission of HTLV-III virus. *The New England Journal of Medicine, 312*, 1325-1326.

Minkoff, H. L. (1987). Care of pregnant women infected with human immunodeficiency virus. *JAMA*, *258*(19), 2714-2717.

Nolan, K. (1989). Ethical issues in caring for pregnant women and newborns at risk for human immunodeficiency virus infection. *Seminars in Perinatology*, *13*(1), 55-65.

Scott, G. B. (1989). Perinatal HIV-1 infection: Diagnosis and management. *Clinical Obstetrics and Gynecology*, *32*(2), 477-484.

Selwyn, P. A., Schoenbaum, E. E., Davenny, K., Robertson, V. J., Feingold, A. R., Shulman, J. F., Mayers, M. M., Klein, R. S., Friedland, G. H., & Rogers, M. F. (1989). Prospective study of human immunodeficiency virus infection and pregnancy outcomes in intravenous drug users. *JAMA*, *261*(9), 1289-1294.

Vogt, M. W., Craven, D. E., Crawford, D. F., Witt, D. J., Byrington, R., Schooley, R. T., & Hirsch, M. S. (1986). Isolation of HTLV-III/LAV from cervical secretions of women at risk for AIDS. *The Lancet*, *1*(8480), 525-527.

Ziegler, J. B., Cooper, D. A., Johnson, R. O., & Gold, J. (1985). Postnatal transmission of AIDS associated retrovirus from mother to infant. *Lancet*, *1*, 896-897.

LISTERIA

Barresi, J. A. (1980). Listeria monocytogenes: A cause of premature labor and neonatal sepsis. *American Journal of Obstetrics and Gynecology*, *136*(3), 410-411.

Bobbit, J. R. (1984). Specific bacterial infections: Group B streptococcus and listeria. In R.K. Creasy & R. Resnik (Eds.), *Maternal-fetal medicine*. Philadelphia: W.B. Saunders.

Boucher, M., & Yonekura, M. (1986). Perinatal listeriosis (Early-onset): Correlation of antenatal manifestations and neonatal outcome. *Obstetrics and Gynecology*, *68*(5), 593-597.

Chapman, S. T. (1986). Bacterial infections in pregnancy. *Clinics in Obstetrics and Gynecology*, *13*(2), 397-416.

Valkenburg, M. H., Essed, G., & Potters, H. (1988). Perinatal listeriosis underdiagnosed as a cause of pre-term labour? *European Journal of Obstetrics, Gynecology, & Reproductive Biology*, 27, 283-288.

MEASLES

Gibbs. R. S., & Sweet, R. L. (1989). Clinical disorders. In R. K. Creasy & R. Resnik (Eds.), *Maternal-fetal medicine* (2nd. ed., pp. 682-683). Philadelphia: W. B. Saunders.

MUMPS

Gibbs. R. S., & Sweet, R. L. (1989). Clinical disorders. In R. K. Creasy & R. Resnik (Eds.), *Maternal-fetal medicine* (2nd. ed., pp. 682-683). Philadelphia: W. B. Saunders.

PARVOVIRUS

Bernstein, I. M., & Capeless, E. M. (1989). Elevated maternal serum alpha feto-protein and hydrops fetalis in association with fetal parvovirus B19 infection. *Obstetrics & Gynecology*, *74*(3, II), 456-457.

Kinney, J. S., & Kumar, M. L. (1988). Should we expand the TORCH concept? *Clinics in Perinatology, 15*(4), 727-745.

Maeda, H., Shimokawa, H., Satoh, S., Nakano, H., & Nunove, T. (1988). Nonimmune hydrops fetalis resulting from intrauterine parvovirus B19 infection: Report of two cases. *Obstetrics & Gynecology, 73*(3,II), 482-485.

Mead, M. (1989). Parvovirus B19 infection and pregnancy. *Contemporary Ob/Gyn, 34*(3), 56-69.

RUBELLA

American College of Obstetricians and Gynecologists (ACOG) (1981). *Rubella: A clinical update* (Technical Bulletin No. 62). Washington, DC: Author.

Centers for Disease Control (CDC) (1989). Rubella vaccination during pregnancy - United States, 1971-1988. *Morbidity and Mortality Weekly Report, 38*(17), 289-293.

Freij, B. J., South, M., & Sever, J. L. (1988). Maternal rubella and the congenital rubella syndrome. *Clinics in Perinatology, 15*(2), 247-257.

Gibbs. R. S., & Sweet, R. L. (1989). Clinical disorders. In R. K. Creasy & R. Resnik (Eds.), *Maternal-fetal medicine* (2nd. ed., pp. 682-683). Philadelphia: W. B. Saunders.

Zeichner, S. L., & Plotkin, S. A. (1988). Mechanisms and pathways of congenital infections. *Clinics in Perinatology, 15*(2),163-189.

SYPHILIS

Centers for Disease Control (CDC) (1987). Increases in primary and secondary syphilis--United States. *Morbidity and Mortality Weekly Report, 36*(25), 393-397.

Centers for Disease Control (CDC) (1989). 1989 sexually transmitted diseases treatment guidelines. *Morbidity and Mortality Weekly Report, 38*(S-8) 5-15.

Chapel, T. A. (1984). Primary and secondary syphilis. *Cutis, 33*, 20-25.

Gibbs, R. S., & Sweet, R. L. (1989). Clinical disorders. In R. K. Creasy & R. Resnik (Eds.), *Maternal-fetal medicine: Principles and practice* (2nd ed., pp. 701-704). Philadelphia: W. B. Saunders.

Main, D. M., & Main, E. K. (1982). Infection during pregnancy. In F. Arias (Ed.), *High risk pregnancy and delivery*. St. Louis: C. V. Mosby.

McPhee, S. J. (1984). Secondary syphilis: Uncommon manifestations a common disease. *The Western Journal of Medicine, 140*(1), 10-20.

Noble, R. C. (1982). *Sexually transmitted diseases* (2nd ed.). Garden City, NJ: Excerpta Medica.

Stewart, T. (1983). Interpreting serologic tests for syphilis. *American Family Physicians, 26*(2), 157-162.

Wendel, G. D. (1988). Gestational and congenital syphilis. *Clinics in Perinatology, 15*(2), 287-303.

TOXOPLASMOSIS

Gibbs, R. S., & Sweet, R. L. (1989). Clinical disorders. In R. K. Creasy & R. Resnik (Eds.), *Maternal-fetal medicine* (2nd ed., pp. 717-719). Philadelphia: W. B. Saunders.

Krick, J. A., & Remington, J. S. (1978). Toxoplasmosis in the adult - an overview. *New England Journal of Medicine, 298*(50).

Sever, J. L. (1990). Toxoplasmosis. *Contemporary Ob/Gyn, 35*(3), 13-17.

U.S. Department of Health and Human Services, Public Health Service, National Institutes of Health (NIH) (1983). *Toxoplasmosis* (Publication No. 83-308). Bethesda, MD: Author.

TUBERCULOSIS--PRIMARY IDENTIFICATION OF CARRIERS

Bush, J. J. (1986). Protocol for tuberculosis screening in pregnancy. *Journal of Obstetric, Gynecologic, and Neonatal Nursing, 15*(3), 225-230.

Summers, L. (1987). Tuberculosis--a persistent health care problem. *Journal of Nurse-Midwifery, 32*(2), 68-78.

VAGINITIS

Bump, R. C., & Buesching, W. J. (1988). Bacterial vaginosis in virginal and sexually active adolescent females: Evidence against exclusive sexual transmission. *American Journal of Obstetrics and Gynecology, 158*(4), 935-939.

Centers for Disease Control (CDC) (1989). Sexually transmitted diseases treatment guidelines. *Morbidity and Mortality Weekly Report.* Atlanta, GA: U.S. Department of Health and Human Services.

Landers, D. V. (1988). The treatment of vaginitis: Trichomonas, yeast, and bacterial vaginosis. *Clinical Obstetrics and Gynecology, 31*(2), 473-479.

Mead, P. B., & Eschenbach, D. A. (moderators) (1989). Vaginitis that fails to respond to treatment. *Contemporary Ob/Gyn, 27*(2), 73-88.

Star, W. L. (1990). *Vaginitis lecture notes.* University of California, San Francisco, School of Nursing.

Wardell, D. W. (1988). Chronic exposure to sexually transmitted diseases. *Nursing Clinics of North America, 23*(4), 947-955.

VARICELLA

Boodley, C. A., & Jaquis, J. L. (1989). Measles, mumps, rubella, and chicken pox in the adult population. *The Nurse Practitioner, 14*(2), 12-22.

Gershon, A. (1988). Chickenpox: How dangerous is it? *Contemporary Ob/Gyn, 31*(3), 41-56.

Horstmann, D. M. (1982). Viral infections. In G. N. Burrow & T. F. Ferris (Eds.), *Medical complications during pregnancy* (2nd ed., pp. 341-343). Philadelphia: W. B. Saunders.

McGregor, J. A., Mark, S., Crawford, G. P., & Levin, M. (1987). Varicalla zoster antibody testing in the care of pregnant women exposed to rubella. *American Journal of Onbstetrics and Gynecology, 157*(2), 281-283.

CHAPTER 8

Abrams. B. (1985a). *How to eat well when you must rest in bed* (Patient handout). San Francisco: University of California, San Francisco, Department of Ob/Gyn.

Abrams, B. (1985b). *Tips for feeding your baby* (Patient handout). San Francisco: University of California, San Francisco, Department of Ob/Gyn.

California Department of Health Services (1989). *Nutrition during pregnancy and the post-partum period: A manual for health care professionals.* Sacramento, CA: Author.

Center for Science in the Public Interest (1985). *Nutrition Action Magazine.* Bonnie Liebman and the Editors.

Committee on Diet and Health, Food and Nutrition Board, National Research Council (1989). *Diet and health: Implications for reducing chronic disease risk (Executive Summary).* Washington, DC: National Academy Press.

Gunderson, E. (1990). Diabetes in pregnancy lecture notes. University of California, San Francisco, School of Nursing.

Gutierrez, Y. (1990a). Maternal and infant nutrition in the fourth trimester. In K. A. May (Ed.), *Comprehensive maternity nursing* (pp. 1135-1164). Philadelphia: J. B. Lippincott Co.

Gutierrez, Y. (1990b). Nutritional aspects of pregnancy. In K. A. May (Ed.), *Comprehensive maternity nursing* (pp. 359-388). Philadelphia: J. B. Lippincott Co.

Kolars, J. C., Levitt, M. D., Aouji, M., & Savaiano, D. A. (1984). Yogurt--an auto-digesting source of lactose. *New England Journal of Medicine, 310*, 1-3.

National Academy of Sciences (1990). *Maternal nutrition.* Washington, DC: National Academy Press.

National Academy of Sciences, National Research Council (1989, October). *Recommended dietary allowances* (10th ed.). Washington, DC: National Academy Press.

Newcomer, A. D., & McGill, D. B. (1984). Clinical importance of lactase deficiency. *New England Journal of Medicine, 310*, 42-43.

San Francisco Department of Public Health (1989). *Perinatal nutrition protocols.* San Francisco: Author.

U.S. Department of Health and Human Services, Public Health Service, National Institutes of Health (1988). *1988 Report of the Joint National Committee on Detection, Evaluation, and Treatment of High Blood Pressure* (Publication No. PHS 88-1088). Washington, DC: U.S. Government Printing Office.

Villar, J., Kestler, E., Castillo, P., & Solomons, NL. (1987). Improved lactose digestion during human pregnancy in primary lactose maldigestion [Abstract]. *American Journal of Clinical Nutrition*, *46*, 528.

Windholz, M. (Ed.) (1976). *Merck index* (9th ed., pp. 210-213). Rahway, NJ: Merck & Co.

Worthington-Roberts, B. S., & Williams, S. R. (1989). *Nutrition in pregnancy and lactation* (4th ed.). St. Louis: Times Mirror/Mosby.

Wytock, D. H., & DiPalma, J. A. (1988). All yogurts are not created equal. *American Journal of Clinical Nutrition*, *47*, 454-457.